# The New Complete
# MEDICAL
# and HEALTH
# ENCYCLOPEDIA

# The New Complete
# MEDICAL
# and HEALTH
# ENCYCLOPEDIA

**EDITED BY**
**Richard J. Wagman, M.D., F.A.C.P.**

*Assistant Clinical Professor of Medicine*
*Downstate Medical Center*
*New York, New York*

**AND BY**
**the J. G. Ferguson Editorial Staff**

## Volume Four

**J. G. FERGUSON PUBLISHING COMPANY/CHICAGO**

Portions of *The New Complete Medical and Health Encyclopedia* have been previously published under the title of *The Complete Illustrated Book of Better Health* and *The Illustrated Encyclopedia of Better Health,* edited by Richard J. Wagman, M.D.

**Editor**

Richard J. Wagman, M.D.,
F.A.C.P.
Assistant Clinical Professor of
  Medicine
Downstate Medical Center
New York, New York

## Contributors to The New Complete Medical and Health Encyclopedia

### Consultant in Surgery

N. Henry Moss, M.D., F.A.C.S.
Associate Clinical Professor of
  Surgery
Temple University Health Sciences
  Center and Albert Einstein
  Medical Center;
Past President, American Medical
  Writers Association;
Past President, New York Academy
  of Sciences

### Consultant in Gynecology

Douglass S. Thompson, M.D.
Clinical Professor of Obstetrics and
  Gynecology and Clinical Associate
  Professor of Community Medicine
University of Pittsburgh School of
  Medicine

### Consultant in Pediatrics

Charles H. Bauer, M.D.
Clinical Associate Professor of
  Pediatrics and Chief of Pediatric
  Gastroenterology
The New York Hospital-Cornell
  Medical Center
New York, New York

### Consultants in Psychiatry

Julian J. Clark, M.D.
Assistant Professor of Psychiatry
                and
Rita W. Clark, M.D.
Clinical Assistant Professor of
  Psychiatry
Downstate Medical Center

### Consulting Editor

Kenneth N. Anderson
Formerly Editor
*Today's Health*

Bruce O. Berg, M.D.
Associate Professor
Departments of Neurology and
  Pediatrics
Director, Child Neurology
University of California
San Francisco, California

D. Jeanne Collins
Assistant Professor
College of Allied Health Professions
University of Kentucky
Lexington, Kentucky

Anthony A. Davis
Vice President and Education
    Consultant
Metropolitan X-Ray and Medical
    Sales, Inc.
Olney, Maryland

Peter A. Dickinson
Editor Emeritus
Harvest Years/Retirement Living

Gordon K. Farley, M.D.
Associate Professor of Child
    Psychiatry
Director, Day Care Center
University of Colorado Medical
    Center

Arthur Fisher
Group Editor
Science and Engineering
Popular Science

Edmund H. Harvey, Jr.
Editor
Science World

Helene MacLean
Medical writer

Ben Patrusky
Science writer

Stanley E. Weiss, M.D.
Assistant Attending Physician, Renal
    Service
Beth Israel Hospital and Medical
    Center, New York

Jeffrey S. Willner, M.D.
Attending Radiologist
Southampton Hospital
Southampton, New York

# Contents

Volume IV

# 35

# Medical Emergencies

Anyone attempting to deal with a medical emergency will do so with considerably more confidence if he has a clear notion of the order of importance of various problems. Over and above all technical knowledge about such things as tourniquets or cardiac massage is the ability of the rescuer to keep a cool head so that he can make the right decisions and delegate tasks to others who wish to be helpful.

## Cessation of Breathing

The medical emergency that requires prompt attention before any others is cessation of breathing. No matter what other injuries are involved, artificial respiration must be administered immediately to anyone suffering from respiratory arrest.

To determine whether a person is breathing naturally, place your cheek as near as possible to the victim's mouth and nose. While you are feeling and listening for evidence of respiration, watch the victim's chest and upper abdomen to see if they rise and fall. If respiratory arrest is indicated, begin artificial respiration immediately.

Time is critical; a human body has only about a four-minute reserve supply of oxygen in its tissues, although some persons have been revived after being submerged in water for ten minutes or more. Do not waste time moving the victim to a more comfortable location unless his position is life threatening.

If more than one person is available, the second person should summon a physician. A second rescuer can also assist in preparing the victim for artificial respiration by helping to loosen clothing around the neck, chest, and waist, and by inspecting the mouth for false teeth, chewing gum, or other objects that could block the flow of air. The victim's tongue must be pulled forward before artificial respiration begins.

Normal breathing should start after not more than 15 minutes of artificial respiration. If it doesn't, you should continue the procedure for at least two hours, alternating, if possible, with other persons to maintain maximum efficiency. Medical experts have defined normal breathing as eight or more breaths per minute; if breathing resumes but slackens to a rate of fewer than eight breaths per minute, or if breathing stops suddenly for more than 30 seconds, continue artificial respiration.

### Mouth-to-Mouth and Mouth-to-Nose Artificial Respiration

Following is a description of the techniques used to provide mouth-to-mouth or mouth-to-nose artificial respiration. These are the preferred

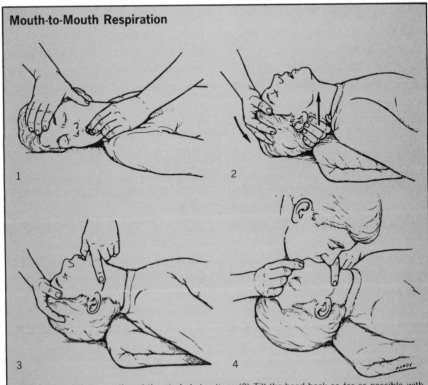

**Mouth-to-Mouth Respiration**

(1) Clear the victim's mouth and throat of obstructions. (2) Tilt the head back as far as possible, with the chin up and neck stretched taut. (3) Insert your thumb between the victim's teeth to pull his lower jaw open. Keep his head pushed back. (4) Pinch the nostrils shut. Open your mouth, take a deep breath, and, placing your mouth firmly against the victim's, blow forcefully. Repeat every 3 or 4 seconds.

methods of artificial respiration because they move a greater volume of air into a victim's lungs than any alternative method.

After quickly clearing the victim's mouth and throat of obstacles, tilt the victim's head back as far as possible, with the chin up and neck stretched to ensure an open passage of air to the lungs. If mouth-to-mouth breathing is employed, pull the lower jaw of the victim open with one hand, inserting your thumb between the victim's teeth, and pinch the nostrils with the other to prevent air leakage through the nose. If using the mouth-to-nose technique, hold one hand over the mouth to seal it against air leakage.

Next, open your own mouth and take a deep breath. Then blow forcefully into the victim's mouth (or nose) until you can see the chest rise. Quickly remove your mouth and listen for normal exhalation sounds from the victim. If you hear gurgling sounds, try to move the jaw higher because the throat may not be stretched open

properly. Continue blowing forcefully into the victim's mouth (or nose) at a rate of once every three or four seconds. (For infants, do not blow forcefully; blow only small puffs of air from your cheeks.)

If the victim's stomach becomes distended, it may be a sign that air is being blown into the stomach; press firmly with one hand on the upper abdomen to push the air out of the stomach.

If you are hesitant about direct physical contact of the lips, make a ring with the index finger and thumb of the hand being used to hold the victim's chin in position. Place the ring of fingers firmly about the victim's mouth; the outside of the thumb may at the same time be positioned to seal the nose against air leakage. Then blow the air into the victim's mouth through the finger-thumb ring. Direct lip-to-lip contact can also be avoided by placing a piece of gauze or other clean porous cloth over the victim's mouth.

## Severe Bleeding

If the victim is not suffering from respiration failure or if breathing has been restored, severe bleeding is the second most serious emergency to attend to. Such bleeding occurs when either an artery or a vein has been severed. Arterial blood is bright red

and spurts rather than flows from the body, sometimes in very large amounts. It is also more difficult to control than blood from a vein, which can be recognized by its dark red color and steady flow.

### Emergency Treatment

The quickest and most effective way to stop bleeding is by direct pressure

on the wound. If heavy layers of sterile gauze are not available, use a clean

## Pressure Points

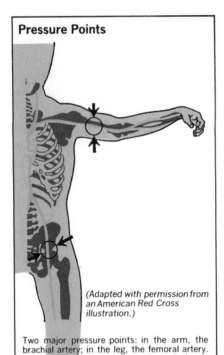

*(Adapted with permission from an American Red Cross illustration.)*

Two major pressure points: in the arm, the brachial artery; in the leg, the femoral artery. Continue to apply direct pressure and elevate the wounded part while utilizing pressure points to stop blood flow.

handkerchief, or a clean piece of material torn from a shirt, slip, or sheet to cover the wound. Then place the fingers or the palm of the hand directly over the bleeding area. The pressure must be *firm and constant* and should be interrupted only when the blood has soaked through the dressing. *Do not remove the soaked dressing.* Cover it as quickly as possible with additional new layers. When the blood stops seeping through to the surface of the dressing, secure it with strips of cloth until the victim can receive medical attention. This procedure is almost always successful in stopping blood flow from a vein.

If direct pressure doesn't stop arterial bleeding, two alternatives are possible: pressure by finger or hand on the pressure point nearest the wound, or the application of a tourniquet. No matter what the source of the bleeding, if the wound is on an arm or leg, elevation of the limb as high as is comfortable will reduce the blood flow.

### Tourniquets

A tourniquet improperly applied can be an extremely dangerous device, and should only be considered for a hemorrhage that can't be controlled in any other way.

It must be remembered that arterial blood flows away from the heart and that venous blood flows toward the heart. Therefore, while a tourniquet placed on a limb between the site of a wound and the heart may slow or stop arterial bleeding, it may actually increase venous bleeding. By obstructing blood flow in the veins beyond the wound site, the venous blood flowing toward the heart will have to exit from the wound. Thus, the proper application of a tourniquet depends upon an understanding and differentiation of arterial from venous bleeding. Arterial bleeding can be recognized by the pumping action of the blood and by the bright red color of the blood.

Once a tourniquet is applied, it should not be left in place for an excessive period of time, since the tissues in the limb beyond the site of the wound need to be supplied with blood.

## Shock

In any acute medical emergency, the

## Pressure Points

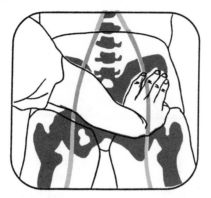

*(Top)* Use the femoral artery for control of severe bleeding from an open leg wound. Place the victim flat on his back, and put the heel of your hand directly over the pressure point. Apply pressure by forcing the artery against the pelvic bone. *(Bottom)* Use the brachial artery for control of severe bleeding from an open arm wound. Apply pressure by forcing the artery against the arm bone. Continue to apply direct pressure over the wound, and keep the wounded part elevated.

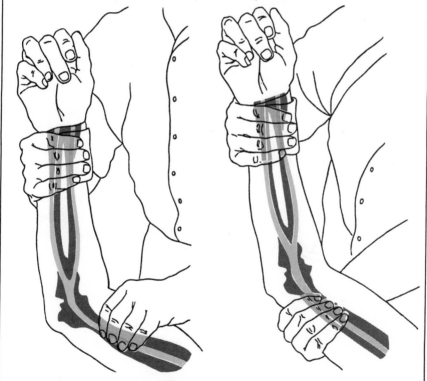

*(Adapted with permission from American Red Cross illustrations.)*

possibility of the onset of shock must always be taken into account, especially following the fracture of a large bone, extensive burns, or serious wounds. If untreated, or if treated too late, shock can be fatal.

## Arterial Bleeding

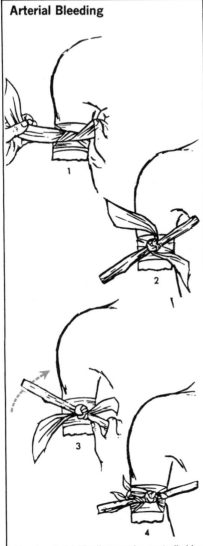

Severe arterial bleeding can be controlled by the correct application of a tourniquet. (1) A long strip of gauze or other material is wrapped twice around the arm or leg above the wound and tied in a half-knot. (2) A stick, called a windlass, is placed over the knot, and the knot is completed. (3) The windlass is turned to tighten the knot and finally, (4) the windlass is secured with the tails of the tourniquet. Improper use of a tourniquet can be very dangerous.

Shock is an emergency condition in which the circulation of the blood is so disrupted that all bodily functions are affected. It occurs when blood pressure is so low that insufficient blood supply reaches the vital tissues.

### Types of Circulatory Shock and Their Causes

- *Low-volume shock* is a condition brought about by so great a loss of blood or blood plasma that the remaining blood is insufficient to fill the whole circulatory system. The blood loss may occur outside the body, as in a hemorrhage caused by injury to an artery or vein, or the loss may be internal because of the blood loss at the site of a major fracture, burn, or bleeding ulcer. Professional treatment involves replacement of blood loss by transfusion.

- *Neurogenic shock,* manifested by *fainting,* occurs when the regulating capacity of the nervous system is impaired by severe pain, profound fright, or overwhelming stimulus. This type of shock is usually relieved by having the victim lie down with his head lower than the rest of his body.

- *Allergic shock,* also called *anaphylactic shock,* occurs when the functioning of the blood vessels is disturbed by a person's sensitivity to the injection of a particular foreign substance, as in the case of an insect sting or certain medicines.

- *Septic shock* is brought on by infection from certain bacteria that release a poison which affects the proper functioning of the blood vessels.

- *Cardiac shock* can be caused by any circumstance that affects the pumping action of the heart.

## Symptoms

Shock caused by blood loss makes the victim feel restless, thirsty, and cold. He may perspire a great deal, and although his pulse is fast, it is also very weak. His breathing becomes labored and his lips turn blue.

## Emergency Treatment

A physician should be called immediately if the onset of shock is suspected. Until medical help is obtained, the following procedures can alleviate some of the symptoms:

**1.** With a minimum amount of disturbance, arrange the victim so that he is lying on his back with his head somewhat lower than his feet. (**Exception:** If the victim's breathing is difficult, or if he has suffered a head injury or a stroke, keep his body flat but place a pillow or similar cushioning material under his head.) Loosen any clothing that may cause constriction, such as a belt, tie, waistband, shoes.

Cover him warmly against possible chill, but see that he isn't too hot.

**2.** If his breathing is weak and shallow, begin mouth-to-mouth respiration.

**3.** If he is hemorrhaging, try to control bleeding.

**4.** When appropriate help and transportation facilities are available, quickly move the victim to the nearest hospital or health facility in order to begin resuscitative measures.

**5.** *Do not* try to force any food or stimulant into the victim's mouth.

# Cardiac Arrest

Cardiac arrest is a condition in which the heart has stopped beating altogether or is beating so weakly or so irregularly that it cannot maintain proper blood circulation.

Common causes of cardiac arrest are heart attack, electric shock, hemorrhage, suffocation, and other forms of respiratory arrest. Symptoms of cardiac arrest are unconsciousness, the absence of respiration and pulse, and the lack of a heartbeat or a heartbeat that is very weak or irregular.

## Cardiac Massage

If the victim of a medical emergency manifests signs of cardiac arrest, he should be given cardiac massage at the same time that another rescuer is administering mouth-to-mouth resuscitation. Both procedures can be carried on in the moving vehicle taking him to the hospital.

It is assumed that he is lying down with his mouth clear and his air passage unobstructed. The massage is given in the following way:

**1.** The heel of one hand with the heel of the other crossed over it should be placed on the bottom third of the breastbone and pressed firmly down with a force of about 80 pounds so that the breastbone moves about two inches toward the spine. Pressure should not be applied directly on the ribs by the fingers.

**2.** The hands are then relaxed to allow the chest to expand.

**3.** If one person is doing both the cardiac massage and the mouth-to-mouth respiration, he should stop the massage after every 15 chest compressions and administer two very quick lung inflations to the victim.

**4.** The rescuer should try to make the rate of cardiac massage simulate restoration of the pulse rate. This is not always easily accomplished, but compression should reach 60 times per minute.

The techniques for administering cardiac massage to children are the same as those used for adults, except that much less pressure should be applied to a child's chest, and, in the case of babies or young children, the pressure should be exerted with the tips of the fingers rather than with the heel of the hand.

### Caution

Cardiac massage can be damaging if applied improperly. Courses in emergency medical care offered by the American Red Cross and other groups are well worth taking. In an emergency in which cardiac massage is called for, an untrained person should seek the immediate aid of someone trained in the technique before attempting it himself.

## Obstruction in the Windpipe

Many people die each year from choking on food; children incur an additional hazard in swallowing foreign objects. Most of these victims could be saved through quick action by nearly any other person, and without special equipment.

Food choking usually occurs because a bite of food becomes lodged at the back of the throat or at the opening of the trachea, or windpipe. The victim cannot breathe or speak. He may become pale or turn blue before collapsing. Death can occur within four or five minutes. But the lungs of an average person may contain at least one quart of air, inhaled before the start of choking, and that air can be used to unblock the windpipe and save the victim's life.

### Finger Probe

If the object can be seen, a quick attempt can be made to remove it by probing with a finger. Use a hooking motion to dislodge the object. Under no circumstances should this method be pursued if it appears that the object is being pushed farther downward rather than being released and brought up.

## Back Blows

Give the victim four quick, hard blows with the fist on his back between the shoulder blades. The blows should be given in rapid succession. If the victim is a child, he can be held over the knee while being struck; an adult should lie face down on a bed or table, with the upper half of his body suspended in the direction of the floor so that he can receive the same type of blows. A very small child or infant should be held upside down by the torso or legs and struck much more lightly than an adult.

## The Heimlich Maneuver

If the back blows fail to dislodge the obstruction, the Heimlich maneuver should be given without delay. (Back blows may loosen the object even if they fail to dislodge it completely; that is why they are given first.) The lifesaving technique known as the *Heimlich maneuver* (named for Dr. Henry J. Heimlich) works simply by squeezing the volume of air trapped in the victim's lungs. The piece of food literally pops out of the throat as if it were ejected from a squeezed balloon.

To perform the Heimlich maneuver, the rescuer stands behind the victim and grasps his hands firmly over the victim's abdomen, just below the victim's rib cage. The rescuer makes a fist with one hand and places his other hand over the clenched fist. Then, the rescuer forces his fist sharply inward and upward against the victim's diaphragm. This action compresses the lungs within the rib cage. If the food does not pop out on the first try, the maneuver should be repeated until the air passage is un-

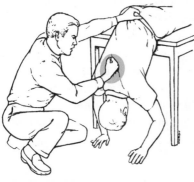

**Back Blows for Treatment of Strangulation**

Children may be placed over the knee and struck sharply between the shoulders.

Adults may be placed over the edge of a table, supported by grasping the waist, and struck sharply between the shoulders with the fist.

## The Heimlich Maneuver

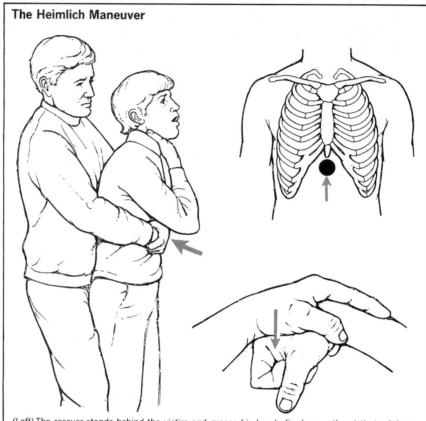

*(Left)* The rescuer stands behind the victim and grasps his hands firmly over the victim's abdomen just below the rib cage *(top right)*. The position of the rescuer's hands and the direction of thrust are shown at the bottom right.

blocked.

When the victim is unable to stand, he should be rolled over on his back on the floor. The rescuer then kneels astride the victim and performs a variation of the Heimlich maneuver by placing the heel of one open hand, rather than a clenched fist, just below the victim's rib cage. The second hand is placed over the first. Then the rescuer presses upward (toward the victim's head) quickly to compress the lungs, repeating several times if necessary.

The Heimlich maneuver has been used successfully by persons who were alone when they choked on food; some pressed their own fist into their abdomen, others forced the edge of a chair or sink against their abdomen.

## Poisoning

In all cases of poisoning, it is imperative to get professional assistance as soon as possible.

Listed below are telephone numbers for Poison Control Centers throughout the United States. These health service organizations are accessible 24 hours a day to provide information on how best to counteract the effects of toxic substances.

In the event of known or suspected poisoning, call the center nearest you immediately. Give the staff member to whom you speak as much information as possible: the name or nature of the poison ingested, if you know; if not, the symptoms manifested by the victim.

If for any reason it is impossible to telephone or get to a Poison Control Center (or a doctor or hospital), follow these two general rules:

**1.** If a strong acid or alkali or a petroleum product has been ingested, dilute the poison by administering large quantities of milk or water. Do not induce vomiting.

**2.** For methanol or related products such as window cleaners, antifreeze, paint removers, and shoe polish, induce vomiting—preferably with syrup of ipecac.

## Calling for Help

Every household should have a card close by the telephone—if possible attached to an adjacent wall—that contains the numbers of various emergency services. In most communities, it is possible to simply dial the operator and ask for the police or fire department. In many large cities, there is a special three-digit number that can be dialed for reaching the police directly.

An ambulance can be summoned either by asking for a police ambulance, by calling the nearest hospital, or by having on hand the telephone numbers of whatever private ambulance services are locally available. Such services are listed in the classified pages of the telephone directory.

Practically all hospitals have emergency rooms for the prompt treatment of accident cases. If the victim is in good enough physical condition, he can be placed in a prone position in a family station wagon for removal to a hospital. However, under no circumstances should a person who has sustained major injuries or who has collapsed be made to sit upright in a car. First aid must be administered to him on the spot until a suitable conveyance arrives.

Every family should find out the telephone number of the nearest Poison Control Center (see section in this chapter) and note it on the emergency number card.

# The Emergency-Free Home

Every year, hundreds of thousands of Americans go to hospital emergency rooms to obtain treatment for injuries or illnesses incurred in their homes. But many of these emergency health problems could have been prevented. In too many cases, no one took action to eliminate home hazards simply because they were easy to overlook or were not readily detectable.

Millions more Americans suffer less serious home injuries and do not go to hospitals. A cut finger, a stubbed toe, a fall that results in a bruise but no broken bones—all these minor accidents and many more occur daily.

With a little forethought, many of these home accidents can be prevented. This chapter provides basic guidelines for home safety.

## Medical Supplies and Equipment

Can you "immunize" your home against accidents, illnesses, and injuries resulting from misuse of medicines and medical equipment? The answer is Yes. The effort to immunize is worth taking, if only for your peace of mind.

## First Aid Needs

The first step toward home safety is preparedness. This means ensuring that basic first aid equipment and medications are in the home, readily available.

Both materials and medicines should be chosen with care. Key considerations are the ages of those who live in the home, special requirements of particular family members, the seasons of the year, and other factors that may suggest a need for certain products or preparations.

First aid supplies should be kept in a medicine cabinet or in a larger storage place such as a bathroom closet or a cabinet beneath a sink. The size of any given item and the available space may determine where each item is stored. Basic first aid items include:

- Assorted bandages
- Sterile gauze pads (for compresses)
- Waterproof adhesive tape
- 3% hydrogen peroxide (for cleaning cuts, wounds)
- 5% hydrocortisone ointment (for local pain, itching)
- Ice pack
- Tweezers (for removing splinters, debris)
- Oral fever thermometer
- Rectal thermometer (for children)
- Heating pad

## Medicines and Medications

With the nondrug necessities stocked, you can turn your attention to such needs as pills, medications, ointments, powders, drugs, and others.

A first rule is: Don't overstock. Many medicine cabinets contain things that only help to delay proper medical attention.

"One such hazardous medicine is syrup of ipecac," according to a medical authority. "A preparation that induces vomiting, it's a basic need in a household with children. But it should never be used unless a physician approves. Use of ipecac after ingestion of some liquids can be very damaging and even fatal."

Leftover antibiotics may present another problem. Because these medications can be costly, many householders keep in their medicine cabinets (or on their dressers or nightstands) any supplies that are left after an initial bout with illness. *Antibiotics should never be used a second time without consulting a physician.*

Taking leftover antibiotics can cause severe allergic reactions. Self-medication may also make it difficult or impossible for a physician to diagnose an illness.

Antibiotics prescribed in series should be taken until the series is completed. As a final rule, no such medications should be passed on to friends or relatives for their use. Borrowed medications could harm, rather than help, the recipient.

What drugs or medications should be in your medicine cabinet? Some basic items are:

- Cold and allergy medications, including an antihistamine, a decongestant, a cough suppressant, an expectorant

- An antacid for indigestion

- An anti-odor foot cream or powder

- An anti-diarrheal medicine

- A laxative

- Eyedrops

- Aspirin or an aspirin-free pain reliever

- Other items as required for chronic conditions.

Here are some additional safety rules regarding medicine cabinets:

- If possible, locate the medicine cabinet in a cool, dry, dark place, out of the reach of children.

- Check the contents periodically and throw away out-of-date or spoiled items (including aspirin that smells like vinegar).

- Remove the cotton from any medicine cabinet containers that may use cotton stoppers (because the cotton can absorb a medication's active ingredients).

- If even one pill in a bottle has deteriorated or spoiled, throw out the entire batch.

- Keep liquids in their amber containers to protect the contents from light.

- To discard medications, flush them down the toilet, then remove the labels on the containers to prevent others from refilling the prescriptions.

- Keep emergency phone numbers (physician, pharmacist, fire, police, and so on; see the list of emergency phone numbers on the inside front cover of this volume) on the medicine cabinet or near it. When in doubt about which medication to use, call a doctor or pharmacist.

## Reducing the Risk of Medicine Poisoning

Following certain safety rules can help ensure against the possibility of medicine poisoning. The rules are most important in homes where there are very young children or very old family members.

Medicines or preparations that are potentially harmful should be kept in a locked cabinet. If there are a number of such preparations in the home, they should probably be kept in a separate, locking storage place. If this is not possible, they should at least be stored out of the reach of young children.

Other safety rules are simply common sense. For example, one should never transfer a medicine into an unlabeled container. Special care should be taken with the dosages of both liquid and solid drugs. Sleeping tablets, tranquilizers, and even aspirin can, if taken in overdose, seriously harm the body.

If you plan to keep old medicine containers, wash them thoroughly and then store them carefully. Otherwise, they should be thrown away. If children resist taking their medicine, parents should never encourage them by pretending that the medicine is candy. Nor should parents rely too heavily on anti-tamper packaging. The shrink-wraps, push-and-turn bottle caps, foil inner seals, and other anti-tamper devices are valuable but not foolproof.

In any case of medicine poisoning, do not wait to seek help. Stay calm, call your physician or the nearest hospital or poison control center, and get instructions on correct procedures. If you take a poisoned family member to a hospital or elsewhere for help, you should bring with you the container(s) from which pills or liquid were taken. Do not administer salt and water to induce vomiting; the mixture is potentially fatal. With a child, a much more reliable method is to put a finger into the youngster's throat if the child is conscious.

## Dangers of Alternative Medicines and Quack Remedies

Americans spend billions of dollars each year on "alternative" medicinal supplies and equipment. In too many cases the quack remedies not only do not help, they may do serious harm.

Examples of items that flood the marketplace but should not be found in your home are numerous. Among the many unproved procedures and preparations are hair analysis and cytotoxic tests for food allergies; oral chelation therapy, with vitamin and mineral capsules or tables for cardiovascular disease; and various "metabolic" programs, "non-toxic holistic medicines," radical dietary changes and regimens, and programs calling for massive doses of vitamins.

Still others include detoxification and drastic "cleansing" enemas, herbal mixtures to be applied to a sore or inflamed area, immune boosters that once were sold as cancer cures and now are promoted as treatments for AIDS, and laetrile, an unproven cancer treatment.

The following guidelines can help protect your family from such noneffective medications:

- Beware of testimonials in ads or on labels that purportedly come from satisfied users.

- Do not believe any promises of "money-back guarantees." They are rarely dependable.

- Be wary of advertising that claims a product is effective against numerous ailments.

- Be wary of promises of a "cure" or of "complete relief" from pain.

- Discount any "FDA-tested" or "FDA-recommended" testimonials. Federal law states that the Food and Drug Administration cannot be mentioned as giving marketing approvals.

- Beware of mentions of "natural" ingredients. The definition of natural is elusive, and the word is often abused.

- Think twice before buying *anything* that is advertised with such terms as these: "amazing," "vanish," "discovery," "breakthrough," "painless," "exclusive," or "instant."

- Finally, warns the FDA, "If the product sounds too good to be true, it probably is."

## Emergency-Proofing Your Home

The modern home is a marvel of time-saving, labor-saving, and comfort-producing devices and appliances. These include such products as space heaters, washers, dryers, refrigerators, gas and electric furnaces, and many others. To a great extent, the hazards that large or small appliances may introduce into your home are associated with fire. But householders should also take precautions against the dangers of electrocution, falls caused by poorly placed electrical cords, and other accident-producers.

Most emergencies arising from appliance use or misuse can be avoided by acting in advance to prevent possible hazards. Household items that are most likely to be hazardous are heating-cooling equipment, cooking equipment, heat tapes and humidifiers, and small electrical appliances.

## Heating-Cooling Equipment

In the first category are furnaces, air conditioners, space heaters, and similar equipment. The primary safety rule with heating equipment is to make sure it is operating properly and efficiently. For furnaces of any kind, an annual checkup—usually in the summer or fall—is advisable. Many homeowners have maintenance policies that include such checkups.

All *space heaters* come with instructions for installation and operation. These instructions should be followed closely. Space heaters should be located so that they have plenty of room around them. They should be placed at a safe distance from all papers, clothing, draperies, furniture, and (if possible) children. Manufacturers' labels usually indicate what the proper clearance is for a particular model.

As with furnaces, space heaters should be kept in good working condition. Missing controls should be replaced; so should missing or defective guards or screens.

*Electric space heaters* should have tip-over shutoff switches that turn off the current if the unit is knocked over. These heaters should also have guards around their coils. The guard can be a wire grille or other protective "fence" that can keep fingers or fabrics away from the heating element.

If an extension cord is used with the space heater, the cord should have a power rating at least as high as the heater's rating. The cord should be in a safe place and out of the reach of children.

An important rule: Do not use a portable electric heater in a bathroom, near a sink, or close to water. This presents the risk of electrocution.

*Gas space heaters* may be vented or unvented. Both kinds need special care and attention.

If a gas space heater is vented, it should be vented correctly. That is, the vent pipe should be properly sized and free of cracks, leaks, and blockages, with tight joints and crack-free heat exchanger (to prevent leakage of carbon monoxide). If in doubt about the venting, call a servicer or your gas supplier.

When using an unvented gas space heater, you should always have a door or window slightly open in the room where the heater is located.

With either kind of gas heater, you should light the match *first* before you turn on the gas for the pilot light. This prevents flareups due to accumulated gas.

*Woodburning, kerosene, or oil space heaters* not only need to be installed properly; it would also be wise to have them inspected by a local fire safety official. Then you should use only the fuel, and in some cases the *grade* of fuel, for which the heater was designed.

The chimney of the heater or stove should be cleaned regularly, once every couple of months at least. In the case of a woodburning heater, it is best to use only paper or wood for kindling. *Never* use gasoline or another flammable or combustible fluid to start a woodburning stoves.

## Cooking Equipment

The U.S. Consumer Product Safety Commission (CPSC) reports that more than 100,000 fires each year are associated with cooking equipment, especially stoves. These fires cause an estimated $300 million in property losses.

Some basic safety precautions can prevent most of these fires. For example, householders can avoid storing flammable or combustible items above the stove. The same applies to potholders, plastic utensils, towels, and other flammable items. Children's favorite foods, including cookies or candy, should never be kept above the range or in its immediate vicinity.

Clothing can be a trap for the unwary. Loose-fitting sleeves should not be worn while cooking. Also, you should never leave a stove unattended, especially when a burner is turned to a high setting.

## Heat Tapes and Humidifiers

Heat tapes and ultrasonic humidifiers can pose home safety and health hazards. Heat tapes, used to keep exposed water pipes from freezing, present fire hazards. Ultrasonic humidifiers filled with tap water may discharge dangerous mineral particles into the air.

*Electric heat tapes,* or pipe heating cables, plug into wall or floor outlets. Once plugged in, they emit heat through their molded plastic insulation. Used in crawl spaces and in the substructures of homes and mobile homes, many tapes remain plugged in year-round. A thermostat in the power supply cord turns the tape on when the temperature falls below a certain level.

Improper installation of heat tapes has become a major cause of home fires in recent years. In many cases, lack of attention to the instructions that come with the product has resulted in faulty installation. Some homeowners lap the tape over itself when winding the tape around the pipe. Others ignore manufacturers' warnings that specific lengths of tape be used to protect pipes of given diameters and lengths.

If your home has heat tapes already installed you should (1) inspect all tapes, or have a licensed electrician inspect them, for proper installation or deteriorated installation; (2) check older tapes for cracks in the plastic insulation or bare wires, and replace worn tapes at once; (3) make certain, if you have plastic pipes, that the tapes you are using are recommended specifically for your kind of plastic piping; and (4) inspect all tapes to make sure none is wrapped over the thermal insulation on a pipe or near flammable objects.

Ultrasonic humidifiers using tap water have been found to spread such impurities as lead, aluminum, asbestos, or dissolved organic gases into the air. All these substances can be health hazards. To avoid such problems, use bottled, demineralized water or install demineralizing filters on your tap-water supply.

Other humidifiers pose no such mineral particle threat.

## Home Electrical Safety

Have you conducted an audit of the connections, cords, gadgets (aside from major appliances), and other electrical equipment in your home? If not, such an audit is virtually a must.

You can start checking all lighting, including bulbs and sockets, all cords and extension cords, and all TV or audio equipment. Bulbs with wattages too high for the size of a fixture may overheat and cause a fire, so you should replace oversized bulbs with others of appropriate wattages. If the correct wattage is not indicated, use a bulb no larger than 60 watts.

Make sure all electrical cords are placed out of traffic areas so that people will not trip or fall over them. Stepping on cords can damage them, too, and produce fire hazards. Also check to make sure that cords do not have furniture resting on them. Cords should not be frayed, should not be wrapped around themselves or any object, and should *never* be attached to walls with nails or staples.

Extension cords should be equipped with safety covers and should never be expected to carry more than their proper loads. Both the cord and the electrical device will normally have electrical ratings.

*Wall outlets and switches* call for special attention. Whether they are in use or not, the same basic safety rules apply. All switches and wall outlets should be checked to make sure they are working properly and fixed if they are not. You can test them by touching: an unusually warm outlet or switch may indicate an unsafe wiring condition. Plugs should fit into outlets snugly, and all outlets should have face plates so that no wiring is exposed.

*Kitchen countertop appliances,* like TVs, radios, and other home entertainment equipment, should be placed so that they remain dry. If they give off heat, as does a toaster, they should have some space to "breathe." Countertop appliances should be unplugged when not in use.

Cords for countertop appliances are critically important. These should never be placed so that they can come into contact with hot surfaces; this applies especially to cords around toasters, ovens, and ranges. The same rule holds where water or wet surfaces are concerned.

Because ground fault circuit interrupters (GFCIs) can prevent many electrocutions, the Consumer Product Safety Commission recommends that all countertop outlets be equipped with them. They should also be used in bathrooms and other areas where there is a risk of electrical shock. Test your GFCIs regularly in accordance with the manufacturers' instructions.

Most current building codes require that bathrooms be equipped with GFCIs. Older homes may not have them.

*Other electrical appliances and equipment* require other kinds of safety care. These items can include hair dryers, curling irons, and electric blankets.

A universal rule is that such devices be unplugged when not in use. Plugged in and allowed to fall into water, they can cause an electrocution. They should also be in good operating condition, with no damaged wiring or other parts.

Do not use portable electric heaters in the bathroom or other rooms where they may come into contact with water. Keep *any* use of electrical devices or appliances in such rooms to a minimum.

*Electric blankets* also have to be used with care. They should be in good condition and have no charred spots on either the upper or the lower blanket surface. Before using them, look for cracks or breaks in wiring, connectors, and plugs.

To prevent overheating, do not cover electric blankets with other blankets, comforters, or other bedding. They should also be used flat, not folded back, and should not be tucked in except in accordance with the manufacturers' instructions.

*Basement, garage, and workshop power tools and outlets* constitute another extremely important area of safety concern. Power tools should have three-pronged plugs to indicate

that they are double insulated. These plugs reduce the risk of electric shock.

Check your fuse box or circuit breaker. A fuse of the wrong size can present a fire hazard. If you do not know what sizes are correct, an electrician can tell you. Your circuit breakers should be "exercised" periodically if they are to remain in good working order. This procedure is simple:

**1.** Turn off your freezer, refrigerator, and air conditioner.

**2.** Flip each circuit breaker off and on three times.

**3.** Turn the appliances back on.

Repeat this routine at least once a year. Also check the GFCIs on your basement, garage, or workshop equipment to make sure they are working properly.

*Receptacles located outdoors* represent a final stage in your electrical audit.

These receptacles or outlets should have waterproof covers that keep water out and prevent malfunctions. The covers should be *closed* when not in use. If your home has no GFCIs on outside receptacles, you should have them installed.

As regards electric lawn movers and other electric garden tools and appliances, the basic rules of safety apply. But remember: extension cords used outside should be specifically designed for such use, or you may be risking a fire or a serious shock.

## Home Fire Prevention and Protection

Many home fires have nothing to do with gadgets or appliances. Both the simplest and the most complex of our daily amenities can be fire hazards. Extremely flammable liquids provide power for our cars. Fabrics and upholstered furniture can ignite and burn. Some of us carry fire sources, matches or cigarette lighters, in our pockets.

In the sections that follow, effort will be made to call attention to the most important of these hazards.

### Matches, Lighters, and Cigarettes

Some prohibitions that help to immunize your home against accidental fires are matters of common sense. Others have more technical origins.

Some 140 young children die each year in fires that they or their friends or siblings started. Children start thousands more home fires while playing with matches or lighters. Thus a basic rule is that children should not have access to either matches or cigarette lighters. Both should be kept out of sight and reach.

Adults should never use either matches or lighters as toys or sources of amusement. Cigarette butts should not be left burning in ashtrays that children can reach.

Ashtray and cigarette discipline is always appropriate. Lighted butts should not be thrown into the trash. A lighted butt can start a major fire. Ashtrays should not be placed on the arms of chairs, where they can be knocked off. As a precaution, check the furniture where smokers have been sitting to make sure that no lighted cigarettes have fallen unnoticed behind or between cushions or under furniture.

In a recent year, 46,700 mattress and bedding fires took some 700 lives. Thus, "No smoking in bed" represents a cardinal rule of home safety.

### Furniture Precautions

Because many home fires start on pieces of furniture, you should take special care when selecting the items you need. In particular, you should look for furniture designed to reduce the likelihood of furniture fires that may be started by cigarettes.

This task has become simpler in recent years. Manufacturers are making upholstered furniture far more fire resistant than they have in the past. All furniture that meets the standards of the Upholstered Furniture Action Council (UFAC) carries a gold-colored tag with red letters that states, "Important Consumer Safety Information from UFAC."

The tag is a form of safety certification that the manufacturer attaches in compliance with UFAC's Voluntary Action Program. "The manufacturer of this furniture," states the tag, "certifies that it is made in accordance with the new, improved UFAC methods, designed to reduce the likelihood of furniture fires from cigarettes."

Other precautions help reduce the risks of injury or death from furniture fires. For example, look for upholstery fabrics made primarily from such thermoplastic fibers as nylon, polyester, acrylic, and olefin. These resist ignition by burning cigarettes better than do rayon or cotton, both cellulose fabrics.

## Flammable Liquids

The federal Hazardous Substances Act establishes three labeling categories for liquid products:

**1.** *Extremely flammable liquids* include gasoline, the white gas commonly used in camping stoves, contact adhesives, and wood stains that produce ignitable vapors at room temperature. Once ignited, the vapors act as wicks to carry the fire to the container of the liquid.

**2.** *Flammable liquids* produce ignitable vapors at higher temperatures. In this group are such liquids as paint thinners, some paints, and automotive products such as brake fluids.

**3.** *Combustible liquids* can be ignited but are less likely to catch fire than the other kinds. This category includes furniture polishes, oil-based paints, fuel oil, diesel oil, and kerosene.

To some extent, you can shop wisely for flammable liquids. You can, for example, buy a product that is least likely to ignite but that still meets your needs. But remember: some products do not carry *flammable* labels because they will not catch fire in liquid form as they come from the container. Some paint strippers belong in this category. Once they are applied, however, they become quite flammable because their flame-suppressant chemicals evaporate.

Use solvent-based products with adequate moving air ventilation, and ventilate the work area. These precautions will keep fumes from building up and igniting. They will also protect you from the toxic effects of invisible and sometimes explosive vapors.

## Wise Use of Flammable Liquids

At one time or another, nearly everyone has to use flammable liquids. Here are some fundamental rules for wise use:

- Never use such liquids near flames or a source of sparks, including pilot lights.

- Use gasoline only as a fuel, not as a cleaning fluid.

- Always shut off power mowers, chain saws, or other gas-powered equipment before refueling them. Refuel outdoors and wait for hot parts to cool before adding fuel.

- Use only liquids identified as *charcoal starters* to get charcoal fires going. Never pour on additional fluid after starting the fire.

## Proper Storage

Gasoline and other extremely flammable liquids should be stored outside your house or apartment, but they should *not* be stored in the trunk of your car. Children should not be able to reach your safe-storage place. For added insurance, lock up all flammable liquids.

Never keep gasoline in glass bottles, plastic jugs, or other makeshift containers. If possible, invest in a gasoline container with such safety features as a pressure release valve or a flame arrester.

## Flammable Fabrics

There are four basic safety principles regarding the flammability of fabrics:

**1.** All fibers used in ordinary clothing can burn. But some catch fire and burn less readily than others. The more-fire-resistant fabrics are fire-resistant cotton, wool, rayon, polyester, and modacrylic. Fabrics that burn most readily are acetate, untreated cotton and rayon, and linen.

**2.** The way in which a fabric is made determines the way it burns. As a rule, heavy, tightly constructed fabrics ignite with difficulty and burn more slowly than fabrics that are light, open, or fuzzy. Once ignited, however, the heavier fabrics burn longer than the lightweights and can cause very serious injuries.

**3.** "Flame resistant" does not mean "noncombustible." The phrase only indicates that a fabric is designed to resist ignition and burning. Under some conditions such fabrics will not only burn; they will be incapable of providing you with protection if you reach into a fireplace, a wood-burning stove, or an oven. To maintain a fabric's flame-resistant qualities, follow the manufacturer's instructions regarding care and cleaning.

**4.** A garment's style has much to do with safety. The safest clothes are those that fit closely, have large neck openings and quick release closures, and are wrap-style.

Remember the three rules for extinguishing a clothing fire:

**1.** Don't run.

**2.** Do try to remove the burning article of clothing.

**3.** If that fails, drop to the floor or ground and roll back and forth.

## Smoke Detectors

There are two basic rules regarding smoke detectors. First, every home should have at least one smoke detector, approved by a recognized national testing laboratory. Second, at least one smoke detector should be placed on each floor of your home.

These rules apply for both ionization and photoelectric detectors. Both types of detectors, if well designed and engineered, are effective. The particular layout of your home may determine whether you need plug-in or battery-powered devices. You may choose to have one or two of each type; both have advantages and disadvantages.

The battery-powered smoke detector can run out of power, usually after about a year. It then gives a warning sound, at which time you need to install new batteries.

The plug-in detector operates like a permanently burning lamp. However, it cannot operate if fire or some other interference breaks the electrical circuit that powers the detector. Other tips:

- Place detectors high up, on a ceiling or wall, close to where people sleep. Otherwise the alarm may not be heard.

- Never place a smoke detector in the kitchen or very near it. Airborne kitchen grease and cooking fumes can easily activate the device, touching off a false alarm.

- Even if a battery-powered detector does not give a signal that its batteries are running down, change the batteries at least once a year.

- With a photoelectric detector, the light source should be replaced as soon as it burns out.

- Test photoelectric detectors regularly with real smoke—from a just-extinguished candle, for example. Test ionization detectors using a *lighted* candle. Test detectors every two to four weeks.

## Fire Extinguishers

Fire extinguishers complement your smoke alarms and should be part of your home "immunization" program. The extinguishers should be kept in areas where fires are most likely to occur: the kitchen, home workshop, or rooms where flammable materials are kept, where people may be smoking, or where there are hazard-producing activities or materials.

Fire extinguishers are rated according to size. A five-pound extinguisher rated ABC (meaning it can be used to fight fires of any kind) is considered minimal for home protection. Many homeowners, however, buy two-and-one-half-pound extinguishers specifically to fight small kitchen fires.

The best protection against home fires may be a common garden hose. Using extensions, it can be made long enough to reach every room in the house. You can also attach nozzles that make it possible to sprinkle, spray, or direct a solid stream. Keep the hose in one place so that it is always ready to use.

## An Escape Plan

Fire causes most home emergencies, but other conditions can be just as disastrous. An accident outside the home may force immediate evacuation; so may natural disasters such as storms or floods.

An escape plan should be part of your program for immunizing your home against emergencies. The plan, in a sense, is an admission that an emergency could occur, but it can save lives by preventing panic.

## For Fires

Your escape plan has to take into consideration the possibility that you may have to evacuate for an hour or several days or longer. In cases of fire, you need to have two exits from each part of the house. You may want to consider installing rope or chain safety ladders outside windows that are too high above the ground for safe jumping. If you live in an apartment, you should obtain escape instructions from your building management or landlord or your local fire department.

Through informal fire drills, you can help to ensure that each member of your household understands the escape plan. You should include small children as part of your escape rehearsals, and the rehearsals should be repeated periodically. Everyone should know where they are to meet to be sure everyone got out safely.

Young children should understand clearly that they have to evacuate when everyone else does. They *must* escape; they cannot hide under a bed or in a closet.

Safe escape may require understanding of the tricks of self- preservation in case of fire. Three rules are critically important:

**1.** *Stay low.* Since most smoke rises, you need to keep low, crawling on hands and knees when necessary, to pass safely through a smoke-filled hallway or room.

**2.** *Feel doors before you open them.* If you find that the door panels, the knob, or the molding surrounding the door are hot to the touch, it may mean that the fire is just outside. Move toward another exit.

**3.** *Use wet cloths.* To avoid excessive smoke inhalation, a major cause of fire-related deaths, you can wet pillow cases, towels, or other fabrics and hold them over your face while you make your way to an exit.

## For Natural Disasters

In case of natural disasters, you may need to obtain accurate, current information as well as warnings, advice, or instructions issued by various agencies. Disregarding such instructions or advice can endanger you and your family.

Your home should be equipped with a battery-powered portable radio. The radio could mean the difference between disaster and survival if your power is interrupted. You should have spare, sealed-in-the-package batteries for the radio. To prolong their lives, you can keep them in a refrigerator freezer.

Other avenues of communication in an emergency are available in most communities in the United States. These include amateur radio, citizens' band (CB) radio, community disaster warnings, special signals and communications methods, and (of course) the telephone.

Amateur radio or "ham" operators have proven to be unusually helpful in emergencies. To locate such an operator in your community, you can inquire among your neighbors or write, enclosing a self-addressed, stamped envelope, to the Amateur Radio Relay League, 225 Main St., Newington, CT 06111.

## Poisonous or Harmful Substances

Each year, more than 100,000 children under the age of five become victims of accidental ingestion of poisonous or harmful substances. These include medicines and such flammable liquids as gasoline, but they can also include a vast range of liquids, solids, and gases that find their ways into the typical home for a variety of purposes.

Substances that require special precautions range from carbon monoxide to spoiled food and from cleaning fluids and detergents to pesticides. Some general guidelines are as follows:

- Bring such substances into your home only if necessary, and then in the smallest possible quantity.

- Keep all products in their original containers, never in containers customarily used for food or drinks.

- If a product comes in a child-re-

sistant container, never transfer it to a container that has no such protection.

- Carefully separate foods from potentially harmful household products.

- After using a product that comes in a child-resistant container, resecure the cap or other closure.

- Make sure that all products that entail any risk or hazard are properly labeled, and turn on lights before using such products.

- Store potentially hazardous products in a separate area from other household products, preferably in a locked cabinet.

Because not all the harmful substances that enter your home have warnings on their containers, your should make it your business to learn whether hazards exist.

### Lead Poisoning

Almost from the beginnings of civilization, people have used lead as a

component in glazing materials for ceramic dishes, bowls, pitchers, plates, and other earthenware. The practice continues today. Many ceramic-ware products sold in the United States are coated with glazes that are applied and fused onto a shaped piece of clay. Cadmium may be used to enhance the vividness of the colors.

Both cadmium and lead are toxic metals. Both can under given conditions leach into foods stored in some glazed ceramic containers.

Since 1971, the FDA has limited the amounts of lead that can leach or soak out of ceramic ware into foods. But cases of lead poisoning and various studies have renewed concerns about lead from all sources and from many different consumer products. These products include the 60 percent of all ceramic foodware imported into the United States from foreign countries.

Lead can, however, invade the home environment in other ways or from other sources. Some paints manufactured before 1978 contained lead (see Lead Poisoning, pp. 163–4). That paint still covers the walls, floors, and furniture of many older apartments and homes. In some communities, water reaches homes by way of old lead service pipes and water system mains.

You can protect yourself and your family against many of the health hazards that lead presents. You can reduce the risks to a safe minimum and avoid the stomach disorders and other problems, including brain damage in severe cases, that lead can produce.

## Ceramic-ware Lead Poisoning

The following precautions can help prevent lead poisoning from ceramic ware:

**1.** *Avoid storing foods in ceramic ware.* Much preferred and far safer are glass or plastic containers. The high acid content of many foods increases the amounts of lead that the food can absorb.

**2.** *Be especially wary of products imported from or bought in foreign countries.* Manufacturers in those countries do not necessarily adhere to high safety standards. You may be wise either to avoid purchasing dinnerware made in other countries or

to use such products for other purposes, such as decoration.

**3.** *Avoid using antiques or collectibles to hold food and vegetables.* They may be family heirlooms, or they may have been bought at garage or rummage sales, antique shops, or flea markets, but ceramic ware of uncertain origin may be dangerous.

**4.** *Beware of ceramic items made by amateurs or hobbyists.* Hobbyists can obtain safe glazes today, but you may not be able to tell whether the maker actually used such a glaze.

You have another choice if you want to use ceramic items to store foods or liquids: you can have your ceramic ware tested by a qualified commercial laboratory. Check your local health department or the telephone book for laboratories in your area.

## Paint Lead Poisoning

Warnings about lead poisoning from paint are directed primarily at the parents of young children. The warnings suggest that parents learn to recognize the symptoms of such poisoning and to consult as quickly as possible with a doctor, local hospital or clinic, or public health department. Delay can, in serious cases, lead to mental retardation, paralysis, and even death.

A difficulty in recognizing paint lead poisoning is that the symptoms are similar to those of many other childhood ailments. A child with lead poisoning may complain of stomachaches or may vomit. Headaches, a loss of appetite, crankiness, and excessive tiredness may be other symptoms. The child may lose interest in normal play.

A second problem is that a child can be poisoned by chewing on or eating dirt, dust, newspapers, some pottery, some furniture, or many other nonfood substances containing lead. But hospital or clinic blood tests for lead poisoning take only minutes. If a high concentration of lead is found in the blood, treatment may be necessary. The standards for treatment of lead poisoning can vary from community to community, so you should follow the directions and guidance of your doctor or local health department.

Depending on your child's age, you may be able to explain that he or she should eat nothing but food. Babysitters should be instructed about lead poisoning hazards and should keep children in their care from eating paint, newspapers, or other nonfood substances.

You can take still more direct action to remove the threat of paint lead poisoning from your home. A key task is to keep your home in good shape, free of water leaks from faulty plumbing, defective roofs, or exterior holes that could admit rain or dampness. Repaint the interior surfaces of your home every four to five years. Here are some further precautions:

**1.** Replaster any plaster walls that may be cracking or peeling.

**2.** Using a broom or stiff brush, remove all the pieces of loose paint from the walls.

**3.** Sweep up and put into a paper bag all the pieces of paint and plaster and place them in a trash can. *Do not burn them.*

**4.** While removing lead-based paint by scraping or sanding, keep children and pregnant women away (preferably outside the home) and take precautions to protect yourself. The dust you raise may be harmful.

## Radon, A Special Case

Radon is a colorless, odorless, radio-active gas that is almost impossible to detect without instruments. It seeps through the crevices or spaces in the soil or rock on which a home is built. It can enter your home through dirt floors, cracks in concrete floors and walls, joints, sumps, floor drains, and the tiny holes or pores in hollow-block walls.

Persons exposed to radon face serious health risks, specifically lung cancer. Also, continued exposure to radon increases the risk of illness. Many persons never realize that the gas is invading their homes.

*Detection* of radon requires special equipment but moderate cost. Two commercially available radon detectors are the charcoal canister and the alpha track detector. The former calls for a test period of three to seven days, and the latter requires two to four weeks. Trained personnel can provide other methods of detection. Reports on measurements of radon gas are made in terms of picocuries per liter (pCi/l).

If you obtain readings of above 1.0 WL (working level) or above 200 pCi/l, take follow-up measurements as quickly as possible.

*Doing it yourself* to close off the radon entry points in your basement begins with caulking. Using urethane or silicone caulk, seal up the gap (if any) between the basement floor and all walls; fill cracks in the mortar joints between concrete blocks; and lay a thick bead of caulk around the perimeter of sump openings. Treated ply-wood or a metal sheet can then be used to cover the sump, with more caulk used as a sealant.

Use ready-mix concrete to seal any large openings around pipes, pipe-chase openings, and spaces along the top rows of concrete-block walls. Inject insulation into the top rows of concrete-block walls before sealing them. Foam backing can be applied before the concrete sealing is applied to pipe-chase openings.

Ventilation supplements your efforts to close all gaps and holes in your basement's floors and walls. Without creating uncomfortable drafts, you can ventilate under your basement slab *if:* (1) you have a continuous slab with no large, unsealed openings to the earth beneath, and (2) there is a sufficiently porous bed under the slab to permit ventilating air to circulate through it. Given both conditions, you can create your own subslab vent system with pipes and a fan; the air intake and exhaust pipes should be located in opposite corners of the basement.

Other methods of ventilating your basement include forced-air systems using fans to maintain a balanced air exchange rate; heat-recovery ventilators that replace radon-tainted air with outside air; and use of a product called Enka-drain, which traps radon in a nylon mesh airspace that is then vented through an exhaust pipe.

Because it is a gas, radon always moves from a higher pressure area (the ground) to a lower-pressure one (your house). That means you have a final alternative to ventilation: pressurize your basement and home by providing outside air supplies for wood stoves, fireplaces, gas dryers, and furnaces.

## The Food Department

Threats to your health can enter your home in a grocery bag. They can develop in your home in the forms of mold or bacteria on food. Poor food handling practices, either inside or outside the home, can contribute to these health hazards. The greatest threats are a lack of sanitation, insufficient cooking, and improper storage (see also "Food Hazards," pp. 967–970).

Bacteria cause about 95 percent of all cases of food poisoning. People can ingest illness-producing bacteria in contaminated foods; the bacteria can then multiply and spread infections in the digestive tract or the bloodstream. Such digestive problems occur most often in warm weather, when food may be taken to picnics or on cookout without proper refrigeration.

Contamination may also take place if parasitic animals such as the roundworm, found sometimes in pork, enter the body. The roundworm produces a disease called trichinosis.

There are four main kinds of bacteria that can contaminate foods and cause diseases: salmonella; "staph," or *staphylococcus aureus;* botulism; and *clostridium perfringens,* which causes diarrhea. However, you can avoid contamination if you take precautions. This is important because the four kinds of bacteria can produce symptoms as mild as an upset stomach or as severe as death, as in the case of botulism.

### Food-Borne Poisons and Allergens

When shopping, you usually have to take on faith the food manufacturer's and the grocer's claims that their food is safe. But you can certainly be selective. You may want to avoid foods that touch off negative or allergic reactions. If certain foods have given you gastrointestinal or other problems in the past, it would be wise to avoid those foods when shopping.

Other factors may guide your shopping choices. You may be dieting; or, you may be trying to "beef up" your diet, for example, to provide more calcium or other minerals. You may have allergies—for example, to sulfites, the additives in many foods that can cause serious or even fatal reactions. Today, the labels on food packaging provide an abundance of dietary information to aid consumers in making choices.

*Buying intelligently* and carefully constitutes your first line of defense against food-borne illness and disease. Here are some guidelines for the conscientious shopper:

- Watch for possible spoilage in everything you buy, and *never* purchase food in a torn package or a dented or bulging can.

- Exercise your right to doubt: check display cases to make sure frozen foods are stored above the frost lines or load lines. Never buy frozen food that has softened.

- Always pick up meat, poultry, and dairy products last when making your grocery rounds.

- Never leave a sackful of groceries in the car on a hot day. Make the grocery store your last stop on the way home, and make sure perishable groceries are wrapped in an insulated bag for the trip home.

- Once home, put everything away quickly in the appropriate storage place, whether refrigerator, freezer, or storage cupboard.

Different foods require different storage methods. The labels on many packaged or canned foods provide instructions for storage procedures.

*Food preparation* under the wrong conditions creates many of the problems that Americans face when they sit down to eat. The wrong conditions range from unclean hands, hair, fingernails, and clothing to failure to wash one's hands thoroughly after using the toilet. You should wash your hands thoroughly after smoking or blowing your nose. You should also wash your hands after handling raw meat, poultry, or eggs and before

working with other foods. Other precautions: Do not use your hands to mix foods; use clean utensils instead. Avoid using the same spoon more than once to taste food while preparing it. Never eat any food directly from the jar or can; this could contaminate the can's contents. Scrub potatoes and other raw foods before cooking them. Carefully clean all utensils, work surfaces, dishes, and kitchen equipment before using them. And drink only pasteurized milk.

It is best to serve foods soon after they are cooked; otherwise, refrigerate them. You can refrigerate hot or warm foods if you are sure they will not raise the refrigerator temperature above 45° F.

The temperatures at which you keep foods affect directly your home's level of food safety. Hot foods should be kept above 140 degrees for safety while cold foods should be stored at 40 degrees or lower. The danger zone in which foods can develop bacteria, sometimes in the space of two or three hours, lies between 60° and 125°. Keeping food warm for several hours in an oven can be hazardous if the oven's temperature is between 60° and 125°.

Some foods require special attention. Eggs, for example, should be used only if they are fresh, clean, uncracked, and odor-free. You may make exceptions if the eggs are unspoiled and if they are to be used in recipes that call for thorough cooking. When serving a dish that has eggs as a major ingredient, cool the dish quickly after it is cooked, preferably in cold water, if it is not to be served hot. Then refrigerate it.

Meat, poultry, and fish are also sensitive. If frozen, they should be thawed in the refrigerator. If you need to thaw these products more quickly, you can place them, sealed in watertight wrappers, in cold water. To cook frozen items of these types, allow about one-and-one-half times the ordinary cooking times for thawed products of the same weight and shape.

Meats, poultry, or fish should be stuffed just before they are cooked, not a day or two ahead of time. The stuffing should reach a temperature of at least 165° F. during cooking. Use reliable timetables or follow package directions when cooking these products, and take extra care with ground meat. Because it is handled several times in packaging, ground meat should be cooked thoroughly and never eaten raw. Some *hams* need to be cooked, and should be if you have any doubt.

Fish, meat, and poultry should be cooked entirely in a single process, not cooked partially one day and then finished on another. Poultry should always be cooked thoroughly. If you store poultry products before the day on which you plan to cook them, you should store the giblets and the rest of the bird separately in the refrigerator. Use the hot dogs and cold meat within a few days after purchasing, and never more than a week later.

*Freezer practices* should be grounded in common sense. A fundamental rule is that freezing does not kill the bacteria in food; it only keeps existing bacteria from multiplying. Thawing enables those bacteria to begin to proliferate again.

Do not refreeze food that has been frozen and thawed. To protect frozen foods, wrap or package each item carefully to keep air away from the product. Different items can be kept safely in a freezing compartment for different periods of time, depending on the product. Label each item with the date it went into the freezer and the type of food.

## Reaching a Physician

Emergencies are usually best handled in a hospital because they are likely to require oxygen, blood transfusions, or other services only a hospital can provide. There are many situations, however, in which a physician's guidance on the phone can be extremely helpful and reassuring.

Because there are times when the family physician may not be available by phone, it's a good idea to ask for the names and phone numbers of physicians who can be called when your own physician can't be reached. In many communities, it is also possible to get the services of a physician by calling the county medical society.

A family on vacation in a remote area or on a cross-country trip by car can be directed to the nearest medical services by calling the telephone operator or the nearest headquarters of the state police.

## Emergency Transport

In the majority of situations, the transfer of an injured person should be handled only by experienced rescue personnel. If you yourself must move a victim to a physician's office or hospital emergency room, here are a few important rules to remember:

**1.** Give all necessary first aid before attempting to move the victim. Do everything to reduce pain and to make the patient comfortable.

**2.** If you improvise a stretcher, be sure it is strong enough to carry the victim and that you have enough people to carry it. Shutters, doors, boards, and even ladders may be used as stretchers. Just be sure that the stretcher is padded underneath to protect the victim and that a blanket or coat is available to cover him and protect him from exposure.

**3.** Bring the stretcher to the victim, not the victim to the stretcher. Slide him onto the stretcher by grasping his clothing or lift him—if enough bearers are available—as shown in the illustration.

**4.** Secure the victim to the stretcher so he won't fall off. You may want to tie his feet together to minimize his movements.

**5.** Unless specific injuries prevent it, the victim should be lying on his back while he is being moved. However, a person who is having difficulty breathing because of a chest injury might be more comfortable if his head and shoulders are raised slightly. A person with a severe injury to the back of his head should be kept lying on his side. In any case, place the patient in a comfortable position that will protect him from further injury.

**6.** Try to transport the patient feet first.

**7.** Unless absolutely necessary, don't try to put a stretcher into a passenger car. It's almost impossible to get the stretcher or injured person into a passenger car without further injuring him. If there is no ambulance,

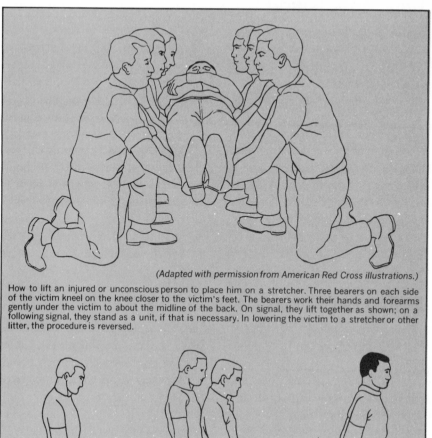

(Adapted with permission from American Red Cross illustrations.)

How to lift an injured or unconscious person to place him on a stretcher. Three bearers on each side of the victim kneel on the knee closer to the victim's feet. The bearers work their hands and forearms gently under the victim to about the midline of the back. On signal, they lift together as shown; on a following signal, they stand as a unit, if that is necessary. In lowering the victim to a stretcher or other litter, the procedure is reversed.

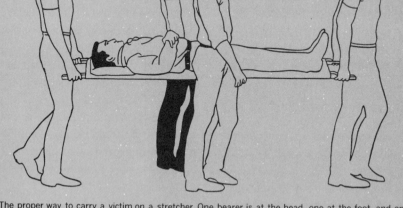

The proper way to carry a victim on a stretcher. One bearer is at the head, one at the foot, and one at either side of the stretcher. The victim should be carried feet first.

a station wagon or truck makes a good substitute.

**8.** When you turn the patient over to a doctor or take him to an emer-gency room of a hospital, give a com-plete account of the situation to the person taking charge. Tell the doctor what you've done for.

# Alphabetic Guide to Medical Emergencies

## Abdominal Wound

Abdominal wounds can result from gunshots during hunting or working with firearms, from falling on a knife or sharp object at home or work, or from a variety of other mishaps ranging from automobile accidents to a mugging attack. Such a wound can be a major emergency requiring surgery and other professional care. Call a physician or arrange for quick transportation to a hospital as quickly as possible.

### Emergency Treatment

If there is severe bleeding, try to control it with pressure. Keep the victim lying on his back with the knees bent; place a pillow, coat, or a similar soft object under the knees to help hold them in the bent position. If abdominal organs are exposed, do not touch them for any reason. Cover the wound with a sterile dressing. Keep the dressing moistened with sterile water or the cleanest water available. Boiled water can be used to moisten the dressing, but be sure it has cooled before applying.

If the victim is to be moved to a hospital or physician's office, be sure the dressing over the wound is large enough and is held in place with a bandage. In addition to pain, you can expect the victim to experience nausea and vomiting, muscle spasms, and severe shock. Make the victim as comfortable as possible under the circumstances; if he complains of thirst, moisten his mouth with a few drops of water, but do not permit him to swallow the liquid.

## Abrasions

### Emergency Treatment

Wash the area in which the skin is scraped or rubbed off with soap and water, using clean gauze or cotton. Allow the abrasion to air-dry, and then cover it with a loose sterile dressing held in place with a bandage. If a sterile dressing is not available, use a clean handerchief.

Change the dressing after the first 24 hours, using household hydrogen peroxide to ease its removal if it sticks to the abrasion because of clotted blood. If the skinned area appears to be accompanied by swelling, or is painful or tender to the touch, consult a physician.

## Acid Burns

Among acids likely to be encountered at work and around the home are sulphuric, nitric, and hydrochloric acids. Wet-cell batteries, such as automobile batteries, contain acid powerful enough to cause chemical destruction of body tissues, and some metal cleaners contain powerful acids.

## Emergency Treatment

Wash off the acid immediately, using large amounts of clean, fresh, cool water. Strip off or cut off any clothing that may have absorbed any of the acid. If possible, put the victim in a shower bath; if a shower is not available, flood the affected skin areas with as much water as possible. However, do not apply water forcefully since this could aggravate damage already done to skin or other tissues.

After as much of the acid as possible has been eliminated by flooding with water, apply a mild solution of sodium bicarbonate or another mild alkali such as lime water. Caution should be exercised, however, in neutralizing an acid burn because the chemical reaction between an acid and an alkali can produce intense heat that would aggravate the injury; also, not all acids are effectively neutralized by alkalis—carbolic acid burns, for example, should be neutralized with alcohol.

Wash the affected areas once more with fresh water, then dry gently with sterile gauze; be careful not to break the skin or to open blisters. Extensive acid burns will cause extreme pain and shock; have the victim lie down with the head and chest a little lower than the rest of the body. As soon as possible, summon a physician or rush the victim to the emergency room of a hospital.

## Aerosol Sprays

Although aerosol sprays generally are regarded as safe when handled according to directions, they can be directed accidentally toward the face with resulting contamination of the eyes or inhalation of the fumes. The pressurized containers may also contain products or propellants that are highly flammable, producing burns when used near an open flame. When stored near heat, in direct sunlight, or in a closed auto, the containers may explode violently.

## Emergency Treatment

If eyes are contaminated by spray particles, flush the eye surfaces with water to remove any particles of the powder mist. Then carefully examine eye surfaces to determine if chemicals appear to be imbedded in the surface of the cornea. If aerosol spray is inhaled, move the patient to a well-ventilated area; keep him lying down, warm, and quiet. If breathing fails, administer artificial respiration. Victims of exploding containers or burning contents of aerosol containers should be given appropriate emergency treatment for bleeding, burns, and shock.

The redness and irritation of eye injuries should subside within a short time. If they do not, or if particles of spray seem to be imbedded in the surface of the eyes, take the victim to an ophthalmologist. A physician should also be summoned if a victim fails to recover quickly from the effects of inhaling an aerosol spray, particularly if the victim suffers from asthma or a similar lung disorder or from an abnormal heart condition.

### Alkali Burns

Alkalis are used in the manufacture of soap and cleaners and in certain household cleaning products. They combine with fats to form soaps and may produce a painful injury when in contact with body surfaces.

### Emergency Treatment

Flood the burned area with copious amounts of clean, cool, fresh water. Put the victim under a shower if possible, or otherwise pour running water over the area for as long as is necessary to dilute and weaken the corrosive chemical. Do not apply the water with such force that skin or other tissues are damaged. Remove clothing contaminated by the chemical.

Neutralize the remaining alkali with diluted vinegar, lemon juice, or a similar mild acid. Then wash the affected areas again with fresh water. Dry carefully with sterile gauze, being careful not to open blisters or otherwise cause skin breaks that could result in infection. Summon professional medical care as soon as possible. Meanwhile, treat the victim for shock.

### Angina Pectoris

Angina pectoris is a condition that causes acute chest pain because of interference with the supply of oxygen to the heart. Although the pain is sometimes confused with ulcer or acute indigestion symptoms, it has a distinct characteristic of its own, producing a feeling of heaviness, strangling, tightness, or suffocation. Angina is a symptom rather than a disease, and may be a chronic condition with those over 50. It is usually treated by placing a nitroglycerine tablet under the tongue.

An attack of acute angina can be brought on by emotional stress, overeating, strenuous exercise, or by any activity that makes excessive demands on heart function.

### Emergency Treatment

An attack usually subsides in about ten minutes, during which the patient appears to be gasping for breath. He should be kept in a semireclining position rather than made to lie flat, and should be moved carefully only in order to place pillows under his head and chest so that he can breathe more easily. A physician should be called promptly after the onset of an attack.

### Animal Bites/Rabies

Wild animals, particularly bats, serve as a natural reservoir of rabies, a disease that is almost always fatal unless promptly and properly treated. But the virus may be present in the saliva of any warm-blooded animal. Domestic animals should be immunized against rabies by vaccines injected by a veterinarian.

Rabies is transmitted to humans by an animal bite or through a cut or scratch already in the skin. The infected saliva may enter through any opening, including the membranes lining the nose or mouth. After an incubation period of about ten days, a person infected by a rabid animal experiences pain at the site of infection, extreme sensitivity of the skin to temperature changes, and painful spasms of the larynx that make it almost impossible to drink. Saliva thickens and the patient becomes restless and easily excitable. By the time symptoms develop, death may be imminent. Obviously, professional medical attention should begin promptly after having been exposed to the possibility of infection.

## Emergency Treatment

The area around the wound should be washed thoroughly and repeatedly with soap and water, using a sterile gauze dressing to wipe fluid away from—not toward—the wound. Another sterile dressing is used to dry the wound and a third to cover it while the patient is taken to a hospital or physician's office. A tetanus injection is also indicated, and police and health authorities should be promptly notified of the biting incident.

If at all possible the biting animal should be indentified—if a wild animal, captured alive—and held for observation for a period of 10 to 15 days. If it can be determined during that period that the animal is not rabid, further treatment may not be required. If the animal is rabid, however, or if it cannot be located and impounded, the patient may have to undergo a series of daily rabies vaccine injections lasting from 14 days for a case of mild exposure to 21 days for severe exposure (a bite near the head, for example), plus several booster shots. Because of the sensitivity of some individuals to the rabies vaccines used, the treatment itself can be quite dangerous.

Recent research, however, has established that a new vaccine called HDCV (human diploid cell vaccine), which requires only six or fewer injections, is immunologically effective and is not usually accompanied by any side effects. The new vaccine has been used successfully on people of all ages who had been bitten by animals known to be rabid.

## Appendicitis

The common signal for approaching appendicitis is a period of several days of indigestion and constipation, culminating in pain and tenderness on the lower right side of the abdomen. Besides these symptoms, appendicitis may be accompanied by nausea and a slight fever. Call a physician immediately and describe the symptoms in detail; delay may result in a ruptured appendix.

## Emergency Treatment

While awaiting medical care, the victim may find some relief from the pain and discomfort by having an ice bag placed over the abdomen. Do not apply heat and give nothing by mouth. A laxative should not be offered.

## Asphyxiation

See GAS POISONING.

## Asthma Attack

### Emergency Treatment

Make the patient comfortable and offer reassurance. If he has been examined by a physician and properly
diagnosed, the patient probably has
an inhalant device or other forms of
medication on his person or nearby.

The coughing and wheezing spell
may have been triggered by the presence of an allergenic substance such
as animal hair, feathers, or kapok in
pillows or cushions. Such items
should be removed from the presence
of the patient. In addition, placing the
patient in a room with high humidity,
such as a bathroom with the shower
turned on, may be helpful.

Asthma attacks are rarely fatal in
young people, but elderly persons
should be watched carefully because
of possible heart strain. In a severe
attack, professional medical care including oxygen equipment may be required.

## Back Injuries

In the event of any serious back injury, call a physician or arrange for
immediate professional transfer of the
victim to a hospital.

### Emergency Treatment

Until determined otherwise by a physician, treat the injured person as a
victim of a fractured spine. If he complains that he cannot move his head,
feet, or toes, the chances are that the
back is fractured. But even if he can
move his feet or legs, it does not necessarily mean that he can be moved
safely, since the back can be fractured
without immediate injury to the spinal
cord.

If the victim shows symptoms of
shock, do not attempt to lower his
head or move his body into the usual
position for shock control. If it is absolutely essential to move the victim
because of immediate danger to his
life, make a rigid stretcher from a
wide piece of solid lumber such as a
door and cover the stretcher with a
blanket for padding. Then carefully
slide or pull the victim onto the
stretcher, using his clothing to hold
him. Tie the body onto the stretcher
with strips of cloth.

## Back Pain

See SCIATICA.

## Black Eye

Although a black eye is frequently regarded as a minor medical problem, it
can result in serious visual problems,
including cataract or glaucoma.

### Emergency Treatment

Inspect the area about the eye for
possible damage to the eye itself,
such as hemorrhage, rupture of the
eyeball, or dislocated lens. Check also
for cuts around the eye that may require professional medical care. Then
treat the bruised area by putting the

victim to bed, covering the eye with a bandage, and applying an ice bag to the area.

If vision appears to be distorted or lacerations need stitching and antibiotic treatment, take the victim to a physician's office. A physician should also be consulted about continued pain and swelling about the eye.

## Black Widow Spider Bites

### Emergency Treatment

Make the victim lie still. If the bite is on the arm or leg, position the victim so that the bite is lower than the level of the heart. Apply a rubber band or similar tourniquet between the bite and the heart to retard venom flow toward the heart. The bite usually is marked by two puncture points. Apply ice packs to the bite. Summon a physician or carry the patient to the nearest hospital.

Loosen the tourniquet or constriction band for a few seconds every 15 minutes while awaiting help; you should be able to feel a pulse beyond the tourniquet if it is not too tight. Do not let the victim move about. Do not permit him to drink alcoholic beverages. He probably will feel weakness, tremor, and severe pain, but reassure him that he will recover. Medications, usually available only to a physician, should be administered promptly.

## Bleeding, Internal

Internal bleeding is always a very serious condition; it requires immediate professional medical attention.

In cases of internal bleeding, blood is sometimes brought to the outside of the body by coughing from the lungs, by vomiting from the stomach, by trickling from the ear or nose, or by passing in the urine or bowel movement.

Often, however, internal bleeding is concealed, and the only symptom may be the swelling that appears around the site of broken bones. A person can lose three or four pints of blood inside the body without a trace of blood appearing outside the body.

### Some Symptoms of Internal Bleeding

The victim will appear ill and pale. His skin will be colder than normal, especially the hands and feet; often the skin looks clammy because of sweating. The pulse usually will be rapid (over 90 beats a minute) and feeble.

### Emergency Treatment

Serious internal bleeding is beyond the scope of first aid. If necessary treat the victim for respiratory and cardiac arrest and for shock while waiting for medical aid.

## Bleeding, Minor

Bleeding from minor cuts, scrapes, and bruises usually stops by itself, but even small injuries of this kind should receive attention to prevent infection.

### Emergency Treatment

The injured area should be washed thoroughly with soap and water, or if possible, held under running water. The surface should then be covered with a sterile bandage.

The type of wound known as a puncture wound may bleed very little, but is potentially extremely dangerous because of the possibility of tetanus infection. Anyone who steps on a rusty nail or thumbtack or has a similar accident involving a pointed object that penetrates deep under the skin surface should consult a physician about the need for antitetanus inoculation or a booster shot.

### Blisters

### Emergency Treatment

If the blister is on a hand or foot or other easily accessible part of the body, wash the area around the blister thoroughly with soap and water. After carefully drying the skin around the blister, apply an antiseptic to the same area. Then sterilize the point and a substantial part of a needle by heating it in an open flame. When the needle has been thoroughly sterilized, use the point to puncture the blister along the margin of the blister. Carefully squeeze the fluid from the blister by pressing it with a sterile gauze dressing; the dressing should soak up most of the fluid. Next, place a fresh sterile dressing over the blister and fasten it in place with a bandage. If a blister forms in a tender area or in a place that is not easily accessible, such as under the arm, do not open it yourself; consult your physician.

The danger from any break in the skin is that germs or dirt can slip through the natural barrier to produce an infection or inflammation. Continue to apply an antiseptic each day to the puncture area until it has healed. If it appears that an infection has developed or healing is unusually slow, consult a doctor. Persons with diabetes or circulatory problems may have to be more cautious about healing of skin breaks than other individuals.

### Blood Blisters

Blood blisters, sometimes called hematomas, usually are caused by a sharp blow to the body surface such as hitting a finger with a hammer while pounding nails.

### Emergency Treatment

Wash the area of the blood blister thoroughly with soap and water. Do not open it. If it is a small blood blister, cover it with a protective bandage; in many cases, the tiny pool of blood under the skin will be absorbed by the surrounding tissues if there is no further pressure at that point.

If the blood blister fails to heal quickly or becomes infected, consult a physician. Because the pool of blood has resulted from damage to a blood vessel, a blood blister usually is more vulnerable to infection or inflammation than an ordinary blister.

### Boils

Boils frequently are an early sign of diabetes or another illness and should be watched carefully if they occur often. In general, they result from germs or dirt being rubbed into the skin by tight-fitting clothing, scratching, or through tiny cuts made during shaving.

## Emergency Treatment

If the boil is above the lip, do not squeeze it or apply any pressure. The infection in that area of the face may drain into the brain because of the pattern of blood circulation on the face. Let a physician treat any boil on the face. If the boil is on the surface of another part of the body, apply moist hot packs, but do not squeeze or press on the boil because that action can force the infection into the circulatory system. A wet compress can be made by soaking a wash cloth or towel in warm water.

If the boil erupts, carefully wipe away the pus with a sterile dressing, and then cover it with another sterile dressing. If the boil is large or slow to erupt, or if it is slow to heal, consult a physician.

## Bone Bruises

### Emergency Treatment

Make sure the bone is not broken. If the injury is limited to the thin layer of tissue surrounding the bone, and the function of the limb is normal though painful, apply a compression dressing and an ice pack. Limit use of the injured limb for the next day or two.

As the pain and swelling recede, cover the injured area with a foam-rubber pad held in place with an elastic bandage. Because the part of the limb that is likely to receive a bone bruise lacks a layer of muscle and fat, it will be particularly sensitive to any pressure until recovery is complete.

## Botulism

The bacteria that produce the lethal toxin of botulism are commonly present on unwashed farm vegetables and thrive in containers that are improperly sealed against the damaging effects of air. Home-canned vegetables, particularly string beans, are a likely source of botulism, but the toxin can be found in fruits, meats, and other foods. It can also appear in food that has been properly prepared but allowed to cool before being served. Examples are cold soups and marinated vegetables.

### Emergency Treatment

As soon as acute symptoms—nausea, diarrhea, and abdominal distress—appear, try to induce vomiting. Vomiting usually can be started by touching the back of the victim's throat with a finger or the handle of a spoon, which should be smooth and blunt, or by offering him a glass of water in which two tablespoons of salt have been dissolved. Call a physician; describe all of the symptoms, which also may include, after several hours, double vision, muscular weakness, and difficulty in swallowing and breathing. Save samples of the food suspected of contamination for analysis.

Prompt hospitalization and injection of antitoxin are needed to save most cases of botulism poisoning. Additional emergency measures may include artificial respiration if regular breathing fails because of paralysis of respiratory muscles. Continue artificial respiration until professional medical care is provided. If other individuals have eaten the contaminated food, they should receive treatment for botulism even if they show no symptoms of the toxin's effects, since symptoms may be delayed by several days.

## Brown House (or Recluse) Spider Bites

### Emergency Treatment

Apply an ice bag or cold pack to the wound area. Aspirin and antihistamines may be offered to help relieve any pain or feeling of irritation. Keep the victim lying down and quiet. Call a physician as quickly as possible and describe the situation; the physician will advise what further action should be taken at this point.

The effects of a brown spider bite frequently last much longer than the pain of the bite, which may be comparatively mild for an insect bite or sting. But the poison from the bite can gradually destroy the surrounding tissues, leaving at first an ulcer and eventually a disfiguring scar. A physician's treatment is needed to control the loss of tissue; he probably will prescribe drugs and recommend continued use of cold compresses. The victim, meanwhile, will feel numbness and muscular weakness, requiring a prolonged period of bed rest in addition to the medical treatments.

## Bruises/Contusions

### Emergency Treatment

Bruises or contusions result usually from a blow to the body that is powerful enough to damage muscles, tendons, blood vessels, or other tissues without causing a break in the skin.

Because the bruised area will be tender, protect it from further injury. If possible, immobilize the injured body part with a sling, bandage, or other device that makes the victim feel more comfortable; pillows, folded blankets, or similar soft materials can be used to elevate an arm or leg. Apply an ice bag or cold water dressing to the injured area.

A simple bruise usually will heal without extensive treatment. The swelling and discoloration result from blood oozing from damaged tissues. Severe bruising can, however, be quite serious and requires medical attention. Keep the victim quiet and watch for symptoms of shock. Give aspirin for pain.

## Bullet Wounds

Bullet wounds, whether accidental or purposely inflicted, can range from those that are superficial and external to those that involve internal bleeding and extensive tissue damage.

## Emergency Treatment

A surface bullet wound accompanied by bleeding should be covered promptly with sterile gauze to prevent further infection. The flow of blood should be controlled as described under "Severe Bleeding" in this chapter. *Don't* try to clean the wound with soap or water.

If the wound is internal, keep the patient lying down and wrap him with coats or blankets placed over and under his body. If respiration has ceased or is impaired, give mouth-to-mouth respiration and treat him for shock. Get medical aid promptly.

### Burns, Thermal

Burns are generally described according to the depth or area of skin damage involved. First-degree burns are the most superficial. They are marked by reddening of the skin and swelling, increased warmth, tenderness, and pain. Second-degree burns, deeper than first-degree, are in effect open wounds, characterized by blisters and severe pain in addition to redness. Third-degree burns are deep enough to involve damage to muscles and bones. The skin is charred and there may be no pain because nerve endings have been destroyed. However, the area of the burn generally is more important than the degree of burn; a first- or second-degree burn covering a large area of the body is more likely to be fatal than a small third-degree burn.

### Emergency Treatment

You will want to get professional medical help for treatment of a severe burn, but there are a number of things you can do until such help is obtained. If burns are minor, apply ice or ice water until pain subsides. Then wash the area with soap and water. Cover with a sterile dressing. Give the victim one or two aspirin tablets to help relieve discomfort. A sterile gauze pad soaked in a solution of two tablespoons of baking soda (sodium bicarbonate) per quart of lukewarm water may be applied.

For more extensive or severe burns, there are three first-aid objectives: (1) relieve pain, (2) prevent shock, (3) prevent infection. To relieve pain, exclude air by applying a thick dressing of four to six layers plus additional coverings of clean, tightly woven material; for extensive burns, use clean sheets or towels. Clothing should be cut away—never pulled—from burned areas; where fabric is stuck to the wound, leave it for a physician to remove later. Do not apply any ointment, grease, powder, salve, or other medication; the physician simply will have to remove such material before he can begin professional treatment of the burns.

To prevent shock, make sure the victim's head is lower than his feet. Be sure that the victim is covered sufficiently to keep him warm, but not enough to make him overheated; exposure to cold can make the effects of shock more severe. Provide the victim with plenty of nonalcoholic liquids such as sweetened water, tea, or fruit juices, so long as he is conscious and able to swallow.

To prevent infection, do not permit absorbent cotton or adhesive tape to touch the wound caused by a burn. Do not apply iodine or any other antiseptic to the burn. Do not open any blisters. Do not permit any unsterile matter to contact the burn area. If possible, prevent other persons from coughing, sneezing, or even breathing toward the wound resulting from a burn. Serious infections frequently develop in burn victims from contamination by microorganisms of the mouth and nose.

## Long-Term Treatment

A highly effective method of treating serious burns involves, first, removal of samples of uninjured skin from victims' bodies. Laboratory workers then "grind up" the healthy skin samples and separate them into groups of cells. Placed in flasks and bathed in a growth-stimulating solution, the cells grow rapidly; while the colonies are small, they double in size every 17 hours. New skin appears. The procedure can be repeated until enough has been grown to cover the burned areas.

Because the "test-tube skin" is developed from samples of a victim's own skin, the body does not reject it. It can be grafted onto a burned area in patches until the entire burn is covered. The new skin has no hair follicles or sweat glands, and is thinner than normal skin. But it offers hope to persons who are hospitalized with burn injuries.

See also CHEMICAL BURNS OF THE EYE.

## Carbuncles

Carbuncles are quite similar to boils except that they usually develop around multiple hair follicles and commonly appear on the neck or face. Personal hygiene is one factor involved in the development of carbuncles; persons apparently susceptible to the pustular inflammations must exercise special care in cleansing areas in which carbuncles occur, particularly if they suffer from diabetes or circulatory ailments.

### Emergency Treatment

Apply moist hot packs to the boil-like swelling. Change the moist hot packs frequently, or place a hot-water bottle on the moist dressing to maintain the moist heat application. Do not handle the carbuncle beyond whatever contact is necessary to apply or maintain the moist heat. The carbuncle should eventually rupture or reach a point where it can be opened with a sterile sharp instrument. After the carbuncle has ruptured and drained, and the fluid from the growth has been carefully cleaned away, apply a sterile dressing.

Frequently, carbuncles must be opened and drained by a physician.

## Cat Scratch Fever

Although the scratch or bite of a house cat or alley cat may appear at first to be only a mild injury, the wound can become the site of entry for a disease virus transmitted by apparently healthy cats. The inflammation, accompanied by fever, generally affects the lymph nodes and produces some aches and pains as well as fatigue. Although the disease is seldom fatal, an untreated case can spread to brain tissues and lead to other complications.

### Emergency Treatment

Wash the scratch thoroughly with water and either soap or a mild detergent. Apply a mild antiseptic such as hydrogen peroxide. Cover with a sterile dressing.

Watch the area of the scratch carefully for the next week or two. If redness or swelling develop, even after the scratch appears healed, consult your physician. The inflammation of the scratch area may be accompanied by mild fever and symptoms similar to those of influenza; in small children, the symptoms may be quite serious. Bed rest and antibiotics usually are prescribed.

### Charley Horse

A charley horse occurs because a small number of muscle fibers have been torn or ruptured by overstraining the muscle, or by the force of a blow to the muscle.

### Emergency Treatment

Rest the injured muscle and apply an ice pack if there is swelling. A compression dressing can be applied to support the muscle. Avoid movement that stretches the muscle, and restrict other movements that make the victim uncomfortable. If pain and swelling persist, call a physician.

During the recovery period, which may not begin for a day or two, apply local heat with a hot water bottle or an electric heating pad, being careful not to burn the victim. A return to active use of the muscle can begin gradually as pain permits.

### Chemical Burns of the Eye

### Emergency Treatment

Flush the victim's eye immediately with large quantities of fresh, clean water; a drinking fountain can be used to provide a steady stream of water. If a drinking fountain is not available, lay the victim on the floor or ground with his head turned slightly to one side and pour water into the eye from a cup or glass. Always direct the stream of water so that it enters the eye surface at the inside corner and flows across the eye to the outside corner. If the victim is unable, because of intense pain, to open his eyes, it may be necessary to hold the lids apart while water pours across the eye. Continue flushing the eye for at least 15 minutes. (An alternate method is to immerse the victim's face in a pan or basin or bucket of water while he opens and closes his eyes repeatedly; continue the process for at least 15 minutes.)

When the chemical has been flushed from the victim's eye, the eye should be covered with a small, thick compress held in place with a bandage that covers both eyes, if possible; the bandage can be tied around the victim's head. **Note:** Apply nothing but water to the eye; do not attempt to neutralize a chemical burn of the eye and do not apply oil, ointment, salve, or other medications. Rush the victim to a physician as soon as possible, preferably to an ophthalmologist.

## Chemicals on Skin

Many household and industrial chemicals, such as ammonia, lye, iodine, creosote, and a wide range of insecticides can cause serious injury if accidentally spilled on the skin.

### Emergency Treatment

Wash the body surface that has been affected by the chemical with large amounts of water. Do not try to neutralize the chemical with another substance; the reaction may aggravate the injury. If blisters appear, apply a sterile dressing. If the chemical is a refrigerant, such as Freon, or carbon dioxide under pressure, treat for frostbite.

If the chemical has splashed into the eyes or produces serious injury to the affected body surface, call a physician. The victim should be watched closely for possible poisoning effects if the chemical is a pesticide, since such substances may be absorbed through the skin to produce internal toxic reactions. If there is any question about the toxicity of a chemical, ask your doctor or call the nearest poison control center.

## Chigger Bites

### Emergency Treatment

Apply ice water or rub ice over the area afflicted by bites of the tiny red insects. Bathing the area with alcohol, ammonia water or a solution of baking soda also will provide some relief from the itching.

Wash thoroughly with soap, using a scrub brush to prevent further infestation by the chiggers in other areas of the body. Rub alcohol over the surrounding areas and apply sulfur ointment as protection against mites that may not have attached themselves to the skin. Continue applications of ice water or alcohol to skin areas invaded by the insects. Clothing that was worn should be laundered immediately.

## Chilblains

### Emergency Treatment

Move the victim to a moderately warm place and remove wet or tight clothing. Soak the affected body area in warm—but not hot—water for about ten minutes. Then carefully blot the skin dry, but do not rub the skin. Replace the clothing with garments that are warm, soft, and dry.

Give the victim a stimulant such as tea or coffee, or an alcoholic beverage, and put him to bed with only light blankets; avoid the pressure of heavy blankets or heavy, tight garments on the sensitive skin areas. The victim should move the affected body areas gently to help restore normal circulation. If complications develop, such as marked discoloration of the skin, pain, or blistering and splitting of the skin, call a physician.

## Cold Sores/Fever Blisters

### Emergency Treatment

Apply a soothing ointment or a medication such as camphor ice. Avoid squeezing or otherwise handling the blisters; moisture can aggravate the sores and hinder their healing. Repeated appearances of cold sores or fever blisters, which are caused by the herpes simplex virus, may require treatment by a physician.

## Concussion

See HEAD INJURIES.

## Contusions

See BRUISES.

## Convulsions

### Emergency Treatment

Protect the victim from injury by moving him to a safe place; loosen any constricting clothing such as a tie or belt; put a pillow or coat under his head; if his mouth is open, place a folded cloth between his teeth to keep him from biting his tongue. Do not force anything into his mouth. Keep the patient warm but do not disturb him; do not try to restrain his convulsive movements.

Send for a physician as quickly as possible. Watch the patient's breathing and begin artificial respiration if breathing stops for more than one minute. Be sure that breathing actually has stopped; the patient may be sleeping or unconscious after an attack but breathing normally.

Convulsions in a small child may signal the onset of an infectious disease and may be accompanied by a high fever. The same general precautions should be taken to prevent self-injury on the part of the child. If placed in a bed, the child should be protected against falling onto the floor. Place him on his side—not on his back or stomach—if he vomits. Cold compresses or ice packs on the back of the neck and the head may help relieve symptoms. Immediate professional medical care is vital because brain damage can result if treatment is delayed.

See also EPILEPTIC SEIZURES.

## Cramps

See MUSCLE CRAMPS.

## Croup

Croup is a breathing disorder usually caused by a virus infection and less often by bacteria or allergy. It is a common condition during childhood, and in some cases, may require brief hospitalization for proper treatment.

The onset of a croup attack is likely to occur during the night with a sudden hoarse or barking cough accompanied by difficulty in breathing. The coughing is usually followed by choking spasms that sound as though the child is strangling. There may also be a mild fever. A physician should be called immediately when these symptoms appear.

## Emergency Treatment

The most effective treatment for croup is cool moist air. Cool water vaporizers are available as well as warm steam vaporizers. Another alternative is to take the child into the bathroom, close the door and windows, and let the hot water run from the shower and sink taps until the room is filled with steam.

It is also possible to improvise a croup tent by boiling water in a kettle on a portable hot plate and arranging a blanket over the back of a chair so that it encloses the child and an adult as well as the steaming kettle. A child should never be left alone even for an instant in such a makeshift arrangement.

If the symptoms do not subside in about 20 minutes with any of the above procedures, or if there is mounting fever, and if the physician is not on his way, the child should be rushed to the closest hospital. Cold moist night air, rather than being a danger, may actually make the symptoms subside temporarily.

## Diabetic Coma and Insulin Shock

Diabetics should always carry an identification tag or card to alert others of their condition in the event of a diabetic coma—which is due to a lack of insulin. They also should advise friends or family members of their diabetic condition and the proper emergency measures that can be taken in the event of an onset of diabetic coma. A bottle of rapid-acting insulin should be kept on hand for such an emergency.

## Emergency Treatment

If the victim is being treated for diabetes, he probably will have nearby a supply of insulin and a hypodermic apparatus for injecting it. Find the insulin, hypodermic syringe, and needle; clean a spot on the upper arm or thigh, and inject about 50 units of insulin. Call a physician without delay, and describe the patient's symptoms and your treatment. The patient usually will respond without ill effects, but may be quite thirsty. Give him plenty of fluids, as needed.

If the victim does not respond to the insulin, or if you cannot find the insulin and hypodermic syringe, rush the victim to the nearest physician's office.

Insulin shock—which is due to a reaction to too much insulin and not enough sugar in the blood—can be treated in an emergency by offering a sugar-rich fluid such as a cola beverage or orange juice. Diabetics frequently carry a lump of sugar or candy that can be placed in their mouth in case of an insulin shock reaction. It should be tucked between the teeth and cheek so the victim will not choke on it.

If you find a diabetic in a coma and do not know the cause, assume the cause is an insulin reaction and treat him with sugar. This will give immediate relief to an insulin reaction but will not affect diabetic coma.

## Diarrhea

### Emergency Treatment

Give the victim an antidiarrheal agent; all drugstores carry medications composed of kaolin and pectin that are useful for this purpose. Certain bismuth compounds also are recommended for diarrhea control.

Put the victim in bed for a period of at least 12 hours and withhold food and drink for that length of time. Do not let the victim become dehydrated; if he is thirsty, let him suck on pieces of ice. If the diarrhea appears to be subsiding, let him sip a mild beverage like tea or ginger ale; cola syrup is also recommended.

Later on the patient can try eating bland foods such as dry toast, crackers, gelatin desserts, or jellied consomme. Avoid feeding rich, fatty, or spicy foods. If the diarrhea fails to subside or is complicated by colic or vomiting, call a physician.

## Dizziness/Vertigo

Emotional upsets, allergies, and improper eating and drinking habits—too much food, too little food, or foods that are too rich—can precipitate symptoms of dizziness. The cause also can be a physical disorder such as abnormal functioning of the inner ear or a circulatory problem. Smoking tobacco, certain drugs such

as quinine, and fumes of some chemicals also can produce dizziness.

### Emergency Treatment

Have the victim lie down with the eyes closed. In many cases, a period of simple bed rest will alleviate the symptoms. Keep the victim quiet and comfortable. If the feeling of dizziness continues, becomes worse, or is accompanied by nausea and vomiting, call a physician.

Severe or persistent dizziness or vertigo requires a longer period of bed rest and the use of medicines prescribed by a physician. While recovering, the victim should avoid sudden changes in body position or turning the head rapidly. In some types of vertigo, surgery is required to cure the disorder.

## Drowning

Victims of drowning seldom die because of water in the lungs or stomach. They die because of lack of air.

### Emergency Treatment

If the victim's breathing has been impaired, start artificial respiration immediately. If there is evidence of cardiac arrest, administer cardiac massage. When the victim is able to breathe for himself, treat him for shock and get medical help.

## Drug Overdose (Barbiturates)

Barbiturates are used in a number of drugs prescribed as sedatives, although many are also available through illegal channels. Because the drugs can affect the judgment of the user, he may not remember having taken a dose and so may take additional pills, thus producing overdose effects.

## Emergency Treatment

If the drug was taken orally, try to induce vomiting in the victim. Have him drink a glass of water containing two tablespoons of salt. Or touch the back of his throat gently with a finger or a smooth blunt object like the handle of a spoon. Then give the victim plenty of warm water to drink. It is important to rid the stomach of as much of the drug as possible and to dilute the substance remaining in the gastrointestinal tract.

As soon as possible, call a physician or get the victim to the nearest hospital or physician's office. If breathing fails, administer artificial respiration.

## Drug Overdose (Stimulants)

Although most of the powerful stimulant drugs, or pep pills, are available only through a physician's prescription, the same medications are available through illicit sources. When taken without direction of a supervising physician, the stimulants can produce a variety of adverse side effects, and when used frequently over a period of time can result in physical and psychological problems that require hospital treatment.

## Emergency Treatment

Give the victim a solution of one ta-

blespoon of activated charcoal mixed with a small amount of water, or give him a glass of milk, to dilute the effects of the medication in the stomach. Then induce vomiting by pressing gently on the back of the throat with a finger or the smooth blunt edge of a spoon handle. Vomiting also may be induced with a solution made of one teaspoonful of mustard in a half glass of water. Do not give syrup of ipecac to a victim who has been taking stimulants.

As soon as possible call a physician or get the victim to the nearest hospital or physician's office. If breathing fails, administer artificial respiration.

## Earaches

An earache may be associated with a wide variety of ailments ranging from the common cold or influenza to impacted molars or tonsillitis. An earache also may be involved in certain infectious diseases such as measles or scarlet fever. Because of the relationship of ear structures to other parts of the head and throat, an infection involving the symptoms of earache can easily spread to the brain tissues or the spongy mastoid bone behind the ear. Call a physician and describe all of the symptoms, including temperature, any discharge, pain, ringing in the ear, or deafness. Delay in reporting an earache to a doctor can result in complications that require hospital treatment.

## Emergency Treatment

This may incude a few drops of warm

olive oil or sweet oil held in the ear by a small wad of cotton. Aspirin can be given to help relieve any pain. Professional medical treatment may include the use of antibiotics.

## Ear, Foreign Body in

### Emergency Treatment

Do not insert a hairpin, stick, or other object in the ear in an effort to remove a foreign object; you are likely to force the object farther into the ear canal. Instead, have the victim tilt his head to one side, with the ear containing the foreign object facing upward. While pulling gently on the lobe of the ear to straighten the canal, pour a little warmed olive oil or mineral oil into the ear. Then have the victim tilt that ear downward so the oil will run out quickly; it should dislodge the foreign object.

Wipe the ear canal gently with a cotton-tipped matchstick, or a similar device that will not irritate the lining of the ear canal, after the foreign body has been removed. If the emergency treatment is not successful, call a physician.

## Electric Shocks

An electric shock from the usual 110-volt current in most homes can be a serious emergency, especially if the person's skin or clothing is wet. Under these circumstances, the shock may paralyze the part of the brain that controls breathing and stop the heart completely or disorder its pumping action.

### Emergency Treatment

It is of the utmost importance to break the electrical contact *immediately* by unplugging the wire of the appliance involved or by shutting off the house current switch. **Do not touch the victim of the shock while he is still acting as an electrical conductor.**

If the shock has come from a faulty wire out of doors and the source of the electrical current can't be reached easily, make a lasso of dry rope on a long sturdy dry stick. Catch the victim's hand or foot in the loop and drag him away from the wire. Another way to break the contact is to cut the wire with a dry axe.

If the victim of the shock is unconscious, or if his pulse is very weak, administer mouth-to-mouth respiration and cardiac massage until he can get to a hospital.

## Epileptic Seizures

Epilepsy is a disorder of the nervous system that produces convulsive seizures. In a major seizure or *grand mal,* the epileptic usually falls to the ground. Indeed, falling is in most cases one of the principal dangers of the disease. Then the epileptic's body begins to twitch or jerk spasmodically. His breathing may be labored, and saliva may appear on his lips. His face may become pale or bluish. Although the scene can be frightening, it is not truly a medical emergency; the afflicted person is in no danger of losing his life.

Emergency Treatment

Make the person suffering the seizure as comfortable as possible. If he is on a hard surface, put something soft under his head, and move any hard or dangerous objects away from him. **Make no attempt to restrain his movements, and do not force anything into his mouth.** Just leave him alone until the attack is over, as it should be in a few minutes. If his mouth is already open, you might put something soft, such as a folded handerchief, between his side teeth. This will help to prevent him from biting his tongue or lips. If he seems to go into another seizure after coming out of the first, or if the seizure lasts more than ten minutes, call a physician. If his lower jaw sags and begins to obstruct his breathing, support of the lower jaw may be helpful in improving his breathing.

When the seizure is over, the patient should be allowed to rest quietly. Some people sleep heavily after a seizure. Others awake at once but are disoriented or confused for a while. Treat the episode in a matter-of-fact way. If it is the first seizure the person is aware of having had, advise him to see his physician promptly.

### Eye, Foreign Body in

Emergency Treatment

Do not rub the eye or touch it with unwashed hands. The foreign body usually becomes lodged on the inner surface of the upper eyelid. Pull the upper eyelid down over the lower lid to help work the object loose. Tears or clean water can help wash out the dirt or other object. If the bit of irritating material can be seen on the surface of the eyeball, try very carefully to flick it out with the tip of a clean, moistened handkerchief or a piece of moistened cotton. Never touch the surface of the eye with dry materials. Sometimes a foreign body can be removed by carefully rolling the upper lid over a pencil or wooden matchstick to expose the object.

After the foreign object has been removed, the eye should be washed with clean water or with a solution made from one teaspoon of salt dissolved in a pint of water. This will help remove any remaining particles of the foreign body as well as any traces of irritating chemicals that might have been a part of it. Iron particles, for example, may leave traces of rust on the eye's surface unless washed away.

If the object cannot be located and removed without difficulty, a small patch of gauze or a folded handkerchief should be taped over the eye and the victim taken to a physician's office—preferably the office of an ophthalmologist. A physician also should be consulted if a feeling of irritation in the eye continues after the foreign body has been removed.

### Fever

Emergency Treatment

If the fever is mild, around 100°F. by mouth, have the victim rest in bed and provide him with a light diet. Watch closely for other symptoms, such as a rash, and any further increase in body temperature. Aspirin usually can be given.

If the temperature rises to 101° F. or higher, is accompanied by pain, headache, delirium, confused behavior, coughing, vomiting, or other indications of a severe illness, call a physician. Describe all of the symptoms in detail, including the appearance of any rash and when it began.

## Fever blisters

See COLD SORES.

## Finger Dislocation

### Emergency Treatment

Call a physician and arrange for inspection and treatment of the injury. If a physician is not immediately available, the finger dislocation may be reduced (put back in proper alignment) by grasping it firmly and carefully pulling it into normal position. Pull very slowly and avoid rough handling that might complicate the injury by damaging a tendon. If the dislocation cannot be reduced after the first try, go through the procedure once more. But do not try it more than twice.

Whether or not you are successful in reducing the finger dislocation, the finger should be immobilized after your efforts until a physician can examine it. A clean flat wooden stick can be strapped along the palm side of the finger with adhesive tape or strips of bandage to hold it in place.

## Fingernail Injuries/Hangnails

### Emergency Treatment

Wash the injured nail area thoroughly with warm water and soap. Trim off any torn bits of nail. Cover with a small adhesive dressing or bandage.

Apply petroleum jelly or cold cream to the injured nail area twice a day, morning and night, until it is healed. If redness or irritation develops in the adjoining skin area, indicating an infection, consult a physician.

## Fish Poisoning

### Emergency Treatment

Induce vomiting in the victim to remove the bits of poisonous fish from the stomach. Vomiting usually can be started by pressing on the back of the throat with a finger or a spoon handle that is blunt and smooth, or by having the victim drink a solution of two tablespoons of salt in a glass of water.

Call a physician as soon as possible. Describe the type of fish eaten and the symptoms, which may include nausea, diarrhea, abdominal pain, muscular weakness, and a numbness or tingling sensation that begins about the face and spreads to the extremities.

If breathing fails, administer mouth-to-mouth artificial respiration; a substance commonly found in poisonous fish causes respiratory failure. Also, be prepared to provide emergency treatment for convulsions.

## Food Poisoning

### Emergency Treatment

If the victim is not already vomiting, try to induce it to clear the stomach. Vomiting can be started in most cases by pressing gently on the back of the throat with a finger or a blunt smooth spoon handle, or by having the patient drink a glass of water containing two tablespoons of salt. If the victim has vomited, put him to bed.

Call a physician and describe the food ingested and the symptoms that developed. If symptoms are severe, professional medical treatment with antibiotics and medications for cramps may be required. Special medications also may be needed for diarrhea caused by bacterial food poisoning.

## Fractures

Any break in a bone is called a fracture. The break is called an *open* or *compound fracture* if one or both ends of the broken bone pierce the skin. A *closed* or *simple fracture* is one in which the broken bone doesn't come through the skin.

It is sometimes difficult to distinguish a strained muscle or a sprained ligament from a broken bone, since sprains and strains can be extremely painful even though they are less serious than breaks. However, when there is any doubt, the injury should be treated as though it were a simple fracture.

### Emergency Treatment

Don't try to help the injured person move around or get up unless he has slowly tested out the injured part of his body and is sure that nothing has been broken. If he is in extreme pain, or if the injured part has begun to swell, or if by running the finger lightly along the affected bone a break can be felt, *do not* move him. Under no circumstances should he be crowded into a car if his legs, hip, ribs, or back are involved in the accident. Call for an ambulance immediately, and until it arrives, treat the person for shock.

### Splinting

In a situation where it is imperative to move someone who may have a fracture, the first step is to apply a splint so that the broken bone ends are immobilized.

Splints can be improvised from anything rigid enough and of the right length to support the fractured part of the body: a metal rod, board, long cardboard tube, tightly rolled newspaper or blanket. If the object being used has to be padded for softness, use a small blanket or any other soft material, such as a jacket.

The splint should be long enough so that it can be tied with a bandage, torn sheet, or neckties beyond the joint above and below the fracture as well as at the site of the break. If a leg is involved, it should be elevated with pillows or any other firm support after the splint has been applied. If the victim has to wait a considerable length of time before receiving professional attention, the splint bandaging should be checked from time to time to make sure it isn't too tight.

In the case of an open or compound fracture, additional steps must be taken. Remove that part of the victim's clothing that is covering the wound. Do not wash or probe into the wound, but control bleeding by applying pressure over the wound through a sterile or clean dressing.

### Frostbite

### Emergency Treatment

Begin rapid rewarming of the affected tissues as soon as possible. If possible, immerse the victim in a warm bath, but avoid scalding. (The temperature should be between 102°F. and 105°F.) Warm wet towels also will help if changed frequently and applied gently. Do not massage, rub, or even touch the frostbitten flesh. If warm water or a warming fire is not available, place the patient in a sleeping bag or cover him with coats and blankets. Hot liquids can be offered if available to help raise the body temperature.

For any true frostbite case, prompt medical attention is important. The depth and degree of the frozen tissue cannot be determined without a careful examination by a physician.

### Gallbladder Attacks

Although gallstones can affect a wide variety of individuals, the most common victims are overweight persons who enjoy rich foods. The actual attack of spasms caused by gallstones passing through the duct leading from the gallbladder to the digestive tract usually is preceded by periods of stomach distress including belching. X rays usually will reveal the presence of gallstones when the early warning signs are noted, and measures can be taken to reduce the threat of a gallbladder attack.

### Emergency Treatment

Call a physician and describe in detail the symptoms, which may include colic high in the abdomen and pain extending to the right shoulder; the pain may be accompanied by nausea, vomiting, and sweating. Hot water bottles may be applied to the abdomen to help relieve distress while waiting for professional medical care. If the physician permits, the victim may be allowed to sip certain fluids such as fruit juices, but do not offer him solid food.

### Gas Poisoning

Before attempting to revive someone overcome by toxic gas poisoning, the most important thing to do is to remove him to the fresh air. If this isn't feasible, all windows and doors should be opened to let in as much fresh air as possible.

Any interior with a dangerous concentration of carbon monoxide or other toxic gases is apt to be highly explosive. Therefore, gas and electricity should be shut off as quickly as possible. **Under no circumstances should any matches be lighted in an interior where there are noxious fumes.**

The rescuer needn't waste time

covering his face with a handkerchief or other cloth. He should hold his breath instead, or take only a few quick, shallow breaths while bringing the victim to the out-of-doors or to an open window.

## Emergency Treatment

Administer artificial respiration if the victim is suffering respiratory arrest. Arrange for medical help as soon as possible, requesting that oxygen be brought to the scene.

## Head Injuries

Accidents involving the head can result in concussion, skull fracture, or brain injury. Symptoms of head injury include loss of consciousness, discharge of a watery or blood-tinged fluid from the ears, nose, or mouth, and a difference in size of the pupils of the eyes. Head injuries must be thought of as serious; they demand immediate medical assistance.

## Emergency Treatment

Place the victim in a supine position, and, if there is no evidence of injury to his neck, arrange for a slight elevation of his head *and* shoulders. Make certain that he has a clear airway and administer artificial respiration if necessary. If vomitus, blood, or other fluids appear to flow from the victim's mouth, turn his head gently to one side. Control bleeding and treat for shock. Do not administer stimulants or fluids of any kind.

## Heart Attack

A heart attack is caused by interference with the blood supply to the heart muscle. When the attack is brought on because of a blood clot in the coronary artery, it is known as *coronary occlusion* or *coronary thrombosis.*

The most dramatic symptom of a serious heart attack is a crushing chest pain that usually travels down the left arm into the hand or into the neck and back. The pain may bring on dizziness, cold sweat, complete collapse, and loss of consciousness. The face has an ashen pallor, and there may be vomiting.

## Emergency Treatment

The victim **must not be moved** unless he has fallen in a dangerous place. If no physician is immediately available, an ambulance should be called at once. No attempt should be made to get the victim of a heart attack into an automobile.

Until help arrives, give the victim every reassurance that he will get prompt treatment, and keep him as calm and quiet as possible. Don't give him any medicine or stimulants. If oxygen is available, start administering it to the victim immediately, either by mask or nasal catheter, depending on which is available.

If the victim is suffering from respiratory arrest, begin artificial respiration. If he is suffering from cardiac arrest, begin cardiac massage.

## Heat Exhaustion

Heat exhaustion occurs when the

body is exposed to high temperatures and large amounts of blood accumulate in the skin as a way of cooling it. As a result, there is a marked decrease in the amount of blood that circulates through the heart and to the brain. The victim becomes markedly pale and is covered with cold perspiration. Breathing is increasingly shallow and the pulse weakens. In acute cases, fainting occurs. Medical aid should be summoned for anyone suffering from heat exhaustion.

### Emergency Treatment

Place the victim in a reclining position with his feet raised about ten inches above his body. Loosen or remove his clothing, and apply cold, wet cloths to his wrists and forehead. If he has fainted and doesn't recover promptly, smelling salts or spirits of ammonia should be placed under his nose. When the victim is conscious, give him sips of salt water (approximately one teaspoon of salt per glass of water), the total intake to be about two glasses in an hour's time. If the victim vomits, discontinue the salt solution.

### Heatstroke/Sunstroke

Heatstroke is characterized by an acutely high body temperature caused by the cessation of perspiration. The victim's skin becomes hot, dry, and flushed, and he may suffer collapse. Should the skin turn ashen gray, a physician must be called immediately. Prompt hospital treatment is recommended for anyone showing signs of sunstroke who has previously had any kind of heart damage.

### Emergency Treatment

The following measures are designed to reduce the victim's body temperature as quickly as possible and prevent damage to the internal organs:

Place him in a tub of very cold water, or, if this is not possible, spray or sponge his body repeatedly with cold water or rubbing alcohol. Take his temperature by mouth, and when it has dropped to about 100°F., remove him to a bed and wrap him in cold, wet sheets. If possible, expose him to an electric fan or an air conditioner.

### Hiccups

### Emergency Treatment

Have the victim slowly drink a large glass of water. If cold water is not effective, have him drink warm water containing a teaspoonful of baking soda. Milk also can be employed. For babies and small children, offer sips of warm water. Do not offer carbonated beverages.

Another helpful measure is breathing into a large paper bag a number of times to raise the carbon dioxide level in the lungs. Rest and relaxation are recommended; have the victim lie down to read or watch television.

If the hiccups fail to go away, and continued spastic contractions of the diaphragm interfere with eating and sleeping, call a physician.

## Insect Stings

Honeybees, wasps, hornets, and yellow jackets are the most common stinging insects and most likely to attack on a hot summer day. Strongly scented perfumes or cosmetics and brightly colored, rough-finished clothing attract bees and should be avoided by persons working or playing in garden areas. It should also be noted that many commercial repellents do not protect against stinging insects.

### Emergency Treatment

If one is stung, the insect's stinger should be scraped gently but quickly from the skin; don't squeeze it. Apply Epsom salt solution to the sting area. Antihistamines are often helpful in reducing the patient's discomfort. If a severe reaction develops, call a physician.

There are a few people who are critically allergic to the sting of wasps, bees, yellow jackets, or fire ants. This sensitivity causes the vocal cord tissue to swell to the point where breathing may become impossible. A single sting to a sensitive person may result in a dangerous drop in blood pressure, thus producing shock. Anyone with such a severe allergy who is stung should be rushed to a hospital immediately.

A person who becomes aware of having this type of allergy should consult with a physician about the kind of medicine to carry for use in a crisis.

## Insulin Shock

See DIABETIC COMA AND INSULIN SHOCK.

## Jaw Dislocation

The jaw can be dislocated during a physical attack or fight; from a blow on the jaw during sports activities; or from overextension of the joint during yawning, laughing, or attempting to eat a large mouthful of food. The jaw becomes literally locked open so the victim cannot explain his predicament.

### Emergency Treatment

Reducing a dislocated jaw will require that you insert your thumbs between the teeth of the victim. The jaw can be expected to snap into place quickly, and there is a danger that the teeth will clamp down on the thumbs when this happens, so the thumbs should be adequately padded with handkerchiefs or bandages. Once the thumbs are protected, insert them in the mouth and over the lower molars, as far back on the lower jaw as possible. While pressing down with the thumbs, lift the chin with the fingers outside the mouth. As the jaw begins to slip into normal position when it is pushed downward and backward with the chin lifted upward, quickly remove the thumbs from between the jaws.

Once the jaw is back in normal position, the mouth should remain closed for several hours while the ligaments recover from their displaced condition. If necessary, put a cravat bandage over the head to hold the mouth closed. If difficulty is experienced in reducing a jaw dislocation, the victim should be taken to a hospital where an anesthetic can be applied.

## Jellyfish Stings

### Emergency Treatment

Wash the area of the sting thoroughly with alcohol or fresh water. Be sure that any pieces of jellyfish tentacles have been removed from the skin. Aspirin or antihistamines can be administered to relieve pain and itching, but curtail the use of antihistamines if the victim has consumed alcoholic beverages. The leg or arm that received the sting can be soaked in hot water if the pain continues. Otherwise, apply calamine lotion.

If the victim appears to suffer a severe reaction from the sting, summon a doctor. The victim may experience shock, muscle cramps, convulsions, or loss of consciousness. Artificial respiration may be required while awaiting arrival of a doctor. The physician can administer drugs to relieve muscle cramps and provide sedatives or analgesics.

## Kidney Stones

### Emergency Treatment

Call a physician if the victim experiences the agonizing cramps or colic associated with kidney stones. Discuss the symptoms in detail with the doctor to make sure the pain is caused by kidney stones rather than appendicitis.

Comforting heat may be applied to the back and the abdomen of the side affected by the spasms. Paregoric can be administered, if available, while waiting for medical care; about two teaspoonsful of paregoric in a half glass of water may help relieve symptoms.

## Knee Injuries

### Emergency Treatment

If the injury appears to be severe, including possible fracture of the kneecap, immobilize the knee. To immobilize the knee, place the injured leg on a board that is about four inches wide and three to four feet in length. Place padding between the board and the knee and between the board and the back of the ankle. Then use four strips of bandage to fasten the leg to the padded board—one at the ankle, one at the thigh, and one each above and below the knee.

Summon a physician or move the patient to a physician's office. Keep the knee protected against cold or exposure to the elements, but otherwise do not apply a bandage or any type of pressure to the knee itself; any rapid swelling would be aggravated by unnecessary pressure in that area. Be prepared to treat the patient for shock.

## Laryngitis

Laryngitis is associated with colds and influenza and may be accompanied by a fever. The ailment can be aggravated by smoking, and it is possible that the vocal cords can be damaged if the victim tries to force the use of his voice while the larynx is swollen by the infection.

### Emergency Treatment

Have the victim inhale the warm

moist air of a steam kettle or vaporizer. A vaporizer can be improvised in an emergency by pouring boiling water into a bowl and forming a "tent" over the steaming bowl with a large towel or sheet, or by placing a large paper bag over the bowl and cutting an opening at the closed end of the bag so the face can be exposed to the steam. The hot water can contain a bit of camphor or menthol, if available, to make the warm moist air more soothing to the throat, but this is not necessary.

Continue the use of the vaporizer for several days, as needed. The victim should not use the vocal cords any more than absolutely necessary. If the infection does not subside within the first few days, a physician should be consulted.

## Leeches

### Emergency Treatment

Do not try to pull leeches off the skin. They will usually drop away from the skin if a heated object such as a lighted cigarette is held close to them. Leeches also are likely to let go if iodine is applied to their bodies. The wound caused by a leech should be washed carefully with soap and water and an antiseptic applied.

## Lightning Shock

### Emergency Treatment

If the victim is not breathing, apply artificial respiration. If a second person is available to help, have him summon a physician while artificial respiration is administered. Continue artificial respiration until breathing resumes or the physician arrives.

When the victim is breathing regularly, treat him for shock. Keep him lying down with his feet higher than his head, his clothing loosened around the neck, and his body covered with a blanket or coat for warmth. If the victim shows signs of vomiting, turn his head to one side so he will not swallow the vomitus.

If the victim is breathing regularly and does not show signs of shock, he may be given a few sips of a stimulating beverage such as coffee, tea, or brandy.

## Motion Sickness

### Emergency Treatment

Have the victim lie down in a position that is most comfortable to him. The head should be fixed so that any view of motion is avoided. Reading or other use of the eyes should be prohibited. Food or fluids should be restricted to very small amounts. If traveling by car, stop at a rest area; in an airplane or ship, place the victim in an area where motion is least noticeable.

Drugs, such as Dramamine, are helpful for control of the symptoms of motion sickness; they are most effective when started about 90 minutes before travel begins and repeated at regular intervals thereafter.

## Muscle Cramps

### Emergency Treatment

Gently massage the affected muscle, sometimes stretching it to help relieve the painful contraction. Then relax the muscle by using a hot water bottle or an electric heating pad, or by soaking the affected area in a warm bath.

A repetition of cramps may require medical attention.

## Nosebleeds

### Emergency Treatment

Have the victim sit erect but with the head tilted slightly forward to prevent blood from running down the throat. Apply pressure by pinching the nostrils; if bleeding is from just one nostril, use pressure on that side. A small wedge of absorbent cotton or gauze can be inserted into the bleeding nostril. Make sure that the cotton or gauze extends out of the nostril to aid in its removal when the bleeding has stopped. Encourage the victim to breathe through the mouth while the nose is bleeding. After five minutes, release pressure on the nose to see if the bleeding has stopped. If the bleeding continues, repeat pressure on the nostril for an additional five minutes. Cold compresses applied to the nose can help stop the bleeding.

If bleeding continues after the second five-minute period of pressure treatment, get the victim to a physician's office or a hospital emergency room.

## Poison Ivy/Poison Oak/ Poison Sumac

### Emergency Treatment

The poison of these three plants is the same and the treatment is identical. Bathe the skin area exposed to poison ivy, poison oak, or poison sumac with soap and water or with alcohol within 15 mintues after contact. If exposure is not discovered until a rash appears, apply cool wet dressings. Dressings can be made of old bed sheets or soft linens soaked in a solution of one teaspoon of salt per pint of water. Dressings should be applied four times a day for periods of 15 to 60 minutes each time; during these periods, dressings can be removed and reapplied every few minutes. The itching that often accompanies the rash can be relieved by taking antihistamine tablets.

Creams or lotions may be prescribed by a physician or supplied by a pharmacist. Do not use such folk remedies as ammonia or turpentine; do not use skin lotions not approved by a physician or druggist. Haphazard application of medications on poison ivy blisters and rashes can result in complications including skin irritation, infection, or pigmented lesions of the skin.

## Rabies

See ANIMAL BITES.

## Rape

Rape has been defined as any unlawful

sexual intercourse or sexual contact by force or threat. Most commonly, men commit rape against women; but homosexual rape involving men only may occur, for example, in a prison.

Of the million or more Americans who are raped each year, one in five is under the age of 12. Boys are the victims of sexual assault as often as girls. In seven to ten percent of all reported adult cases, men are the victims.

### Emergency Response

The victim of rape may not always be able to help him- or herself. Because violence may accompany the rape, the victim may find it impossible to seek help at once. But where possible, the recommended course of action is to go to a hospital for physical examination. Reporting to a hospital in itself may reduce the feelings of shock, depression, anxiety, and revulsion that generally follow a sexual assault. The physical examination that takes place at the hospital may produce evidence that could be important in a court trial if the rapist is later apprehended. Victims are also advised to report the rape to the police as soon as possible.

For additional information on ways to avoid rape and what to do if it occurs, see "The Rape Victim" in Ch. 25, *Women's Health.*

### Sciatica/Lower Back Pain

Although lower back pain is frequently triggered by fatigue, anxiety, or by strained muscles or tendons, it may be a symptom of a slipped or ruptured disk between the vertebrae or of a similar disorder requiring extensive medical attention.

### Emergency Treatment

Reduce the pressure on the lower back by having the victim lie down on a hard flat surface; if a bed is used there should be a board or sheet of plywood between the springs and mattress. Pillows should be placed under the knees instead of under the head, to help keep the back flat. Give aspirin to relieve the pain, and apply heat to the back. Call a physician if the symptoms do not subside overnight.

### Scorpion Stings

### Emergency Treatment

Apply ice to the region of the sting, except in the case of an arm or leg, in which event the limb may be immersed in ice water. Continue the ice or ice-water treatment for at least one hour. Try to keep the area of the sting at a position lower than the heart. No tourniquet is required. Should the breathing of a scorpion sting victim become depressed, administer artificial respiration. If symptoms fail to subside within a couple of hours, notify a physician, or transfer the victim to a doctor's office or hospital.

For children under six, call a physician in the event of any scorpion sting. Children stung by scorpions may become convulsive, and this condition can result in fatal exhaustion unless it receives prompt medical treatment.

## Snakebites

Of the many varieties of snakes found in the United States, only four kinds are poisonous: copperheads, rattlesnakes, moccasins, and coral snakes. The first three belong to the category of pit vipers and are known as *hemotoxic* because their poison enters the bloodstream. The coral snake, which is comparatively rare, is related to the cobra and is the most dangerous of all because its venom is *neurotoxic*. This means that the poison transmitted by its bite goes directly to the nervous system and the brain.

### How to Differentiate among Snakebites

Snakes of the pit viper family have a fang on each side of the head. These fangs leave characteristic puncture wounds on the skin in addition to two rows of tiny bites or scratches left by the teeth. A bite from a nonpoisonous snake leaves six rows—four upper and two lower—of very small bite marks or scratches and no puncture wounds.

The marks left by the bite of a coral snake do not leave any puncture wounds either, but this snake bites with a chewing motion, hanging on to the victim rather than attacking quickly. The coral snake is very easy to recognize because of its distinctive markings: wide horizontal bands of red and black separated by narrow bands of yellow.

### Symptoms

A bite from any of the pit vipers produces immediate and severe pain and darkening of the skin, followed by weakness, blurred vision, quickened pulse, nausea, and vomiting. The bite of a coral snake produces somewhat the same symptoms, although there is less local pain and considerable drowsiness leading to unconsciousness.

If a physician or a hospital is a short distance away, the patient should receive professional help *immediately.* He should be transported lying down, either on an improvised stretcher or carried by his companions—with the wounded part lower than his heart. He should be advised to move as little as possible.

### Emergency Treatment

If several hours must elapse before a physician or a hospital can be reached, the following procedures should be applied promptly:

**1.** Keep the victim lying down and as still as possible.

**2.** Tie a constricting band *above* the wound between it and the heart and tight enough to slow but not stop blood circulation. A handkerchief, necktie, sock, or piece of torn shirt will serve.

**3.** If a snakebite kit is available, use the knife it contains; otherwise, sterilize a knife or razor blade in a flame. Carefully make small cuts in the skin where the swelling has developed. Make the cuts along the length of the limb, not across or at right angles to it. The incisions should be shallow because of the danger of severing nerves, blood vessels, or muscles.

**4.** Use the suction cups in the snakebite kit, if available, to draw out as much of the venom as possible. If suction cups are not available, the venom can be removed by sucking it out with the mouth. Although snake venom is not a stomach poison, it should not be swallowed but should be rinsed from the mouth.

**5.** This procedure should be continued for from 30 to 60 minutes or until the swelling subsides and the other symptoms decrease.

**6.** You may apply cold compresses to the bite area while waiting for professional assistance.

**7.** Treat the victim for shock.

**8.** Give artificial respiration if necessary.

## Splinters

### Emergency Treatment

Clean the area about the splinter with soap and water or an antiseptic. Next, sterilize a needle by holding it over an open flame. After it cools, insert the needle above the splinter so it will tear a line in the skin, making the splinter lie loose in the wound. Then, gently lift the splinter out, using a pair of tweezers or the point of the needle. If tweezers are used, they should be sterilized first.

Wash the wound area again with soap and water, or apply an antiseptic. It is best to cover the wound with an adhesive bandage. If redness or irritation develops around the splinter wound, consult a physician.

## Sprains

A sprain occurs when a joint is wrenched or twisted in such a way that the ligaments holding it in position are ruptured, possibly damaging the surrounding blood vessels, tendons, nerves, and muscles. This type of injury is more serious than a strain and is usually accompanied by pain, sometimes severe, soreness, swelling, and discoloration of the affected area. Most sprains occur as a result of falls, athletic accidents, or improper handling of heavy weights.

### Emergency Treatment

This consists of prompt rest, the application of cold compresses to relieve swelling and any internal bleeding in the joint, and elevation of the affected area. Aspirin is recommended to reduce discomfort. If the swelling and soreness increase after such treatment, a physician should be consulted to make sure that the injury is not a fracture or a bone dislocation.

## Sting Ray

### Emergency Treatment

If an arm or leg is the target of a sting ray, wash the area thoroughly with salt water. Quickly remove any pieces of the stinger imbedded in the skin or flesh; poison can still be discharged into the victim from the sting-ray sheath. After initial cleansing of an arm or leg sting, soak the wound with hot water for up to an hour. Apply antiseptic or a sterile dressing after the soak.

Consult a physician after a stingray attack. The physician will make a thorough examination of the wound to determine whether stitches or antibiotics are required. Fever, vomiting, or muscular twitching also may result from an apparently simple leg or arm wound by a sting ray.

If the sting occurs in the chest or abdomen, the victim should be rushed to a hospital as soon as possible because such a wound can produce convulsions or loss of consciousness.

## Strains

When a muscle is stretched because of misuse or overuse, the interior bundles of tissue may tear, or the tendon that connects it to the bone may be stretched. This condition is known as strain. It occurs most commonly to the muscles of the lower back when heavy weights are improperly lifted, or in the area of the calf or ankle as the result of a sudden, violent twist or undue pressure.

### Emergency Treatment

Bed rest, the application of heat, and gentle massage are recommended for back strain. If the strain is in the leg, elevate the limb to help reduce pain and swelling, and apply cold compresses or an ice bag to the area. Aspirin may be taken to reduce discomfort.

In severe cases of strained back muscles, a physician may have to be consulted for strapping. For a strained ankle, a flexible elastic bandage can be helpful in providing the necessary support until the injured muscle heals.

## Stroke

Stroke, or apoplexy, is caused by a disruption of normal blood flow to the brain, either by rupture of a blood vessel within the brain or by blockage of an artery supplying the brain. The condition is enhanced by hardening of the arteries and high blood pressure, and is most likely to occur in older persons. A stroke usually occurs with little or no warning and the onset may be marked by a variety of manifestations ranging from headache, slurred speech, or blurred vision, to sudden collapse and unconsciousness.

### Emergency Treatment

Try to place the victim in a semireclining position, or, if he is lying down, be sure there is a pillow under his head. Avoid conditions that might increase the flow of blood toward the head. Summon a physician immediately. Loosen any clothing that may be tight. If the patient wears dentures, remove them.

Before professional medical assistance is available, the victim may vomit or go into shock or convulsions. If he vomits, try to prevent a backflow of vomitus into the breathing passages. If shock occurs, do not place the victim in the shock position but do keep him warm and comfortable. If convulsions develop, place a handkerchief or similar soft object between the jaws to prevent tongue biting.

## Sty on Eyelid

Sties usually develop around hair follicles because of a bacterial infection. Like cold sores, they are most likely to develop in association with poor health and lowered resistance to infection.

### Emergency Treatment

Apply warm, moist packs or compresses to the sty for periods of 15 to 20 minutes at intervals of three or four hours. Moist heat generally is more penetrating than dry heat.

The sty should eventually rupture and the pus should then be washed carefully away from the eye area. If the sty does not rupture or is very painful, consult a physician. Do not squeeze or otherwise handle the sty except to apply the warm moist compresses.

## Sunburn

### Emergency Treatment

Apply cold wet compresses to help relieve the pain. Compresses can be soaked in whole milk, salt water, or a solution of cornstarch mixed with water. The victim also may get some relief by soaking in a bathtub filled with plain water. Soothing lotions, such as baby oil or a bland cold cream, can be applied after carefully drying the skin. Don't rub the burn area while drying. Avoid the use of "shake" lotions, like calamine, which may aggravate the burn by a drying action. The victim should, of course, avoid further exposure to sunlight.

If pain is excessive, or extensive blistering is present, consult a physician. Avoid application of over-the-counter topical anesthetics that may cause allergic skin reactions.

A severe or extensive sunburn is comparable to a second-degree thermal burn and may be accompanied by symptoms of shock; if such symptoms are present the victim should be treated for shock. See also BURNS, THERMAL.

## Sunstroke

See HEATSTROKE.

## Tick Bites

### Emergency Treatment

Do not try to scrape or rub the insect off the skin with your fingers; scraping, rubbing, or pulling may break off only part of the insect body, leaving the head firmly attached to the skin. Rubbing also can smear disease organisms from the tick into the bite. To make the tick drop away from the skin, cover it with a heavy oil, such as salad, mineral, or lubricating oil. Oil usually will block the insect's breathing pores, suffocating it. If oil is not readily available, carefully place a heated object against the tick's body; a lighted cigarette or a match that has been ignited and snuffed out can serve as a hot object.

Carefully inspect the bite area to be sure that all parts of the tick have been removed. Use a pair of tweezers to remove any tick parts found. Then carefully wash the bite and surrounding area with soap and water and apply an antiseptic. Also, wash your hands and any equipment that may have come in contact with the tick. Consult a physician if symptoms of tick fever or tularemia, such as unexplained muscular weakness, occur following a bite.

## Toothaches

### Emergency Treatment

Give an adult one or two aspirin tablets; a young child should be given no more than one-half of an adult tablet. The aspirin should be swallowed with plenty of water. Do not let it dissolve in the mouth or be held near the aching tooth. Aspirin becomes effective as a painkiller only after it has gone through the digestive tract and into the bloodstream; if aspirin is held in the mouth, it may irritate the gums.

Oil of cloves can be applied to the aching tooth. Dip a small wad of cotton into the oil of cloves, then gently pack the oil-soaked cotton into the tooth cavity with a pair of tweezers. Do not let the tweezers touch the tooth.

If the jaw is swollen, apply an ice bag for periods of 15 minutes at a time, at intermittent intervals. Never apply heat to a swollen jaw when treating a toothache. Arrange to see your dentist as soon as possible.

## Tooth, Broken

### Emergency Treatment

Apply a few drops of oil of cloves to the injured tooth to help relieve pain. If oil of cloves is not available, give an adult one to two regular aspirin tablets. One-half of a regular tablet can be given to a young child.

Make an emergency filling from a wad of cotton containing a few drops of oil of cloves. An emergency filling also can be made from powdered chalk; it is important to protect the cavity from infection while providing pain relief.

If the tooth has been knocked out of the socket, retrieve the tooth, because it can be restored in some cases. Do not wash the tooth; ordinary washing can damage dental tissues. A dentist will take care of cleaning it properly. Wrap the tooth in a damp clean handkerchief or tissue or place the tooth in a container of slightly salty warm water for the trip to the dentist.

## Unconsciousness

Unconsciousness is the condition that has the appearance of sleep, but is usually the result of injury, shock, or serious physical disturbance. A brief loss of consciousness followed by spontaneous recovery is called *fainting*. A prolonged episode of unconsciousness is a *coma*.

### Emergency Treatment

Call a physician at once. If none is available, get the victim to the nearest hospital. If the loss of consciousness is accompanied by loss of breathing, begin mouth-to-mouth respiration. If the victim is suffering cardiac arrest, administer cardiac massage. Don't try to revive the victim with any kind of stimulant unless told to do so by a physician.

# 36

# Commonly Prescribed Generic Drugs

| Name | Action | Prescribed for |
|---|---|---|
| **Trade Names** | **(CD = combined drug)** | |
| **Acetaminophen** | Believed to reduce concentration of chemicals involved in production of pain, fever, and inflammation (analgesic; antipyretic) | Relief of mild to moderate pain; reduction of fever |
| Anacin-3<br>Datril<br>Tylenol<br>Acetaco (CD)<br>Algisin (CD)<br>Amacodone (CD)<br>Amaphen (CD)<br>Anoquan (CD)<br>Bancap (CD)<br>Capital (CD)<br>Chlorzone Forte<br>  (CD) | Codalan (CD)    Duradyne (CD)<br>Co-Gesic (CD)  Empracet (CD)<br>Compal (CD)    Esgic (CD)<br>Comtrex (CD)   Excedrin (CD)<br>Congesprin (CD) Hycomine<br>Co-Tylenol (CD)   (CD)<br>Darvocet-N (CD) Hyco-Pop (CD)<br>Dia-Gesic (CD)  Korigesic (CD)<br>Dolacet (CD)   Lorcet (CD)<br>Dolprn (CD)    Midrin (CD)<br>Dorcol (CD)    Migralam (CD)<br>Dristan (CD)   Pacaps (CD) | Parafon Forte  Sinubid (CD)<br>  (CD)         Sinutab (CD)<br>Percocet (CD)  Stopayne (CD)<br>Percogesic (CD) Supac (CD)<br>Penaphen (CD)  Talacen (CD)<br>Phenate (CD)   Two-Dyne (CD)<br>Phrenilin (CD)  Tylox (CD)<br>Protid (CD)    Vanquish (CD)<br>Repan (CD)    Vicodin (CD)<br>Sinarest (CD)  Wygesic (CD)<br>Sine-Aid (CD)<br>Singler (CD) |
| **Amitriptyline** | Believed to restore to normal levels the constituents of brain tissue that transmit nerve impulses (antidepressant) | Relief of emotional depression; gradual improvement of mood |
| Elavil<br>Endep<br>Etrafon (CD) | Limbitral (CD)<br>Triavil (CD) | |
| **Ampicillin** | Interferes with ability of susceptible bacteria to produce new protective cell walls as they grow and multiply (antibiotic) | Elimination of infections responsive to action of this drug |
| Amcill<br>Omnipen<br>Polycillin | Principen<br>SK-Ampicillin | |

| Name | Action | Prescribed for |
|------|--------|----------------|
| **Trade Names** | **(CD = combined drug)** | |

| Name | Action | Prescribed for |
|------|--------|----------------|
| **Antacids** (Aluminum Hydroxide) (Calcium Carbonate) (Sodium Bicarbonate) | Neutralizes stomach acid; reduces action of digestive enzyme pepsin (relief from gastric hyperacidity) | Relief of heartburn, sour stomach, acid indigestion, and discomfort associated with peptic ulcer, gastritis, esophagitis, hiatal hernia |

| | | | | | |
|--|--|--|--|--|--|
| Absorbable: Sodium bicarbonate: | Alka-Seltzer Brioschi Bromo-Seltzer | Less absorbable: Aluminum | hydroxide: Amphojel Calcium | carbonate: Alka-2 Amitone | |

| Name | Action | Prescribed for |
|------|--------|----------------|
| **Aspirin** (Acetylsalicylic Acid) | Dilates blood vessels in skin, thus hastening loss of body heat (antipyretic); reduces tissue concentration of inflammation and pain (analgesic; antirheumatic) | Reduction of fever; relief of mild to moderate pain and inflammation; prevention of blood clots, as in phlebitis, heart attack, stroke |

| | | | | |
|--|--|--|--|--|
| Bayer Easprin Empirin Eneaprin St. Joseph's Children's Aspirin Verin Zorpin | A.P.C. (CD) Alka-Seltzer (CD) Anacin (CD) Ascriptin (CD) Axotal (CD) Buff-A Comp (CD) Bufferin (CD) Congespirin (CD) | Cosprin (CD) Darvon with A.S.A. (CD) Darvon-N with A.S.A (CD) Dia-Gesic (CD) Dolprn #3 (CD) Equagesic (CD) | Excedrin (CD) 4-Way Cold Tablets (CD) Fiorinal (CD) Hyco-Pap (CD) Midol (CD) Norgesic (CD) Percodan (CD) | Robaxisal (CD) Saleto (CD) Soma Compound (CD) Supac (CD) Synalgos-DC (CD) Talwin (CD) Vanquish (CD) |

| Name | Action | Prescribed for |
|------|--------|----------------|
| **Atropine** (Belladonna, Hyoscyamine) | Prevents stimulation of muscular contractions and glandular secretions in organ involved (antispasmodic [anticholinergic]) | Relief of discomfort associated with excessive activity and spasm of digestive tract; irritation and spasm of lower urinary tract; painful menstruation |

| | | | |
|--|--|--|--|
| Antrocol (CD) Arco-Lase Plus (CD) Bellergal (CD) | Donnagel-PG (CD) Donnatal (CD) Donnatal | Extendtabs (CD) Donnazyme (CD) Festalan (CD) Ru-Tuss (CD) | Trac-Tabs 2X (CD) SK-Diphenoxylate (CD) | Urised (CD) Wigraine-PB (CD) |

| Name | Action | Prescribed for |
|------|--------|----------------|
| **Bendroflumethiazide** | Increases elimination of salt and water (diuretic); relaxes walls of smaller arteries, allowing them to expand; combined effect lowers blood pressure (antihypertensive) | Elimination of excessive fluid retention (edema); reduction of high blood pressure |

| | | | |
|--|--|--|--|
| Naturetin | Corzide (CD) | Rautrax-N (CD) | Rauzide (CD) |

| Name | Action | Prescribed for |
|------|--------|----------------|
| **Brompheniramine** | Blocks action of histamine after release from sensitized tissue cells, thus reducing intensity of allergic response (antihistamine) | Relief of symptoms of hay fever (allergic rhinitis) and of allergic reactions of skin (itching, swelling, hives, rash) |

| | | | |
|--|--|--|--|
| Dimetane Veltane | Bromfed (CD) Bromphen (CD) | Dimetapp (CD) Dura Tap-PD (CD) | E.N.T. Syrup (CD)  S-T Decongest (CD) Poly-histine-DX(CD) Tamine S.R. (CD) |

| Name | Action | Prescribed for |
|------|--------|----------------|
| **Butabarbital** | Believed to block transmission of nerve impulses (hypnotic; sedative) | Low dosage: relief of moderate anxiety or tension (sedative effect); higher dosage: at bedtime to induce sleep (hypnotic effect) |

| | | | |
|--|--|--|--|
| Buticaps | Butisol | Pyridium (CD) | Quibron Plus (CD) |

| Name | Action | Prescribed for |
|---|---|---|
| **Trade Names** | **(CD = combined drug)** | |
| **Caffeine** | Constricts blood vessel walls; increases energy level of chemical systems responsible for nerve tissue activity (cardiac, respiratory, psychic stimulant) | Prevention and early relief of vascular headaches such as migraine; relief of drowsiness and mental fatigue |
| No-Doz<br>A.P.C. (CD)<br>Amaphen (CD)<br>Anacin (CD)<br>Anoquan (CD) | Buff-A Comp (CD)    Esgic (CD)<br>Cafergot (CD)    Excedrin Extra<br>Cafetrate-PB (CD)    Strength (CD)<br>Compal (CD)    Fiorinal (CD)<br>Dia-Gesic (CD)    Korigesic (CD) | Maximum    Two-Dyne (CD)<br>   Strength    Vanquish (CD)<br>   Midol (CD)    Wigraine (CD)<br>Migralam (CD)<br>Pacaps (CD) |
| **Carisoprodol** | Believed to block transmission of nerve impulses and/or to produce a sedative effect (muscle relaxant) | Relief of discomfort caused by spasms of voluntary muscles |
| Rela<br>Soprodol<br>Soma (CD) | Soma Compound<br>   (CD) | |
| **Chloral Hydrate** | Believed to affect wake-sleep centers of brain (hypnotic) | Low dosage: relief of mild to moderate anxiety or tension (sedative effect); higher dosage: at bedtime to relieve insomnia (hypnotic effect) |
| Noctec<br>SK-Chloral<br>   Hydrate | | |
| **Chloramphen-icol** | Prevents growth and multiplication of susceptible bacteria by interfering with formation of their essential proteins (antibiotic) | Elimination of infections responsive to action of this drug |
| Chloromycetin<br>Ophthochlor<br>Ophthocort | | |
| **Chlordiaze-poxide** | Believed to reduce activity of some parts of limbic system (tranquilizer) | Relief of mild to moderate anxiety and tension without significant sedation |
| Libritabs<br>Librium<br>SK-Lygen | Clipoxide (CD)<br>Librax (CD) | |
| **Chlorpheniramine** | Blocks action of histamine after release from sensitized tissue cells, thus reducing intensity of allergic response (antihistamine) | Relief of symptoms of hay fever (allergic rhinitis) and of allergic reactions of skin (itching, swelling, hives, rash) |
| Chlor-Trimeton<br>Polaramine<br>Teldrin | | |
| **Chlorpromazine** | Believed to inhibit action of dopamine, thus correcting an imbalance of nerve impulse transmission thought to be responsible for certain mental disorders (antiemetic; tranquilizer) | Relief of severe anxiety, agitation, and psychotic behavior |
| Thorazine | | |

| Name | Action | Prescribed for |
|------|--------|----------------|
| **Trade Names** | **(CD = combined drug)** | |
| **Codeine** | Believed to affect tissue sites that react specifically with opium and its derivatives (antitussive; narcotic analgesic) | Relief of moderate pain; control of coughing |

A.P.C. with Codeine (CD)
Acetaco (CD)
Actifed with Codeine (CD)
Amaphen with Codeine (CD)
Anacin-3 with Codeine (CD)
Ascriptin with Codeine (CD)
Bancap c̄ Codeine (CD)
Bromanyl (CD)

Bromphen DC (CD)
Buff-A Comp No. 3 (CD)
Capital with Codeine (CD)
Codalan (CD)
Codimal PH (CD)
Conex with Codeine (CD)
Deproist (CD)
Dimetane-DC (CD)
Dolprn #3 (CD)

Empirin with Codeine (CD)
Fiorinal with Codeine (CD)
Guiatuss A-C (CD)
Iophen-C (CD)
Naldecon-CX (CD)
Novahistine DK (CD)
Nucofed (CD)
Pediacof (CD)
Phenaphen with Codeine (CD)

Phenergan with Codeine (CD)
Phrenilin with Codeine (CD)
Robitussin A-C (CD)
Ru-Tuss (CD)
Soma Compound (CD)
Stopayne (CD)
Triafed-C (CD)
Triaminic with Codeine (CD)
Tussar (CD)

Tylenol with Codeine (CD)

| Name | Action | Prescribed for |
|------|--------|----------------|
| **Dexamethasone** | Believed to inhibit several tissue mechanisms that induce inflammation (adrenocortical sterioid [anti-inflammatory]) | Symptomatic relief of inflammation (swelling, redness, heat, pain) |
| Decadron<br>Dalalone<br>Dexasone | Hexadrol<br>Neodecadron | |
| **Dextroamphet-amine**<br>(d-Amphetamine) | Increases release of nerve impulse transmitter (central stimulant); this may also improve concentration and attention span of hyperactive child (primary calming action unknown); alters chemical control of nerve impulse transmission in appetite control center of brain (appetite suppressant [anorexiant]) | Reduction or prevention of sleep epilepsy (narcolepsy); reduction of symptoms of abnormal hyperactivity (as in minimal brain dysfunction); suppression of appetite in management of weight reduction |
| Dexedrine | Obetrol                Biphetamine (CD) | |
| **Diazepam** | Believed to reduce activity of some parts of limbic system (tranquilizer) | Relief of mild to moderate anxiety and tension without significant sedation |
| Valium | | |
| **Dicyclomine** | Believed to produce a local anesthetic action that blocks reflex activity responsible for spasm (antispasmodic) | Relief of discomfort from muscle spasm of the gastrointestinal tract |
| Bentyl | | |
| **Digitoxin** | Increases availability of calcium within the heart muscle, thus improving conversion of chemical energy to mechanical energy; slows pacemaker and delays transmission of electrical impulses (digitalis preparations [cardiotonic]) | Improvement of heart muscle contraction force (as in congestive heart failure); correction of certain heart rhythm disorders |
| Crystodigin | Purodigin | |
| **Digoxin** | Same as above | Same as above |
| Lanoxicaps | Lanoxin | |

| Name | Action | Prescribed for |
|---|---|---|
| **Trade Names** | **(CD = combined drug)** | |
| **Diphenhydramine** | Blocks action of histamine after release from sensitized tissue cells, thus reducing intensity of allergic response (antihistamine) | Relief of symptoms of hay fever (allergic rhinitis) and of allergic reactions of skin (itching, swelling, hives, rash) |
| Allerdryl<br>Benadryl<br>Ambenyl (CD) | Benylin (CD)          Dytuss (CD)<br>Bromanyl (CD)      Ziradryl (CD) | |
| **Doxylamine** | Same as above | Same as above |
| Unisome<br>  Nighttime<br>Cremacoat 4<br>  (CD)<br>Nyquil (CD) | | |
| **Ephedrine** | Blocks release of certain chemicals from sensitized tissue cells undergoing allergic reaction; relaxes bronchial muscles; shrinks tissue mass (decongestion) by contracting arteriole walls in lining of respiratory passages (adrenergic [bronchodilator]) | Prevention and symptomatic relief of bronchial asthma; relief of congestion of respiratory passages |
| Efed II (Yellow)<br>Primatene Mist<br>Bronkaid (CD)<br>Bronkolixir (CD) | Bronkotabs (CD)     Mudrane (CD)<br>Derma Medicone-     Nyquil (CD)<br>  HC (CD)           Primatene (CD)<br>Marax (CD)          Quadrinal (CD) | Quelidrine (CD)     T.E.H. (CD)<br>Quibron Plus (CD)  T-E-P (CD)<br>Rynatuss (CD)      Theozine (CD)<br>Tedral (CD)         Wyanoids (CD) |
| **Ergotamine** | Constricts blood vessel walls, thus relieving excessive dilation that causes pain of vascular headaches (migraine analgesic [vasoconstrictor]) | Prevention and early relief of vascular headaches such as migraines or histamine headaches |
| Cafetrate-PB<br>Ergomar<br>Ergostat | Medihaler          Bellergal (CD)<br>  Ergotamine       Cafergot (CD)<br>Wigrettes           Wigraine (CD) | |
| **Erythrityl Tetranitrate** | Acts directly on muscle cells to produce relaxation which permits expansion of blood vessels, thus increasing supply of blood and oxygen to heart | Management of pain associated with angina pectoris (coronary insufficiency) |
| Cardilate | | |
| **Erythromycin** | Prevents growth and multiplication of susceptible bacteria by interfering with formation of their essential proteins (antibiotic) | Elimination of infections responsive to action of this drug |
| A/T/S<br>E.E.S.<br>E-Mycin<br>Eryc | Eryderm          Erythrocin<br>Erymax           Ethril<br>Eryped           Ilosone<br>Ery-Tab          Ilotycin | Pediamycin        SK-Erythromycin<br>Staticin/T-Stat    Pediaxole (CD)<br>Wyamycin E<br>Wyamycin S |
| **Estrogens**<br>(Estrogenic<br>Substances)<br>Conjugated<br>Estrogens,<br>Esterified<br>Estrogens<br>(Estrone and<br>Equilin) | Prepares uterus for pregnancy or induces menstruation by cyclic increase and decrease in tissue stimulation; when taken regularly, blood and tissue levels increase to resemble those during pregnancy, thus preventing pituitary gland from producing hormones that induce ovulation; reduces frequency and intensity of menopausal symptoms (female sex hormone) | Regulation of menstrual cycle; prevention of pregnancy; relief of symptoms of menopause |
| Conjugated<br>  Estrogens<br>Estrocon | Estratab          Menrium (CD)<br>Premarin          Milprem (CD)<br>Estratest (CD) | |

| Name | Action | | Prescribed for | |
|---|---|---|---|---|
| **Trade Names** | **(CD = combined drug)** | | | |
| **Griseofulvin** | Believed to prevent growth and multiplication of susceptible fungus strains by interfering with their metabolic activities (antibiotic; antifungal) | | Elimination of fungus infections responsive to actions of this drug | |
| Fulvicin-U/F<br>Fulvicin P/G<br>Grifulvin V | Grisactin<br>Gris-PEG | | | |
| **Hydralazine** | Lowers pressure of blood in vessels by causing direct relaxation and expansion of vessel walls—mechanism unknown (antihypertensive) | | Reduction of high blood pressure | |
| Apresoline<br>Apresazide (CD)<br>Apresoline-Esidrex (CD)<br>H-H-R (CD) | Ser-Ap-Es (CD)<br>Serpasil-Apresoline (CD)<br>Unipres (CD) | | | |
| **Hydrochlorothiazide** | Increases elimination of salt and water (diuretic); relaxes walls of smaller arteries, allowing them to expand; combined effect lowers blood pressure (antihypertensive) | | Elimination of excessive fluid retention (edema); reduction of high blood pressure | |
| Esidrix<br>HydroDIURIL<br>Oretic<br>Thiuretic<br>Aldactazide (CD) | Aldoril (CD)<br>Apresazide (CD)<br>Apresoline-Esidrix (CD)<br>Dyazide (CD) | Esimil (CD)<br>H-H-R (CD)<br>Hydropres (CD)<br>Hydroserpine (CD) | Inderide (CD)<br>Maxzide (CD)<br>Moduretic (CD)<br>SK-Hydrochlorothiazide | Spironazide (CD)<br>Timolide (CD)<br>Unipres (CD) |
| **Hydrocortisone** (Cortisol) | Believed to inhibit several tissue mechanisms that induce inflammation (adrenocortical steroid [anti-inflammatory]) | | Symptomatic relief of inflammation (swelling, redness, heat, pain) | |
| Aeroseb-HC<br>Alphaderm<br>Carmol HC<br>Cortef<br>Cortril<br>Cort-Dome<br>Cortifair<br>Eldecort | F-E-P<br>Hydrocortone<br>Hytone<br>Penecort<br>Pro-Cort<br>Synacort<br>Texacort<br>Vanoxide-HC | Vioform-<br>  Hydrocortisone<br>VōSoL HC<br>Allersone (CD)<br>Corticaine (CD)<br>Cortisporin (CD)<br>Derma-Sone (CD)<br>Di-Hydrotic (CD) | Hill Cortac (CD)<br>Hysone (CD)<br>Iodo-Cortifair (CD)<br>Octicair (CD)<br>Otic-HC (CD)<br>Oticol (CD)<br>Otobiotic (CD) | Otocort (CD)<br>Pedi-Cort V (CD)<br>Pyocidin-Otic (CD)<br>Vytone (CD) |
| **Hydroxyzine** | Believed to reduce excessive activity in areas of brain that influence emotional health (antihistamine; tranquilizer) | | Relief of anxiety, tension, apprehension, and agitation | |
| Atarax<br>Durrax<br>Nevcalm | T.E.H.<br>Theozine | Vistaril<br>Marax (CD) | | |
| **Insulin** | Facilitates passage of sugar through cell wall to interior of cell (hypoglycemic) | | Control of diabetes | |
| Humulin N<br>Humulin R<br>Iletin I | Iletin II<br>Insulatard NPH<br>Lente Insulin | Mixtard<br>Novolin L<br>Novolin N | Novolin R<br>NPH Insulin<br>Regular Insulin | Semilente Insulin<br>Ultrlente Insulin |
| **Isonizaid** | Believed to interfere with several metabolic activities of susceptible tuberculosis organisms (antibacterial; tuberculostatic) | | Prevention and treatment of tuberculosis | |
| INH<br>Nydrazid<br>Rifamate (CD) | | | | |

## Commonly Prescribed
## Generic Drugs

| Name | Action | Prescribed for |
|------|--------|----------------|
| **Trade Names** | **(CD = combined drug)** | |
| **Isopropamide** | Prevents stimulation of muscular contraction and glandular secretion in organ involved (antispasmodic [anticholinergic]) | Relief of discomfort from excessive activity and spasm of digestive tract |
| Darbid<br>Combid (CD)<br>Ornade (CD) | Prochlor-Iso (CD)<br>Pro-Iso (CD) | |
| **Isoproterenol/<br>Isoprenaline** | Dilates bronchial tubes by stimulating sympathetic nerve terminals (Isoproterenol: adrenergic [bronchodilator]; Isoprenaline: sympathomimetic) | Management of acute bronchial asthma, bronchitis, and emphysema |
| Aerolone<br>Isuprel<br>Medihaler-Iso<br>Norisodrine<br>Vapo-Iso | Duo-Medihaler<br>  (CD)<br>Isuprel Com-<br>  pound (CD) | |
| **Isosorbide<br>Dinitrate** | Acts directly on muscle cells to produce relaxation which permits expansion of blood vessels, thus increasing supply of blood and oxygen to heart (coronary vasodilator) | Management of pain associated with angina pectoris (coronary insufficiency) |
| Dilatrate<br>Iso-Bid | Isochron          Isotrate<br>Isordil             Sorate | Sorbide<br>Sorbitrate |
| **Levodopa** | Believed to be converted to dopamine in brain tissue, thus correcting a dopamine deficiency and restoring more normal balance of chemicals responsible for transmission of nerve impulses (anti-Parkinsonism) | Management of Parkinson's disease |
| Larodopa<br>Sinemet | | |
| **Liothyronine (T-3)** | Increases rate of cellular metabolism and makes more energy available for biochemical activity (thyroid hormone) | Correction of thyroid hormone deficiency (hypothyroidism) |
| Cytomel<br>Euthroid (CD)<br>Thyrolar (CD) | | |
| **Lithium** | Believed to correct chemical imbalance in certain nerve impulse transmitters that influence emotional behavior (antidepressant) | Improvement of mood and behavior in chronic manic-depression |
| Eskalith<br>Libalith-S<br>Lithane | Lithobid<br>Lithotabs | |
| **Meclizine** | Blocks transmission of excessive nerve impulses to vomiting center (antiemetic) | Management of nausea, vomiting, and dizziness associated with motion sickness |
| Antivert<br>Bonine<br>Ru-Vert-M | | |
| **Meperidine/<br>Pethidine** | Believed to increase chemicals that transmit nerve impulses (narcotic analgesic) | Relief of moderate to severe pain |
| Demerol<br>Mepergan (CD) | | |

| Name | Action | Prescribed for |
|------|--------|----------------|
| **Trade Names** | **(CD = combined drug)** | |
| **Meprobamate** | Not known (tranquilizer) | Relief of mild to moderate anxiety and tension (sedative effect); relief of insomnia resulting from anxiety and tension (hypnotic effect) |
| Equanil<br>Miltown<br>SK-Bamate<br>Tranmep | Deprol (CD)          PMB (CD)<br>Equagesic (CD)      Pathibamate (CD)<br>Mepro Compound<br>  (CD) | |
| **Methacycline** | Prevents growth and multiplication of susceptible bacteria by interfering with formation of their essential proteins (antibiotic) | Elimination of infections responsive to action of this drug |
| Rondomycin | | |
| **Methadone** | Believed to increase chemicals that transmit nerve impulses (narcotic analgesic) | Treatment of heroin addiction; sometimes for relief of moderate to severe pain |
| Dolophine | | |
| **Methyclothiazide** | Increases elimination of salt and water (diuretic); relaxes walls of smaller arteries, allowing them to expand; combined effect lowers blood pressure (antihypertensive) | Elimination of excess fluid retention (edema); reduction of high blood pressure |
| Aquatensen<br>Enduron | Diutensen (CD)<br>Enduronyl (CD) | |
| **Methylphenidate** | Believed to increase release of nerve impulse transmitter, which may also improve concentration and attention span of hyperactive child (primary action unknown) (central stimulant) | Management of fatigue and depression; reduction of symptoms of abnormal hyperactivity (as in minimal brain dysfunction) |
| Ritalin | | |
| **Nicotinic Acid/<br>Niacin** | Corrects a deficiency of nicotinic acid in tissues; dilation of blood vessels is believed limited to skin—increased blood flow within head has not been demonstrated; reduces initial production of cholesterol and prevents conversion of fatty tissue to cholesterol and triglycerides (vitamin B-complex component; cholesterol reducer) | Management of pellagra; treatment of vertigo, ringing in ears, premenstrual headache; reduction of blood levels of cholesterol and triglycerides |
| Nico-400<br>Nicobid | Nicolar          Cardioguard (CD)<br>Nicotinex Elixir    Lipo-Nicin (CD) | |
| **Nitrofurantoin** | Believed to prevent growth and multiplication of susceptible bacteria by interfering with function of their essential enzyme systems (antibacterial) | Elimination of infections responsive to action of this drug |
| Furadantin<br>Macrodantin | | |
| **Nitroglycerin** | Acts directly on muscle cells to produce relaxation which permits expansion of blood vessels, thus increasing supply of blood and oxygen to heart (coronary vasodilator) | Management of pain associated with angina pectoris (coronary insufficiency) |
| Nitrobid<br>Nitrodisc<br>Nitro-Dur | Nitroglyn        Nitrong<br>Nitrol            Nitrospan<br>Nitrolin          Nitrostat | Transderm-Nitro<br>Tridil |

**Commonly Prescribed**
**Generic Drugs**

| Name | Action | Prescribed for |
|---|---|---|
| **Trade Names** | **(CD = combined drug)** | |
| **Nystatin** | Prevents growth and multiplication of susceptible fungus strains by attacking their walls and causing leakage of internal components (antibiotic; antifungal) | Elimination of fungus infections responsive to action of this drug |
| Korostatin  Mycostatin | Nilstat  Nystex | O-V Statin  Mycolog (CD) | Myco-Triacet (CD)  Nystraform (CD)  Mytrex (CD)  Nyst-olone (CD) |
| **Oral Contraceptives** | Suppresses the two pituitary gland hormones that produce ovulation (oral contraceptives) | Prevention of pregnancy |
| Ovcon  Brevicon  Demulen  Enovid-E | Loestrin  LO/Ovral  Micronor  Medicon | Nordette  Norinyl  Norlestrin  Nor-Q.D. | Ortho-Novum  Ovrette  Ovulen  Tri-Norinyl |
| **Oxycodone** | Believed to affect tissue sites that react specifically with opium and its derivatives (narcotic analgesic) | Relief of moderate pain; control of coughing |
| Percocet (CD)  Percodan (CD)  SK-Oxycodone  with Acetaminophen (CD) | SK-Oxycodone  with Aspirin  (CD)  Tylox (CD) | |
| **Oxytetracycline** | Prevents growth and multiplication of susceptible bacteria by interfering with their formation of essential proteins (antibiotic) | Elimination of infections responsive to action of this drug |
| Oxymycin  Terramycin  Urobiotic (CD) | | |
| **Papaverine** | Causes direct relaxation and expansion of blood vessel walls, thus increasing volume of blood which increases oxygen and nutrients (smooth muscle relaxant; vasodilator) | Relief of symptoms associated with impaired circulation in extremities and within brain |
| Cerespan  Pavabid  Pavatym | | |
| **Paregoric** (Camphorated Tincture of Opium) | Believed to affect tissue sites that react specifically with opium and its derivatives to relieve pain; its active ingredient, morphine, acts as a local anesthetic and blocks release of chemical that transmits nerve impulses to muscle walls of intestine (antiperistaltic) | Relief of mild to moderate pain; relief of intestinal cramping and diarrhea |
| Donnagel-PG  (CD)  Parepectolin (CD) | | |
| **Penicillin G** | Interferes with ability of susceptible bacteria to produce new protective cell walls as they grow and multiply (antibiotic) | Elimination of infections responsive to action of this drug |
| Bicillin C-R  Crysticillin | Pentids  Pfizerpen | SK-Penicillin G  Wycillin | |
| **Penicillin V** | Same as above | Same as above |
| Betapen-VK  Pen-Vee K  Ledercillin | Robicillin VK  SK-Pencillin VK | V-Cillin K  Veetids | |

| Name | Action | Prescribed for |
|---|---|---|
| **Trade Names** | **(CD = combined drug)** | |
| **Pentaerythritol Tetranitrate** | Acts directly on muscle cells to produce relaxation which permits expansion of blood vessels, thus increasing supply of blood and oxygen to heart (coronary vasodilator) | Management of pain associated with angina pectoris (coronary insufficiency) |
| Duotrate<br>Pentritol | Peritrate<br>Miltrate (CD) | |
| **Pentobarbital** | Believed to block transmission of nerve impulses (hypnotic; sedative) | Low dosage: relief of mild to moderate anxiety or tension (sedative effect); higher dosage: at bedtime to induce sleep (hypnotic effect) |
| Nembutal<br>Wigraine P-B (CD)<br>WANS (CD) | | |
| **Phenacetin (Acetophenetidin)** | Believed to reduce concentration of chemicals involved in production of pain, fever, and inflammation (analgesic; antipyretic) | Relief of mild to moderate pain; reduction of fever |
| A.P.C. (CD)<br>Bromo-Seltzer (CD) | Empirin Compound (CD) | Percodan (CD)<br>Sinubid (CD) | |
| **Phenazopyridine** | Acts as local anesthetic on lining of lower urinary tract (urinary-analgesic) | Relief of pain and discomfort associated with acute irritation of lower urinary tract as in cystitis, urethritis, and prostatitis |
| Pyridium<br>Azo Gantanol (CD) | Thiosulfil-A (CD)<br>Urobiotic (CD) | |
| **Pheniramine** | Blocks action of histamine after release from sensitized tissue cells, thus reducing intensity of allergic response (antihistamine) | Relief of symptoms of hay fever (allergic rhinitis) and of allergic reactions of skin (itching, swelling, hives, and rash) |
| Triaminic<br>Citra Forte (CD)<br>Dristan (CD)<br>Fiogesic (CD) | Poly-Histine-D (CD)<br>Robitussin AC (CD) | Ru-Tuss with Hydrocodone (CD)<br>S-T Forte (CD) | Triaminicin (CD)<br>Tussagesic (CD)<br>Tussirex (CD) |
| **Phenobarbital/ Phenobarbitone** | Believed to block transmission of nerve impulses (anticonvulsant; hypnotic; sedative) | Low dosage: relief of mild to moderate anxiety or tension (sedative effect); higher dosage: at bedtime to induce sleep (hypnotic effect); continuous dosage: prevention of epileptic seizures (anticonvulsant effect) |
| SK-Phenobarbital<br>Solfoton<br>Antispasmodic Capsules (CD) | Antrocol (CD)<br>Arco-Lase Plus (CD)<br>Bronkolixir (CD)<br>Bronkotabs (CD) | Chardonna-2 (CD)<br>Mudrane (CD)<br>Mudrane GG (CD)<br>Phazyme-PB (CD)<br>Primatene (CD) | Pro-Banthine with Phenobarbital (CD)<br>Quadrinal (CD)<br>T-E-P (CD) |
| **Phentermine** | Believed to alter chemical control of nerve impulse transmitter in appetite center of brain (appetite suppressant [anorexiant]) | Suppression of appetite in management of weight reduction |
| Adipex-P<br>Fastin | Ionamin<br>Oby-Trim | Teramine<br>Tora | |
| **Phenylbutazone** | Believed to suppress formation of chemical involved in production of inflammation (analgesic; anti-inflammatory; antipyretic) | Symptomatic relief of inflammation, swelling, pain, and tenderness associated with arthritis, tendinitis, bursitis, superficial phlebitis |
| Azolid<br>Butazolidin | | |

| Name | Action | Prescribed for |
|---|---|---|
| **Trade Names** | **(CD = combined drug)** | |

| Name | Action | Prescribed for |
|---|---|---|
| **Phenylephrine** | Shrinks tissue mass (decongestion by contracting arteriole walls in lining of nasal passages, sinuses, and throat, thus decreasing volume of blood (decongestant [sympathomimetic]) | Relief of congestion of nose, sinuses, and throat associated with allergy |

| | | | |
|---|---|---|---|
| Bromphen (CD) | Dristan, Advanced | 4-Way Nasal Spray (CD) | P-V-Tussin (CD) | Sinarest (CD) |
| Codimal (CD) | Formula (CD) | Histalet (CD) | Pediacof (CD) | Singlet (CD) |
| Comhist (CD) | Dura-Tap/PD (CD) | Histaspan-D (CD) | Phenergan VC (CD) | S-T Decongest (CD) |
| Congespirin (CD) | Dura-Vent/PD (CD) | Histor-D (CD) | Protid (CD) | S-T Forte (CD) |
| Coryban-D Cough Syrup (CD) | E.N.T. (CD) | Hycomine (CD) | Quelidrine (CD) | Tamine S.R. (CD) |
| Dallergy (CD) | Entex (CD) | Korigesic (CD) | Ru-Tuss (CD) | Tussar DM (CD) |
| Dimetapp (CD) | Extendryl (CD) | Naldecon (CD) | Rynatan (CD) | Tussirex (CD) |
| Donatussin (CD) | | Neo-Synephrine (CD) | Rynatuss (CD) | Tympagesic (CD) |

| Name | Action | Prescribed for |
|---|---|---|
| **Phenylpropanol-amine** | Same as above | Same as above |

| | | | |
|---|---|---|---|
| Help | Bromphen (CD) | Dehist (CD) | Histalet (CD) | Rhinolar (CD) |
| Propagest | Codimal Expectorant (CD) | Dexatrim (CD) | Hycomine (CD) | Ru-Tuss (CD) |
| Rhindecon | Comtrex (CD) | Dieutrim (CD) | Korigesic (CD) | S-T Decongest (CD) |
| Alka-Seltzer Plus (CD) | Conex (CD) | Dimetane (CD) | Kronohist (CD) | S-T Forte (CD) |
| Allerest (CD) | Congesprin (CD) | Dimetapp (CD) | Naldecon (CD) | Sinubid (CD) |
| Appedrine, Maximum Strength (CD) | Contac (CD) | Dura-Tapp/PD (CD) | Nolamine (CD) | Sinulin (CD) |
| Bayer Children's Cold Tablets (CD) | Control (CD) | Dura-Vent (CD) | Ornacol (CD) | Sinutab (CD) |
| | Coryban-D (CD) | Dura-Vent/A (CD) | Ornade (CD) | Tamine S.R. (CD) |
| Bayer Cough Syrup for Children (CD) | CoTylenol Children's Liquid (CD) | E.N.T. (CD) | Phenate (CD) | Tavist-D (CD) |
| | Cremacoat 3 (CD) | Entex (CD) | Poly-Histine (CD) | Triaminic (CD) |
| | | 4-Way (CD) | Prolamine, Extra Strength (CD) | Triaminicin (CD) |
| | | Fiogesic (CD) | Quadrahist (CD) | Triaminicol (CD) |
| | | Heat & Chest (CD) | Resaid (CD) | Tuss-Ade (CD) |
| | | | Rescaps (CD) | Tuss-Ornade (CD) |

| Name | Action | Prescribed for |
|---|---|---|
| **Phenytoin** (formerly Diphenyl-hydantoin) | Believed to promote loss of sodium from nerve fibers, thus lowering their excitability and inhibiting spread of electrical impulse along nerve pathways (anticonvulsant) | Prevention of epileptic seizures |
| Dilantin | | |

| Name | Action | Prescribed for |
|---|---|---|
| **Pilocarpine** | Lowers internal eye pressure (antiglaucoma [miotic]) | Management of glaucoma |
| Almocarpine Isopto Carpine Pilocar | | |

| Name | Action | Prescribed for |
|---|---|---|
| **Potassium** | Maintains and replenishes potassium content of cells (potassium preparations) | Management of potassium deficiency |
| Kaon    K-Lor    Klorvess<br>Kay Ciel    Kaochlor    Pima Syrup | | |

| Name | Action | Prescribed for |
|---|---|---|
| **Prednisolone** | Believed to inhibit several mechanisms that induce inflammation (adrenocortical steroid [anti-inflammatory]) | Symptomatic relief of inflammation (swelling, redness, heat, and pain) |
| Delta-Cortef    Metimyd<br>Hydeltra-T.B.A.    Metreton<br>Predate | | |

| Name | Action | Prescribed for |
|---|---|---|
| **Prednisone** | Same as above | Same as above |
| Deltasone    SK-Prednisone<br>Liquid Pred    Sterapred | | |

| Name | Action | Prescribed for |
|------|--------|----------------|
| **Trade Names** | **(CD = combined drug)** | |
| **Probenecid** | Reduces level of uric acid in blood and tissues; prolongs presence of penicillin in blood (antigout [uricosuric]) | Management of gout |
| Benemid<br>SK-Probenecid<br>ColBENEMID<br>(CD) | Col-Probenecid<br>(CD)<br>Polycillin-PRB<br>(CD) | |
| **Promethazine** | Blocks action of histamine after release from sensitized tissue cells, thus reducing intensity of allergic response (antihistamine); blocks transmission of excessive nerve impulses to vomiting center (antiemetic); action producing sedation and sleep is unknown (sedative) | Relief of symptoms of hay fever (allergic rhinitis) and of allergic reactions of skin (itching, swelling, hives, rash); prevention and management of nausea, vomiting, and dizziness associated with motion sickness; production of mild sedation and light sleep |
| Phenergan<br>Promet<br>Remsed | Mepergan (CD)<br>Synalgos-DC (CD) | |
| **Propantheline** | Prevents stimulation of muscular contraction and glandular secretion within organ involved (antispasmodic [anticholinergic]) | Relief of discomfort associated with excessive activity and spasm of digestive tract |
| Norpanth<br>Pro-Banthine<br>SK-Propantheline | | |
| **Propoxyphene** | Increases chemicals that transmit nerve impulses, somehow contributing to the analgesic effect (analgesic) | Relief of mild to moderate pain |
| Darvon<br>Darvon-N<br>Darvocet-N (CD)<br>Darvon Compound (CD) | Lorcet (CD)<br>SK-65 APAP (CD)<br>SK-65 Compound<br>(CD)<br>Wygesic (CD) | |
| **Pseudoephedrine**<br>(Isoephedrine) | Shrinks tissue mass (decongestion) by contracting arteriole walls in lining of nasal passages, sinuses, and throat, thus decreasing volume of blood (decongestant [sympathomimetic]) | Relief of congestion of nose, throat, and sinuses associated with allergy |
| Sudafed<br>Actifed (CD)<br>Ambenyl-D (CD)<br>Anafed (CD)<br>Anamine (CD)<br>Brexin (CD)<br>Bromfed (CD)<br>Cardec DM (CD) | Chlorafed (CD)   Dimacol (CD)<br>Codimal-L.A. (CD) Dorcol (CD)<br>Congess SR & JR  Extra-Strength<br> (CD)            Sine-Aid (CD)<br>CoTylenol Cold  Fedahist (CD)<br> Medication    Gunifed (CD)<br> (CD)          Histalet (CD)<br>Deconamine (CD) Isoclor (CD) | Kronofed-A (CD)  Respaire-SR (CD)<br>Novafed (CD)    Robitussin-DAC<br>Novahistine     (CD)<br> (CD)          Sine-Aid (CD)<br>Nucofed (CD)   Triafed (CD)<br>Phenergan (CD)  Tussend Expecto-<br>Poly-Histine-DX  rant (CD)<br> (CD)         Zephrex (CD) |
| **Pyrilamine/**<br>**Mepyramine** | Blocks action of histamine after release from sensitized tissue cells, thus reducing intensity of allergic response (antihistamine) | Relief of symptoms of hay fever (allergic rhinitis) and of allergic reactions of skin (itching, swelling, hives, and rash) |
| Albatussin (CD)<br>Citra Forte (CD)<br>Codimal (CD)<br>4-Way Nasal<br> Spray (CD) | Fiogesic (CD)    Poly-Histine-D<br>Histalet (CD)    (CD)<br>Kronohist (CD)  Primatene-M (CD)<br>Mydol PMS (CD) Ru-Tuss (CD)<br>P-V-Tussin (CD)  Triaminic (CD) | Triaminicin (CD)<br>Triaminicol (CD)<br>WANS (CD) |

## Commonly Prescribed
## Generic Drugs

| Name | Action | Prescribed for |
|---|---|---|
| Trade Names | (CD = combined drug) | |
| **Quinidine** | Slows pacemaker and delays transmission of electrical impulses (cardiac depressant) | Correction of certain heart rhythm disorders |
| Cardioquin<br>Cin-Quin<br>Duraquin | Quinaglute     Quinora<br>Quinidex     SK-Quinidine | |
| **Rafampin** | Prevents growth and multiplication of susceptible tuberculosis organisms by interfering with enzyme systems involved in formation of essential proteins (antibiotic; tuberculostatic) | Treatment of tuberculosis |
| Rifadin<br>Rimactane | | |
| **Reserpine** | Relaxes blood vessel walls by reducing availability of norepinephrine (antihypertensive; tranquilizer) | Reduction of high blood pressure |
| Sandril<br>Serpasil<br>SK-Resperine<br>Chloroserpine (CD) | Demi-Regroton (CD)  Hydro-Fluserpine (CD)<br>Diupres (CD)  Hydromox R (CD)<br>Diutensen-R (CD)  Hydropres (CD)<br>H-H-R (CD) | Hydroserpine (CD)  Salutensin (CD)<br>Metatensin (CD)  Ser-Ap-Es (CD)<br>Naquival (CD)  Unipres (CD)<br>Regrotin (CD) |
| **Secobarbital** | Believed to block transmission of nerve impulses (hypnotic; sedative) | Low dosage: relief of mild to moderate anxiety or tension (sedative effect); higher dosage: at bedtime to induce sleep (hypnotic effect) |
| Seconal<br>Tuinal (CD) | | |
| **Sulfamethoxazole** | Prevents growth and multiplication of susceptible bacteria by interfering with their formation of folic acid (antibacterial) | Elimination of infections responsive to action of this drug |
| Gantanol<br>Azo Gantanol (CD) | Bactrim (CD)  Septra (CD)<br>Cotrim (CD)  Sulfatrim (CD) | |
| **Sulfisoxazole** | Same as above | Same as above |
| Gantrisin<br>SK-Soxazole<br>Azo Gantrisin (CD)<br>Pediazole (CD) | | |
| **Tetracycline** | Prevents growth and multiplication of susceptible bacteria by interfering with their formation of essential proteins (antibiotic) | Elimination of infections responsive to action of this drug |
| Achromycin V<br>Cyclopar<br>Panmycin<br>Robitet<br>SK-Tetracycline | Topicycline<br>Sumycin<br>Achrostatin V (CD)<br>Mysteclin-F (CD) | |
| **Theophylline**<br>(Aminophylline, Oxtriphylline) | Reverses constriction by increasing activity of chemical system within muscle cell that causes relaxation of bronchial tube (bronchodilator) | Symptomatic relief of bronchial asthma |
| Accurbron<br>Bronkodyl<br>Constant-T<br>Elixicon<br>LABID<br>Lodrane<br>Respbid | Somophyllin  Theon<br>Sustaire  Theo-Organidin<br>Synophylate  Theophyl<br>Theobid  Aerolate (CD)<br>Theoclear  Amesec (CD)<br>Theo-Dur  Aquaphyllin (CD)<br>Theolair  Brondecon (CD) | Bronkolixir (CD)  Quibron (CD)<br>Bronkotabs (CD)  Slo-bid (CD)<br>Elixophyllin (CD)  Slo-Phyllin (CD)<br>Marax (CD)  T.E.H. (CD)<br>Mudrane (CD)  T-E-P (CD)<br>Primatene (CD)  Tedral (CD)<br>Quadrinal (CD)  Theozine (CD) |

| Name | Action | Prescribed for |
|------|--------|----------------|
| **Trade Names** | **(CD = combined drug)** | |
| **Thyroid** (Thyroid Preparations) | Makes more energy available for biochemical activity and increases rate of cellular metabolism by altering processes of cellular chemicals that store energy (thyroid hormones) | Correction of thyroid hormone deficiency (hypothyroidism) |
| Armour Thyroid  Cytomel | Euthroid  Proloid  Levothroid  S-P-T | Synthroid  Thyrolar |
| **Thyroxine (T-4)** | Same as above | Same as above |
| Choloxin  Euthroid | Levothroid  Synthroid  L-Thyroxine  Thyrolar (CD) | |
| **Tolbutamide** | Stimulates secretion of insulin by pancreas (hypoglycemic) | Correction of insulin deficiency in adult diabetes |
| Orinase | | |
| **Tridihexethyl** | Prevents stimulation of muscular contraction and glandular secretion in organ involved (antispasmodic [anticholinergic]) | Relief of discomfort from excessive activity and spasm of digestive tract |
| Pathilon  Milpath (CD)  Pathibamate (CD) | | |
| **Trimethoprim** | Prevents growth and multiplication of susceptible organisms by interfering with formation of proteins (antibacterial) | Elimination of infections responsive to action of this drug |
| Proloprim  Trimpex | Bactrim (CD)  Septra (CD)  Cotrim (CD)  Sulfatrim (CD) | |
| **Triprolidine** | Blocks action of histamine after release from sensitized tissue cells, thus reducing intensity of allergic response (antihistamine) | Relief of symptoms of hay fever (allergic rhinitis) and of allergic reactions of skin (itching, swelling, hives, and rash) |
| Actidil  Actifed (CD)  Actifed-C (CD) | Triafed (CD)  Trifed (CD) | |
| **Vitamin C** (Ascorbic Acid) | Believed to be essential to enzyme activity involved in formation of collagen; increases absorption of iron from intestine and helps formation of hemoglobin and red blood cells in bone marrow; inhibits growth of certain bacteria in urinary tract; enhances effects of some antibiotics (vitamin) | Prevention and treatment of scurvy; treatment of some types of anemia; maintenance of acid urine |
| Cetane  Cevalin | | |

# 37
# Physical Fitness

## The Target: Total Fitness

Total fitness has been described in many ways. Most aptly, perhaps, it involves looking your best, feeling your best, and performing to the best of your ability. In the totally fit body stamina, strength, and flexibility have been brought to peak levels of development.

Total fitness may mean different things to different people. The level of fitness that a person can achieve varies with his or her physical or medical history. The level also depends on the person's height, weight, age, musculature, body type, and other characteristics. Thus, total fitness for any individual is the highest level of fitness to which that person can go, given the limitations imposed by the various factors.

Physicians and fitness experts agree that movement of some kind is mandatory for anyone who wants to achieve total fitness. Movement in the form of a planned, timed, repetitive program of exercise brings the human body to the goal of fitness in the shortest possible time.

Total physical fitness has many aspects. It calls for adequate rest and relaxation and it requires proper nutrition. The totally fit person has to follow sound health practices and have good dental and health care. Otherwise, fitness may prove difficult or impossible to achieve.

In broader terms, fitness brings many advantages and benefits to various aspects of a person's life. Fitness enhances an individual's ability to work with endurance and vigor and to enjoy work and leisure activities. A person who achieves total fitness can usually avoid undue fatigue, so that he or she has energy left for hobbies, recreation, and for meeting unforeseen emergencies.

# Getting Started

Starting your fitness program may call for resolution of some final questions. Got a place in which to work out? Know what you're going to wear? Need any special equipment?

Think of a few other things. The process of warming up and cooling down. The problems of pain and strain, especially at the beginning—problems such as shin splints, which you may remember from college or high school.

You'll want to have these and other items clear in your mind. The questions of where to exercise, when during the day and week, what to wear, and how vigorously to exercise trouble many persons starting out on their self-tailored fitness programs. This is natural; the questions are important. The program has to fit into your life. It has to be practical.

## The Where

We are talking, obviously, of the person who has decided on a personalized program that can be carried out alone. However, the person may not have decided on a place to do his or her exercises. One useful guideline to follow is to choose a space, or develop one, that ensures that the program can be "lived with." Designers of fitness programs suggest that the following three basic provisions should be made if you plan to work out at home.

### Find Enough Space

Floor exercises and weight lifting take a floor area measuring approximately 7.5 by 10.5 feet. A larger area would, of course, be welcome. But to avoid bouncing off the walls you should have the space indicated. The height of the ceiling does not matter unless a trapeze or rings are to be installed. In either case the exercise area would require an 11-foot ceiling. For all other purposes, a ceiling clearance of eight feet is adequate.

### Set Up a Mirror

A mirror set up close to the exercise area expands the space in a visual sense. More importantly, the mirror makes it possible for the person to check the accuracy of his or her exercise positions and routines when working out alone. If possible, the mirror should be six feet high by three feet wide so that it provides a full-length view.

**Creating Your Own Exercise Equipment**

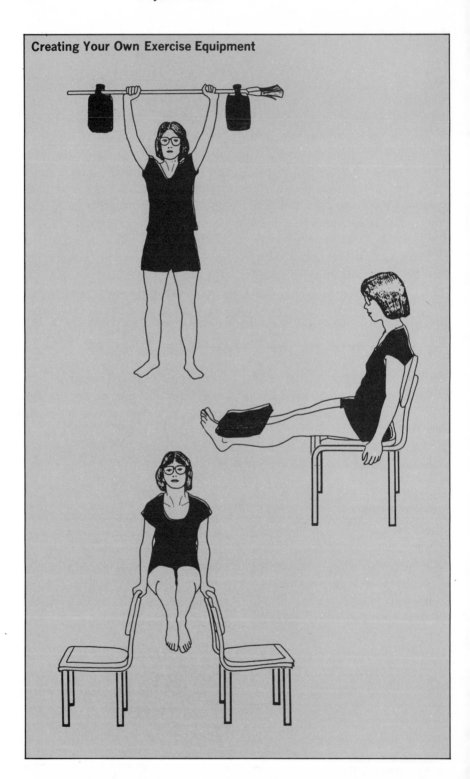

## Ensure Safety Underfoot

Because slippery floors can present major safety hazards, the footing should be tested and retested for safety. Carpeting helps unless the exercise program includes dance routines. In general, a tightly woven, looped-pile, industrial-grade carpeting is recommended. This kind of carpeting has one major advantage over cut-pile—shag or velvet surface—carpeting: the looped-pile type is more durable. Just incidentally, the looped-pile type is cheaper.

## Special Equipment

Keeping a program simple ordinarily rules out expensive equipment. But some equipment will make it possible to add the spice of variety to the program. For example, barbells may help to make flexibility an easily achieved goal.

One or two exercise mats provide the base for many lying-down exercises. Mats can be purchased from sporting goods stores, ordered from mail-order houses, or made at home out of 1.5-inch foam rubber. If made at home, the mats can be covered with a fabric that goes with the room. The material may be terry cloth, vinyl-coated fabric, canvas, or some other type that is soft, easily washed or wiped off, and durable.

If the mat has a line running down its center lengthwise, it will make body alignment a simple task. The line can be made out of a similar fabric of a different color from the mat covering proper.

The mat or mats should be sized to fit the individual's body. The perfect mat is somewhat longer than the user is tall, and wide enough to provide protection against bumps and bruises. That means it should be wider than a line drawn from heel to heel when the person lies flat and stretches both legs as far apart as possible. Another way to measure the ideal mat width is to lie flat and extend the elbows as far as possible straight out from the shoulders. The points reached by the elbows indicate a good width. The good mat has plenty of "give." It also springs back into position when pressure is removed.

Choosing and arranging permanent equipment may take a little thought. With care and planning, the room's appearance need not really suffer. Equipment may come in chrome, steel, or natural wood.

## Handling Space Problems

Got a space problem? No room at all for privacy while charging through a workout? No place to install and use an exercycle or treadmill? Think a minute.

Can space be created? If the exercise equipment had to be stored, where would it go? Can that storage space be turned into an exercise area? A separate room isn't necessarily the only solution. Closets may be useful in solving the no-space problem. A walk-in closet may serve as a special niche for some types of equipment. A two-foot-deep enclosure can be created along a wall by installing folding doors; some equipment can then be hidden behind the barrier. When the doors are opened, presto! The area becomes a miniature gym.

Because exercise equipment has to be ready for use without much advance preparation, it may be desirable to feature it as part of the overall layout. An exercycle may be placed in a corner in a cleared space. A set of barbells may rest on a simple bench that holds them in notches for safety. Ballet bars may double as towel bars when not serving their fitness functions. For real permanence and solidity, exercise benches might be recessed into the walls. They could be covered with throws when not in use.

## Homemade Equipment

If, on the other hand, Spartan simplicity is preferable, formal equipment may be dispensed with totally. Many exercises can be performed without any equipment at all. For example, various sets of exercises have been designed for practice in the shower, sitting down at the work desk, or standing up in an ordinary room. More on that later.

Many household items can be converted to exercise props. Weights can be made out of plastic dish detergent or bleach containers. The containers need only be filled with sand or water. If desired, the weights can be attached to the ends of a bar made of a broom or mop handle. Numerous heavy objects such as ski boots, tele-phone books, or bricks wrapped in towels can also be incorporated into exercise routines.

A little creativity can turn other everyday items into perfectly adequate fitness equipment. A length of clothesline makes an admirable jump rope. Two solid chairs of the same size can be placed back to back a couple of feet apart to form parallel bars. A heavy towel, held with arms spread an appropriate distance, can be used to provide both variable resistance and a massaging effect. Different exercises to increase endurance, equilibrium, speed, suppleness, strength, and coordination have been devised utilizing lengths of cloth.

## Time Out for Exercise

Some trial and error may be necessary in determining the amount of time needed for exercising. At first, repetitions should be in short series, after which the principle of overload dictates a gradual step-up. Particularly at the beginning, those who have not exercised much for years should consider cowardice the better part of fitness valor. Instead of starting with 45-minute sessions that include a mile run, a 30-minute session including a run of a block or two may be adequate. Once it has been established that such minimal achievement levels do not cause overstrain, the program's general shape should be maintained until the specific short-term goals have been reached.

For those in better condition, a faster start is more appropriate. Again, the rule requiring regularity in all the basic phases of the program should be observed.

## Some Important Factors

Mealtimes should be carefully considered in scheduling the daily exercise round. Most authorities believe that engaging in vigorous exercise within an hour before or after a meal may interfere with the digestive processes. That suggests that the exercise time should start at least an hour to an hour and one-half after eating. Conversely, one should allow at least an hour between an exercise session and the next meal.

Some other factors are important. Exercise taken immediately before bedtime may interfere with relaxation, and sleep, through stimulation of the adrenalin flow. Late-evening exercise should, in fact, be followed by an hour or so period of winding down.

At other times of the day the winddown period may be somewhat shortened, and may often be dispensed with altogether.

A psychological element appears to enter into the choice of time during the day. Many persons feel that by scheduling the fitness session in the early morning, they can "get it over with" and thus avoid having other responsibilities of the day interfere with exercising. Others prefer the noon hour. Some like the later afternoon, when the exercise round provides a break in the day's routine. The late-day session acts as a kind of afterwork, before-dinner tonic for many persons.

## The Systematic Approach

An orderly, systematic approach to exercising calls for establishing a special time during the day for working on fitness. The principle of repetitiveness and its corollary—overload—are also founded on the idea of system and regularity.

Most fitness authorities even suggest that system ought to govern the order in which exercises are taken. One version of an exercise circuit for ten different parts of the body is illustrated here. Each person has options here: depending on personal fitness goals, other exercises may be more appropriate for the same circuit.

The systematic approach should also govern decisions on the numbers of repetitions for each exercise. Exercise patterns to be presented later will be accompanied by specification of typical repetition cycles for each exercise.

## The Sweater Myth

For decades people have been donning sweaters after heavy exercise. The name sweater, in fact, has obvious origins. The sweater began as a means of keeping the body warm and covered once it had become hot and sweaty.

Unless exposure to inclement weather is a problem, or the individual has particular reasons for putting on a sweater at the end of a hot workout, the sweater myth is just that. Under normal temperature, weather, and other conditions, the sweater simply prolongs the body's hot state. That helps not at all.

Some stiffness can, of course, result from exercise. But wearing a sweater is not the way to prevent that. Stiffness usually has its sources in the body's condition—or lack of it.

## Physical Activity and Fatigue

The advice that counsels moderation in launching a fitness program or in starting new phases of it has a sound basis in physiology. The purpose is to avoid excessive fatigue. Muscular fatigue is defined as stimulation of a muscle or group of muscles beyond their ability to recover. A second type of fatigue affects the entire body. Known as physical fatigue, this form can be regarded as normal after physical exercise if it does not suggest undue stress.

## Planning a Level of Intensity

Keep in mind that a flexible plan may call for different adjustments under different circumstances. It may indicate sometimes that it is best to terminate the day's activities. On other occasions it may require elimination of some exercises and continuation with others.

- Your knee begins to bother you. You drop the exercises calling for knee exertion and retain those that don't.

- You get a "stitch" in your side. Because it hurts continually, you decide to downplay those exercises—for that day—that produce or exacerbate the discomfort.

- While running in place, you find yourself troubled by shin splints, those pains along the sides of the shin bones. You stop running and turn to something else.

Flexibility can exist alongside dedication to a program. As common sense dictates, the individual should sometimes slow down or blow the whistle completely on some exercises. Even Napoleon retreated now and then.

Another important principle should be noted: the individual will build and take to a fitness program most readily if he believes it will do him some good. And if he has faith and confidence in it, he is likely to stay with the program over the long haul.

## Climbing the Fitness Ladder

Three stages of fitness have been identified. The individual who stays with an intelligently devised program moves through beginning, intermediate, and advanced stages. These have been termed by some authorities the low, medium, and excellent stages or phases. Some experts add a fourth level: the elite stage at which a person finds himself able to take part in highly competitive and demanding athletic activities.

## The Exercise Tolerance Factor

Fatigue places basic strictures on the human body. Exercise tolerance refers to an individual's ability to take part in a demanding sport or game, jog, do a series of exercises, or engage in some other activity without reaching the undue fatigue stage.

At the start-up stage of a fitness program, the beginner should make certain that all the exercises selected are adjusted to his or her own exercise tolerance level. That adjustment has both positive and negative sides: the exercises should not be too difficult, nor should any be chosen that do not make the body work sufficiently hard. Exercises that are too easy will not produce fitness and should be eliminated or made more difficult. Pulse rate provides a good indication of whether the body is being asked to do an appropriate amount of work.

Decreased heart rate usually comes with advancing age. At the same time the older person has decreased work capacity or exercise tolerance. But age is only one villain producing the decreased work capacity. Reduced elasticity in the blood vessels also affects physical performance.

## Warm-up and Cool-down

The rules for warm-up and cool-down are simple. A gradual progression in intensity of exertion should introduce the fitness session. At the end of the session there should be a tapering-off period, during which the body returns to normal. Actually, authorities disagree to some extent on the need for a warm-up and cool-down. But most feel that a preexercise warm-up should be mandatory for everyone taking part in demanding exercises. For those who have not exercised seriously for a long time and who are restarting, the warm-up should last 10 to 15 minutes. For those in better condition, the warm-up can be shorter, even as little as four or five minutes.

An effective warm-up period has several physiological effects. For one thing, it stretches ligaments. The warm-up also raises body temperature and increases cardiovascular activity. In all such ways the warm-up prepares the body for exercise.

### Warm-up: What and How?

The warm-up begins, for best results, with light, rhythmical exercises performed at a slow pace. Stretching and deep breathing both loosen the muscles and increase the body's oxygen supply. Stretching also makes deeper breathing possible.

Most sets of warm-up exercises include about four or five very simple movements. The body should be sweating lightly when the set is done. A typical group of four exercises is shown.

**1.** The *deep-breathing* exercise requires that you rise on your toes, inhaling deeply at the same time. First extend your arms straight out to the side. While breathing in and rising on your toes, raise your arms from shoulder level until your hands come together over your head. That position should be held for a moment or two. Then lower your arms to your sides and exhale while returning to the flat-footed standing position. Six to a dozen repetitions will suffice.

**2.** The *arm rotation* exercise calls again for extension of your arms straight out to the sides from your shoulders. The hands are then rotated in circles about a foot in diameter. Your hands should describe 20 circles while rotating forward and 20 more while rotating in the other direction.

**3.** In the *body rotation* exercise, after placing your feet wide apart and bending forward at the waist, rotate your body from the belt up in slow circles. The upper body should describe circles large enough to stretch all the affected muscles. You can rotate five times in one direction, five more in the other.

**4.** In the *bend and bounce*, bend far over with your legs spread apart. Try to touch your fingers to the ground three times in front of your right foot, then three times in front of the left. The touching should be done with downward bouncing motions of the body. The beginner may want to

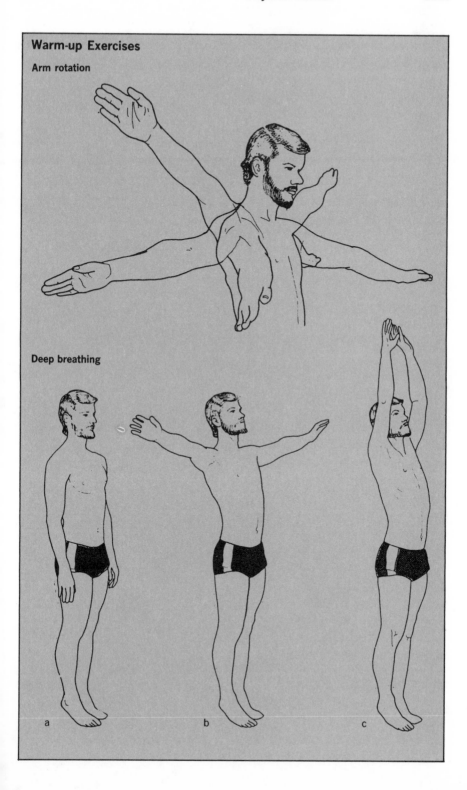

## Warm-up Exercises

### Arm rotation

### Deep breathing

a          b          c

## Warm-up Exercises

### Body rotation

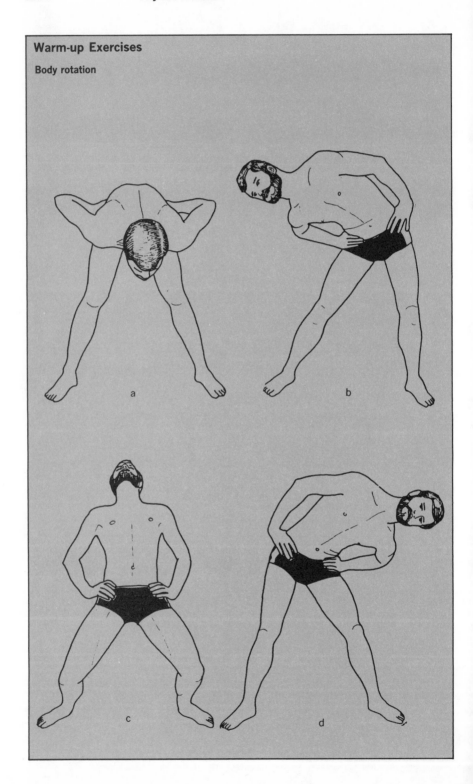

# Warm-up Exercises

## Bend and bounce

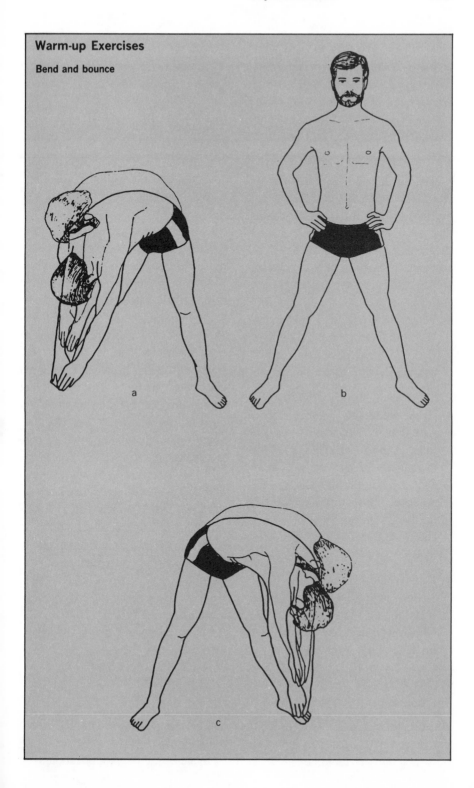

bend without touching the ground at all—just bouncing and bending low. The bend and bounce should stretch the back muscles. The tension on the muscles should be increased daily until flexibility returns.

The same warm-up series can include other exercises designed to get the feet in tune with the body. This final set of movements helps prevent the damage that can be inflicted on the feet by neglect or a premature start on the exercise program proper.

- While sitting, pick up a dozen marbles with the toes of the right foot. Drop each marble in turn into a container. The procedure is repeated with the other foot.

- Again while sitting on the floor, with one leg crossed over the other at the knee, take hold of the toes of the upper leg with both hands. Using that pressure as resistance, try to curl your toes as hard as you can. The exercise should be repeated with the other foot.

- Again while seated on the floor, flex one leg at the knee and place that foot on the floor. Hold the other leg straight out with the toes pointed, and describe a full circle

with the foot. Repeat this exercise 10 times with each foot.

- Standing with your hands on your hips, rise up on tiptoe, then lower yourself to the floor quickly. The exercise should be repeated 10 times in the early sessions, then increased to 20 or more times for later warm-ups.

Note that you can invent your own warm-up exercise routine. It should, if possible, parallel the exercises that you will be performing in the main fitness activity. Indeed, warm-up movements may be identical to those later exercises, particularly where sports are concerned. The handball player warms up with throwing exercises and special shots. The tennis player warms up by rallying easily until his muscles are completely ready for the sometimes violent demands of the regular game.

Those who decide to create their own warm-up routines should keep in mind the basic characteristics of any satisfying set of exercises. Whole-body activity such as running in place or jumping is usually included in a warm-up. The warm-up set should also exercise each of the major body areas: trunk and hips; arms and shoulders; neck; legs and knees; and ankle and foot.

## The Cool-off

If a careful warm-up helps prevent muscle soreness, what does the cool-off period do? Can't you just lie down

and let the sweat dry until you go to the shower?

In answer to the first question, the

cool-down period allows the blood to be gradually redistributed in the normal resting pattern. The body temperature returns to normal. Your heart rate goes back to normal.

The answer to the second question is No. The best procedure is to keep moving for at least several minutes after vigorous exercise. You are trying to get your breathing and heart rate back to normal. You want your body literally to cool down.

Why not just lie down—or sit down—to cool off? An abrupt and complete cessation of the exercise reduces the flow of venous blood to the heart. A complete stop may also de-crease the heart stroke volume. The heart may have to work much harder to maintain an adequate blood flow. Thus abruptly terminating exercise may lead to dizziness, fainting, shock, or other strain on the heart. Most heart attacks that afflict older persons in exercise situations take place during the postexercise period.

The ideal cool-down exercise is slow jogging or walking. At the same time the subject should swing his or her arms. Once the pulse rate has reached about 120—a ten-second count of 20—the readjustment has been largely accomplished.

## Showers, Saunas, and Steam Baths

Hot showers, saunas, and steam baths also are not recommended for the immediate postexercise period. The hot shower, sauna, or steam bath merely adds strain. While they can be enjoyable and relaxing, be sure to wait until the body has returned completely to normal before indulging in them.

Ice-cold showers present their own dangers. Ice-cold water flowing over the chest increases the blood pressure. It also raises the heart rate and cardiac output. While a healthy individual can tolerate the additional load, a person with cardiovascular problems could experience difficulties. Such a person may or may not know of his condition; the ice-cold shower would take its toll in either case.

The need to shower after heavy exercise cannot, of course, be minimized. A noted educator once stated that a social gap exists between those who bathe daily and those who do not. The gap would widen if the shower were not a post exercise priority. But the shower water should have a moderate temperature—about 70 degrees. At that temperature the shower tones the skin while also cleaning.

Some experts recommend a warm shower followed by a cool one. The warm shower opens the skin pores; the cool one closes them. Medical authorities agree generally that the practice has merit for persons in good health.

# Living with Stress

## Ten Ways to
## Get a Handle on Stress

Exercise is a key method of working off stress and tension. But there are many other useful approaches to managing these problems. Ten ways to cope are:

**1.** *"Blow off steam!"* When angry or upset, or when feeling any kind of stress or tension, it's wise to engage in some kind of physical activity. You can garden, jog, play tennis, lift weights, or walk. Virtually any kind of physical activity provides an outlet for the "fight" impulse—as contrasted with a "flight" urge—thus relieving mental or emotional stress.

**2.** *Talk it out:* Is there someone in your life whom you trust and respect? That person may be the one to sit down and "talk it out" with. The person need not be close; it could be a clergyman, a physician, a teacher, a counselor. Professional listeners like psychologists and guidance counselors may be the answer.

**3.** *Accept what you cannot change:* Many problems lie beyond our powers of control. These the individual has to accept—at least until they can be changed. Why spin your wheels? Why beat your head against a brick wall? Even a padded brick wall?

**4.** *Avoid self-medication:* The person who treats himself or herself with medications in hopes of relieving the distress of stress may have a fool for a patient. Many agents and chemicals, including alcohol, may seem to alleviate stress, but they do not help you to adjust to the stress itself. Also, many such substances are habit-forming and should not be taken without a doctor's prescription or approval.

**5.** *Get enough sleep and rest:* Lack of sleep and rest can reduce your ability to deal with the stress that invades every life at one time or another. Most people need seven to eight hours of sleep in every 24-hour day. If stress interferes with sleep, a physician should be consulted.

**6.** *Balance work and recreation:* "All work and no play can make you the richest man in the graveyard." On the way there, you may become a nervous wreck. Because the mind needs recreation just as the body does, you should include some time off in your schedule. Loafing may do it if no other kind of recreation is possible.

**7.** *Help someone:* Doing things for others provides a genuine stress reducer. In many cases stress involves overconcentration on oneself and one's problems. Doing something for someone else helps you to get your mind off your problems as it gets your mind off yourself—and you may win a new friend.

**8.** *Take one thing at a time:* Tackling a dozen tasks at once usually means that none of them will get done right. If you can, line them up either in writing or in your mind and take one at a time.

**9.** *Give in now and then:* A common source of the stress experienced by many people is other people. One possible solution is to give in now and then; try to relax and enjoy your own defeat or change of mind. Stress may fly out the window.

**10.** *Make yourself available:* Does stress hit you when you are feeling bored, left out of life, mired in the slow track? The answer may be to go where the action is. Make yourself available to those who may be able to involve you in an interesting way—in life, in activities, in cultural programs, in whatever you find exciting or important. To withdraw with your stress and feel sorry for yourself is the worst response.

Stress and tension are normal parts of life. But many persons can combat and even eliminate them through regular exercise. Although the program that the fitness novice draws up will generally be geared to the achievement of other goals, elimination of stress should be a by-product of the exercises.

## The Physiological Effect

Stress and tension in the human body encourage the production of adrenaline. Exercise counteracts stress and tension in at least three ways:

- It helps the body to distribute the stress effects over a wider area. That in turn removes the danger that the stress may have a disproportionately damaging effect on one body part, such as the heart. Approached sensibly, exercise thus lessens the danger that a heart attack may follow a stressful situation.

- Exercise also strengthens the body as a whole and its vital organs in particular. The organs can then better withstand the effects of stress.

- Exercise literally "works off" the stress by attacking the physiological and emotional symptoms. Vigorous exercise can often reduce stress to pleasant, normal, physical fatigue.

## Sleep

Sleep is the body's key mechanism for combating fatigue. Like exercise, sleep helps to reduce or eliminate tension. But healthy, sound sleep may elude persons suffering from prolonged stress. In a state of moderate fatigue resulting from exercise, by contrast, the body normally finds sleep a welcome refreshment.

The consensus among physicians today is that vitamins and tranquilizers are almost never the right answers to severe fatigue, nor are alcohol and sleeping pills. Caffeine can be counterproductive to the point where the body cannot really relax. Too much caffeine may even cause anxiety symptoms and an increase in stress and tension.

Curiously, most persons require less—not more—sleep once they have begun an exercise program. The reasons may be psychological or physical or both; physicians are not certain. Those who find it difficult to fall asleep while pursuing an exercise program should examine their schedules. Strenuous exercises shortly before bedtime can interfere with sleep more than help it.

## Muscle-Relaxing Techniques

Muscular tension accompanies psychological stress. The causes of the stress may differ, ranging from fear to worry to anger and frustration, but the muscular tension is always there. The muscle tone or tonus increases beyond the normally low level of contraction.

Exercises designed to reduce muscular tension can have a therapeutic effect on one's emotional state. The basic concept in all the various techniques for reducing stress through

exercise is to reduce tension by depressing muscular activity and by degrees induce a state of relaxation. The exercises incidentally contribute to total fitness, but generally to a minor degree.

Rhythmic exercises for the trunk help to reduce tension and build muscles. These exercises also contribute to improved circulation. Other types of muscle-relaxing exercises help to improve breathing.

## Regional Relaxation

Muscle-relaxing exercises are effective in reducing tension because the mind can affect or control groups of muscles even though the causes of stress may not be reachable—or even recognizable. Learning to relax controllable muscles, the individual can attack first the muscular tension, then the psychological stress that undergirds it. "Uncontrollable tensions" thus come under the influence of the mind. The source of the stress may

or may not be still at work; the exercise nonetheless relieves the symptoms that it has caused.

For the purpose of relieving muscular tension, the person first concentrates on muscle regions or groups. Effort is then exerted to recognize voluntary muscle contractions. In one muscle group after another, the levels of voluntary contraction are progressively lowered. With practice, the subject's perceptions of his own muscular state improves. Eventually he can identify and eliminate any slightest degree of in voluntary muscle tension of any kind in any part of the body.

Often, a kind of meditational relaxation takes place. The subject gradually and for short periods achieves a state of high concentration. Nagging life-problems are—briefly—forgotten.

Tension-reducing exercises fall into a basic pattern. To a large extent, they take their cues from the model developed in 1929 by Dr. Edmund Jacobson. In this model, a formal training method for teaching a person to relax groups of muscles at will, the subject consciously alternates contracting with relaxing various muscle groups at maximum, half-strength, and very slight levels of intensity.

Patterned methods of relaxing muscles should be practiced five or ten minutes a day. They can become part of an exercise program, or they can be completely separate. They do, after all, have their own rationale.

One set of exercises for relaxation of muscle groups follows:

## Relaxation Breathing

Lying on your back on the floor, bend your knees so that your feet can rest flat. While taking a deep breath, let both the chest and the abdominal wall rise and expand. The breath should be held for a few seconds. Then expel it through your mouth with a rush. Repeat the exercise four or five times at regularly spaced intervals.

## Arm Tension

Standing erect, swing both arms forward and back, then side to side. At the same time the arms should be allowed to drop during the swings; the hands should brush your thighs at each pass. Keeping the shoulders low and as relaxed as possible, repeat several times.

Next, sit on the edge of a chair and clench one hand tightly. The hand is kept clenched while the arm is swung vigorously in wide circles. Repeat the movement with the other arm.

## Leg Tension

While sitting on the edge of a table, swing your legs freely backward and forward, bending at the knee. Try to keep your legs moving in rhythm.

## Stomach Tension

In a kneeling position, lower your body so that your feet are under your hips. Extend your arms over your head and clasp your hands. Then swing your trunk down to one side and around. At the same time swing your arms in a wide circle over your head until you come up on the other side.

For an alternative stomach relaxer, stand with your buttocks against a wall. With feet spread apart and a few inches from the wall, bend your body forward and let it sway from side to side. Keep arms and head loose.

## Relaxation for the Neck Muscles

With your head forward and lowered, back straight, and shoulders loose, turn your head first to one side and then the other. Your chin should touch first one collarbone and then the other. Movements should be slow and rhythmic.

## Stretching and Pulling

The personal war against stress, tension, and fatigue ought to take posture and working positions into account. For example, the secretary who has to sit for long periods while working may want special exercises to counter back fatigue, aching muscles, and even headaches. The train conductor who has to stand for long periods may utilize similarly patterned exercises.

One six-part set of simple tension and fatigue-combating exercises calls for stretching and pulling motions:

**1.** *Shoulder/head pull:* In a sitting or standing position, place your arms behind your back. The left hand grasps the back of the right. The hands are pressed against the buttocks. Push your hands downward slowly, at the same time pulling the shoulders back and the shoulder blades down. The head should be tilted as far back as possible. Next,

pull your shoulders forward and your shoulder blades up. Bring the head forward as far as possible. Repeat the exercise two or three times.

**2.** *Shoulder shrug:* In a sitting or standing position, hold your arms at your sides. Slowly pull your shoulders up and back as far as possible while holding the head upright. Finally, let the shoulders drop into a normal, completely relaxed position.

**3.** *Shoulder roll:* Again while sitting or standing with your arms at your sides and your head upright, pull your shoulders forward and down. Then push them back as far as you can. Finally let them drop into the normal, relaxed position.

**4.** *Back fold and unfold:* Sitting or standing, hold your arms relaxed at your sides. Go through two or three twisting, bending movements. Then bend far forward and gradually compress your body into a ball shape. The head should be dropped and the back rounded, with the arms hanging loosely. Straighten the spine slowly and by degrees—the lower back first, then the upper back. Try to be aware of each vertebra as you work your way upwards. The shoulders, chest, and head follow into the starting position. Repeat two or three times. If done in a standing position, this exercise can pay an added dividend. Simply stand with the knees bent slightly to relieve tension in the backs of the legs.

**5.** *Foot stretch and pull:* Sitting on the floor or on the edge of a chair, with your legs extended straight out, curl your toes under slowly. Straighten the feet as far as they will go. Then turn your toes back toward your face as far as possible while spreading your toes at the same time. Release and let your feet relax. Repeat two or three times.

**6.** *Foot roll:* Rotate the feet at the ankle while sitting as in step 5. Rotate slowly, first clockwise, then counterclockwise. Stretch the feet as far as possible. Repeat two or three times.

The stretching and pulling exercises, or variations on them, can be used during the warm-up part of an exercise session. The stretchers and pullers promote flexibility while preparing the muscles, joints, and ligaments for the more strenuous exercise which follows.

## Body Problems

If you encounter physical problems at any time during your workout, it may be desirable to modify what you are doing. Dr. Lenore Zohman, a prominent exercise cardiologist, and her associates have summarized some possible body problems into two categories:

### The Stop Exercising Group

(See a physician before resuming):

- Abnormal heart activity, including such signs and symptoms as irregular pulse (missed beats or extra beats), fluttering, jumping or palpitations in the throat, a sudden burst of rapid heartbeats, or a sudden slowdown in a rapid pulse rate.

- Pain or pressure in the center of the chest, arm, or throat during or immediately after exercise.

- Dizziness, light-headedness, a sudden lack of coordination, confusion, cold sweating, glassy stare, pallor, "blueness," or fainting.

- Illness, in particular a viral infection, which can lead to myocarditis, a viral infection of the heart muscle. Exercise should, in fact, be avoided during and immediately following an illness.

### The Attempt Self-Correction Group

• Persistent rapid pulse for five to ten minutes or more. Self-correction technique: reduce the intensity of the activity, raising heart rate to a lower level, then move on to higher levels of activity at a slower rate. Consult a physician if the problem persists.

• Nausea or vomiting after exercise. Self-correction technique: reduce the intensity of the endurance exercise and lengthen the cool-down period. Avoid eating for at least two hours before the exercise period.

• Extreme breathlessness after exercise. Self-correction technique: reduce the intensity of the exercise. If the condition persists, consult a doctor.

• Prolonged fatigue for up to 24 hours following exercise. Self-correction technique: if the condition persists, reduce the intensity of the exercise and of the total workout session. If those corrective methods fail, see a physician.

## Local Complaints

Many local complaints can afflict the person starting out on a full-scale program. By being careful and taking precautions, you can minimize adverse effects. In many cases they can be eliminated entirely.

Some of the best measures for combating local body problems resulting from exercise or participation in sports have already been described. They include provision of sensible clothing and shoes and the warm-up and cool-down periods. Specific problems such as the following may call for other corrective or curative measures.

### Achilles Tendon Pains or Injuries

This runner's problem, like so many others having to do with the lower extremities, is usually caused by improper footwear. Shoes that lack heel wedges or that rub against the Achilles tendon may be the culprits. The only remedy is total rest and applications of ice (and the purchase of good shoes). Preventive methods include adequate warm-up, part of which should be a heel-stretching exercise.

### Ankle Problems

Ankle problems, afflicting primarily those who take part in sports that require quick changes of direction, should receive immediate attention if they are at all serious. An ankle sprain should be placed in ice at once. A physician should examine a serious sprain. Prevention should begin with protecting the ankle and the sur- rounding muscles by wearing high-top gym or basketball shoes or by taping. Both methods may be used together.

## Athlete's Foot

Clean socks and shoes do the most to prevent athlete's foot, which is caused by a fungus that develops between the toes. Symptoms are itching, burning, and scaling skin; the problem may lead to serious infec- tions. Preventive methods include careful drying between the toes after showering and airing both the shoes and feet. Sprinkling powder between the toes will also help.

## Blisters

Prevention should start with the proper footwear and socks. Socks should be snug enough to remain in place and not "bunch up." If blisters appear anyway, they should be cleaned with an antiseptic solution and covered with light gauze. Growth of an incipient blister may be halted if gauze is taped over the irritated spot.

## Bone Bruises

Where handball players may acquire bone bruises on their hands, participants in other sports activities may experience them on the bottoms of their feet. The cause is usually a single blow or other severe trauma to the flesh and bone. Applying ice and providing padding over the bruised area should help. Appropriate foot- wear, including protective inner soles, serves to prevent foot bruises. Handball players who continue to play after incurring bone bruises may find that the condition persists long after it should have disappeared. The cause in such cases is repeated blows to the bruised area.

## Knee Problems

Because the knee performs such a crucial role in so many different types of exercise and sports activities, it sees extensive use. Joggers and runners in particular develop knee complaints. Most of them can avoid difficulties by wearing the proper footwear and running on soft, level surfaces. Grass or a cinder track is usually the most comfortable. Staying away from sharp turns should also help. A physician should be consulted if knee problems persist.

## Muscle Cramps

While the specific causes of muscle cramps have proved difficult to pinpoint, they appear to result usually from salt and potassium imbalances in muscles. The cramps are involuntary muscle spasms, or contractions. Stretching and massage usually relieve the problem. Preventive measures include adequate warm-up, replacement of the potassium and salt lost in sweating, and stretching during the cool-down period.

## Muscle Soreness

Sore muscles, usually encountered at the start of a fitness program, virtually dictate that the beginner go slowly. Progressing slowly and steadily from a very moderate start through the upper level of a program should reduce or eliminate soreness. Thorough warm-ups and cool-downs are mandatory. Massage and warm baths should help to relieve soreness when it appears.

## Shin Splints

Shin splints are pains that appear along the sides of the shinbone, or tibia. The causes vary and include lowered arches, tearing in a muscle where it attaches to the bone, irritated membranes, hairline fractures of the bone, and others. Running or jogging on hard surfaces, such as streets, and improper running techniques may bring on shin splints. Rest represents the only real cure, but the pains can be alleviated by wrapping or taping the leg.

What do you do when a jogging or running program has to be suspended because of problems in or injuries to a lower extremity? One possibility is to continue the program by cycling, using a regular bicycle or an exercycle. The program can then be continued and fitness maintained.

# Starting With Some Easy Exercises

Feel like starting slowly? A lot of people don't launch a full-scale program all at once. Rather, they test themselves, try out some simple exercises, stay with those on some kind of schedule for two to six weeks or longer, depending on how they take to their newly exercise-oriented lifestyle, and make sure they are enjoying the whole thing. Others integrate the simple exercises into full-scale programs from the beginning.

A simple preliminary program can introduce the neophyte to the world of exercise. A couple of simple rules will be useful. First, the exercise should feel good while you are doing it. The feeling should persist after the exercise is over.

Starting slowly ensures that the Great Resolution that has brought you to a total fitness program will not die a horrible death. If the road to perdition is paved with good intentions, the road to fitness is flooded with them.

## Five-Minute Routines

Five-minute routines can be devised that give a person a wide-awake start to the day or help fill in the waiting period just before Aunt Sally arrives for lunch; they can utilize the desk in the study as a prop, or be performed propless in a standing, sitting, or prone position. A four- or five- or six-minute routine can be performed in an odd moment during a busy workday— at home, at the office—wherever the time and privacy are available.

Five-minute routines may look like warm-up exercises, but they are simpler. They stretch muscles and tendons without preparing the body to spring into the high gear of strenuous activity. They bring major muscle groups into action, but in a relaxed way, thereby inducing a general feeling of relaxation. By calling on different parts of the body for gentle exertion, short routines may warm the body, but they should not work up a heavy sweat.

In brief, instituting a short, standardized routine lays the groundwork for the more formal exercise in a total fitness program that will follow. Once that program starts, five-minute routines can still be part of your day, testimony to the fact that exercise has indeed become part of your lifestyle.

## "Quick-time" Wake-up and Relaxer Routines

The "quick-time" routines are designed for use in the morning and evening. The morning set stretches the muscles that may have become cramped during sleep, placing major emphasis on the legs, hips, and balance. The evening set is intended to help the body to unwind gently and prepare for sleep.

### The Wake-up Routine

The morning routine awakens the body and readies it for the day's mental and physical challenges through seven separate exercises—or several of the seven, according to choice.

**1.** *Side stretch:* Lying flat on your back with arms stretched out above the head, slide the right knee up and at the same time extend the left arm as far as possible. The whole left side of the body should be stretched. Reverse, using the left knee and the right arm. Repeat eight to ten times with both sides.

**2.** *Heel haul:* Sitting up, stretch the legs out in front of the body. Leaning forward, grasp the heels, or the legs as close as possible to the heels, and pull the torso toward the knees. Bend the knees slightly if necessary. The back should be rounded, the toes pointed up and, if you are bending your knees, slightly to the side. Let go and sit up, straightening the spine, then repeat, grasping the heels and pulling forward again. Repeat eight to ten times.

**3.** *Knee bounce:* Sitting up straight, spread your legs and place the soles of the feet together. They need not fit flat against each other. Now gently bounce the knees toward the floor 16 times. Lower the torso over the still-joined feet, then straighten. Repeat five to ten times.

**4.** *Sky reach:* Sit on the floor with your feet apart as far as they will go. Reach for the sky with first the right arm, then the left. You should feel the pull on the muscles of the back and sides down to your hips. Repeat 16 times on each side.

**5.** *Forward reach:* In the seated, legs-spread position, slowly lower the chest toward the floor. At the same time place the hands on the floor directly in front of you and push them out ahead of the lowering upper body. Try to achieve a good stretch. In that position, bounce the torso very gently eight to ten times.

**6.** *Torso bend:* From the same beginning position on the floor, bend the torso gently to the right, at the same time reaching over the head with the left arm. The right arm moves toward the left knee. Gently straighten and bend eight to ten times. Reverse side and repeat.

**7.** *Knee tug:* Lying on your back with your toes pointing up, pull the left knee up toward the chest. Hold that position, gently tugging at the knee with both hands four times in a bouncing motion. Grasping your leg at the ankle or calf, pull it out straight so that your foot is over your head, keeping the other leg straight. Gently pull for eight counts. Next grasp the ankle of the upward-stretched leg and bend it gently out to the side. Hold for eight counts. Repeat with the other leg.

## The Relaxer Routine

The evening routine includes six exercises. You should maintain breathing at a regular, relaxed pace, and exhale through the mouth.

**1.** *Sky reach #2:* While sitting on a chair with the ankles crossed, stretch arms overhead. Reach first with one arm, repeating 16 times, then with the other for another 16 repetitions.

**2.** *Rollover:* Lying flat on your back with your arms at your sides, raise both legs straight up, pointing your toes. Bring the legs back over your head with your knees straight, then—if you can—press your toes to the floor and support your back with your hands. Hold until you have counted to 16. Collapse your legs around your ears and hold for another 16-count. Roll back to the supine position.

**3.** *Modified push-up:* Lie facedown on the floor, then place your hands on the floor and support your upper body on hands and knees. Keeping your back and elbows straight, tilt your chin up and your head back gently. Bend the knees and bounce the toes upward toward your head eight times.

**4.** *Slow knee pull:* While sitting on a chair, cross the right leg over the left and gently pull the right knee toward the chest. Hold for a 16-count. Reverse and repeat with the left leg.

**5.** *Leg extensor:* Lying on your back with your knees drawn up, bounce your right leg up toward your chest four times. Then extend the leg upward, grasping the ankle or calf, and bounce the leg toward your head eight times. Repeat with the left leg.

**6.** *Crouch-and-breathe:* Starting from a kneeling position, crouch down in a ball on the floor, right ear to the floor and knees drawn up under you. Breathe in deeply through your nose. Exhale slowly through your mouth. Repeat three times. Turn the head to the other side and repeat.

## Muscle Locators

If you find it difficult to come up with enough valuable exercises to fill a half-hour to 45 minutes three times a week, why not select some "muscle locators" for the central part (between warm-up and cool-down) of the session? In this section, we will offer two approaches to a set of basic exercises. You may wish to choose some favorites to program into your fitness schedule. By making the selection yourself, you ensure that the program's personalized character will be maintained.

Use caution when performing some of the muscle locators on the Phillips-Hatch list, particularly half sit-ups and squats.

Simplicity characterizes the 11 basic muscle locators. They are:

**1.** *Side bends:* Standing with your feet wide apart, knees slightly bent, lean first to the right, then to the left. Keep your hips as stationary as possible. Starting with ten bends to each side in the first week, increase the number as directed until you are doing 30 in the fifth week.

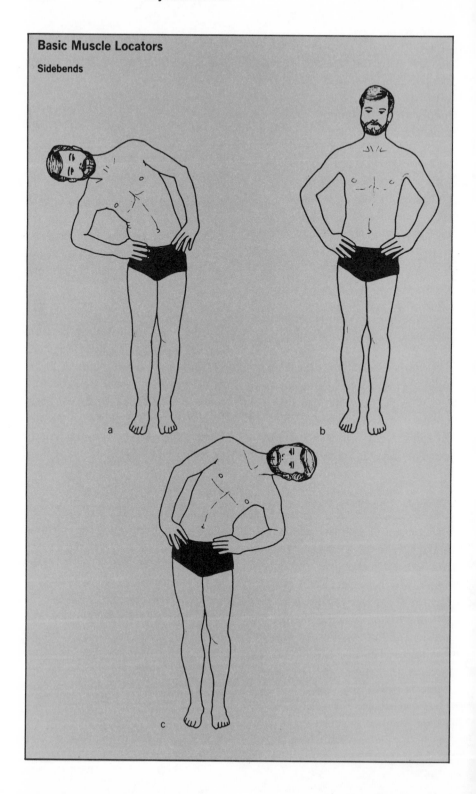

**Basic Muscle Locators**

Sidebends

## Basic Muscle Locators

**Good mornings**

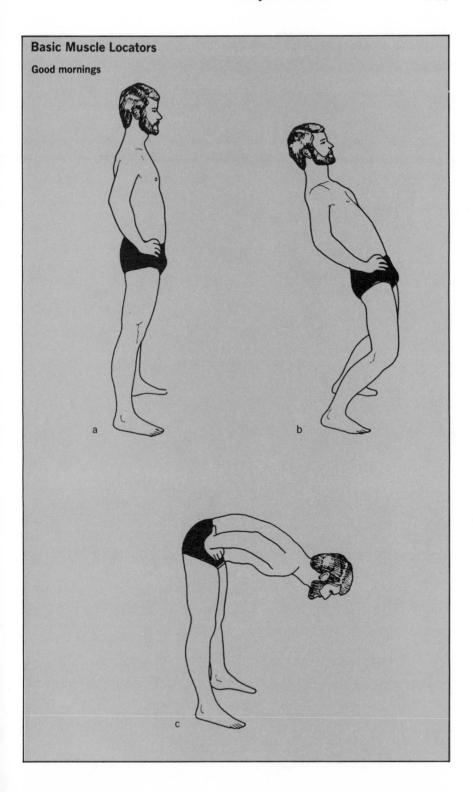

**Basic Muscle Locators**

Squats

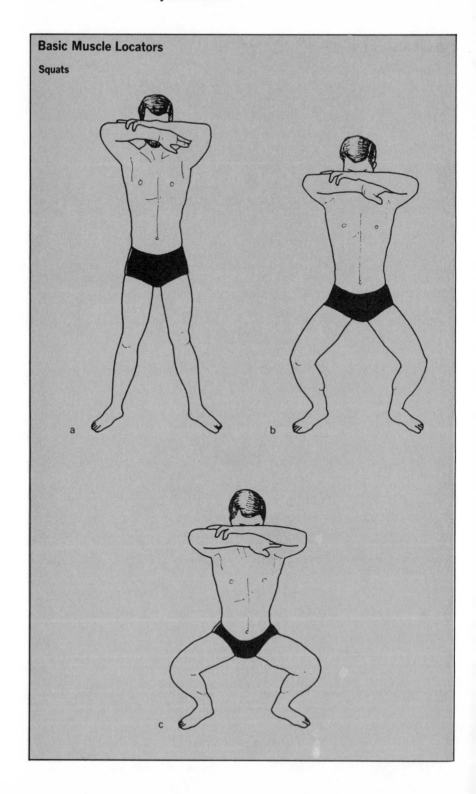

## Basic Muscle Locators

**Seated stretch**

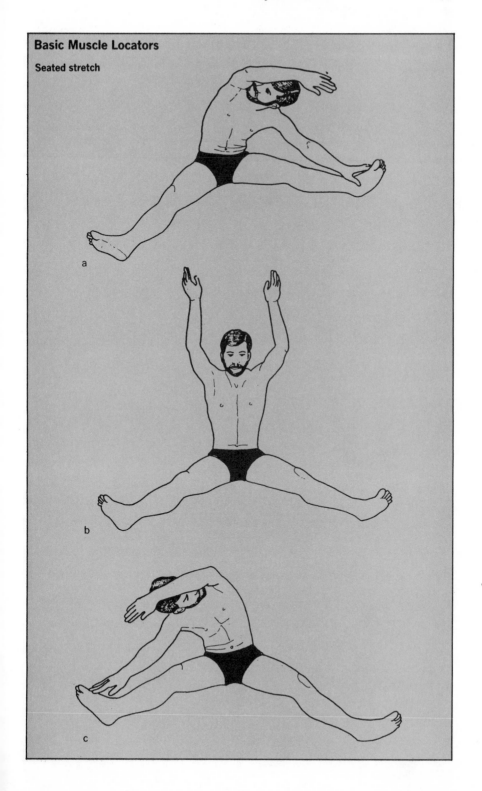

a

b

c

## Basic Muscle Locators

**Curl-ups**

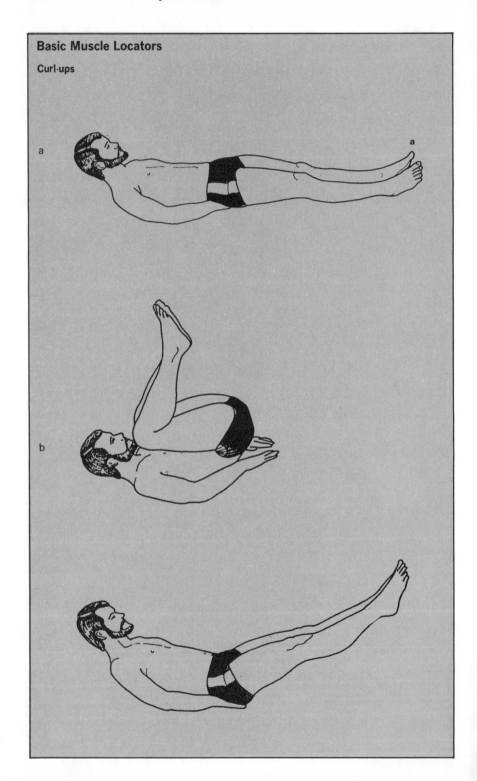

**Basic Muscle Locators**

Scissors

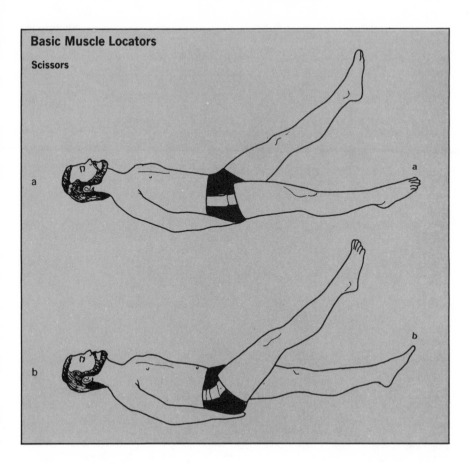

**2.** *Good mornings:* Starting again with feet wide apart, knees bent slightly, lean forward. Keep your hips as stationary as possible. Straighten up and then arch gently backward. Repeat as directed.

**3.** *Seated stretch:* Seated on the floor, spread your legs as far apart as possible. With your right hand on your left knee, try to touch your left toes with your left hand. At the same time, bring your nose close to your knee. In the first week repeat five times, then reverse for five on the right side.

**4.** *Feet raisers:* Lying on the floor with your hands under your buttocks,

palms down, lift your head off the floor. With your legs straight and toes pointed, lift your legs off the floor to an angle of about 45 degrees. Lower your legs.

**5.** *Curl-ups:* Lying on your back with your hands under your buttocks and head slightly raised off the floor, bring your knees up under your chin. Straighten your legs out until they are hovering at a 45-degree angle from your body. Lower your legs and repeat as directed.

**6.** *Scissors:* Again lying on your back, hold up your legs at an angle of 20 to 30 degrees from your body.

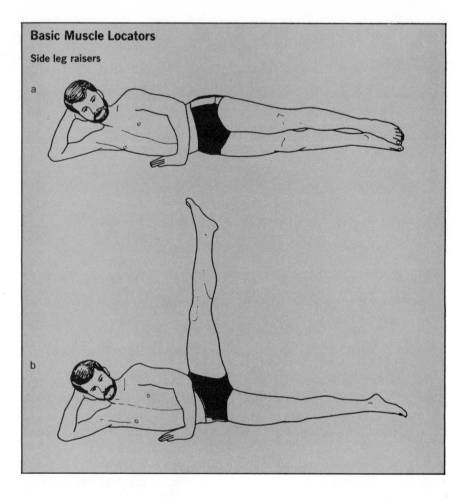

**Basic Muscle Locators**

Side leg raisers

a

b

Keep your hands under your bottom. Work your legs like a pair of scissors, crisscrossing them repeatedly.

**7.** *Half sit-ups:* The half sit-up is the same as the whole, but it is not completed. Lie on the floor, knees up, with your hands on your thighs, then sit up to an angle of 45 degrees. Try not to move your legs or hips. As you sit up, bring your head down toward your chest.

**8.** *Side leg raisers:* Lying on your side and balancing yourself by holding one hand on the floor, prop your head up on your other hand. Lift your top leg as high as possible for the specified number of times, then lie on your opposite side and lift the other leg the same number.

**9.** *Simple press-ups:* standing with your back straight and your bottom tucked in, lean forward, placing your hands on a table edge. Still keeping your back straight, lower yourself down to the table. If the "simple" press-up is too simple, try a regular push-up.

**10.** *Squats:* Standing with your

## Basic Muscle Locators

### Hip kicks

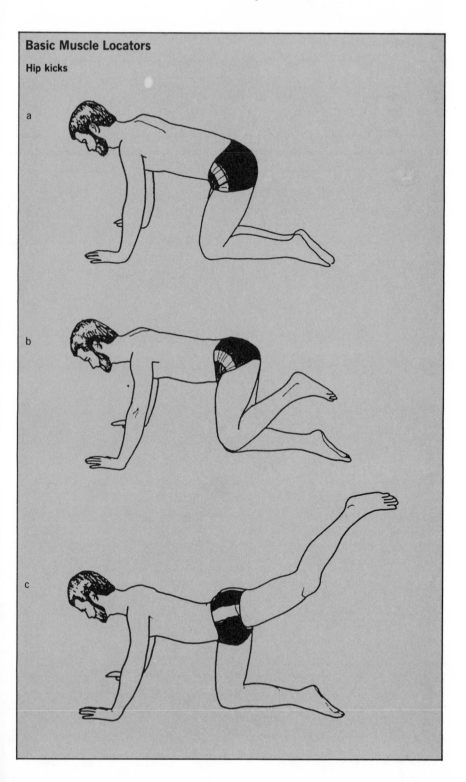

# Basic Muscle Locators

### Simple press-ups

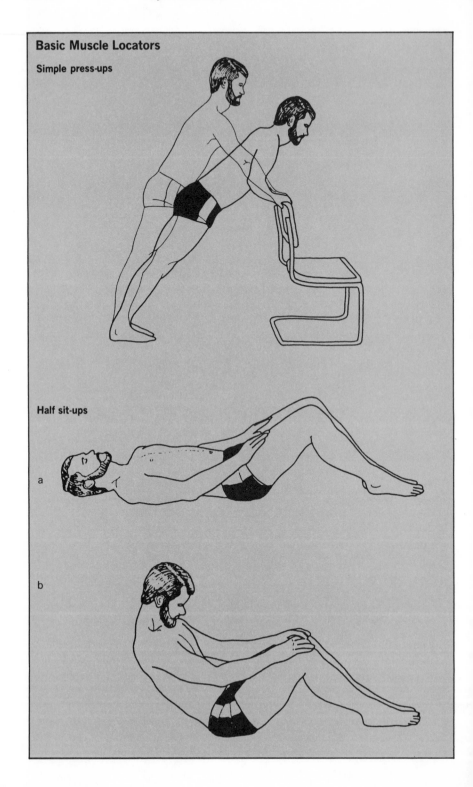

### Half sit-ups

a

b

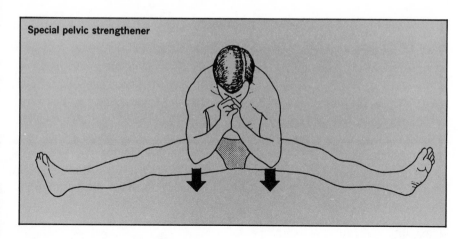

Special pelvic strengthener

feet 15 to 20 inches apart, and with a one- or two-inch block under each heel, bend your knees to a full squatting position. Keep your back as straight as possible at all times and hold your arms folded at shoulder level. Remember the caveat about deep knee bends that involve bringing

your buttocks all the way down to your heels.

**11.** *Hip kicks:* Kneeling on all fours, bring one knee forward off the floor and toward your face. Now push that leg straight back and upward as high as you can. Repeat with the other leg.

## Sitting, Towel, and Other Exercise Routines

As emphasized earlier, a basic exercise program can include a variety of supplementary movements and exercises that add zest. Additional exercises can also be practiced separately from regular exercise sessions and under the most informal of cir-

cumstances: when taking a shower, toweling off after the shower, sweeping the floor with a broom, and in other situations. Any of these can be programmed into the basic fitness schedule without difficulty.

### Sitting-down Exercises

With no more special equipment than a sturdy, dependable chair, you can do at least ten different exercises. For some of the exercises you will need a

chair with arms. Each of these movements contributes in its own way to your basic program.

## Cardiorespiratory Endurance Exercises

Two of the special chairborne exercises contribute to cardiorespiratory endurance.

**1.** Sitting in your chair, stretch your arms out straight in front at shoulder level. Holding your arms in that position, stand up. Do not use your arms. While standing, inhale deeply. Sit down, then exhale. Repeat the exercise 20 to 30 times at a moderate pace.

**2.** Sitting on the chair, breathe deeply, at the same time bending your knees and hugging them so that your feet leave the floor. Exhale, then let go of your knees, bringing your feet down to the floor and pushing your bent elbows back. Gently arch your spine while inhaling. Repeat 20 to 30 times.

## Flexibility and Balance Exercises

Six other exercises utilizing a chair contribute to flexibility and balance.

**1.** Sitting on the chair, inhale deeply and bend forward to touch the floor. Let your breath out as you bend. Straighten up. Bring one arm up and back and let the other swing down and back, gently stretching your shoulders and spine as you inhale. Repeat 15 to 20 times.

**2.** Start by kneeling sideways on the chair seat on your left knee, with the right hand holding the back of the chair and the left arm dangling down. Raise and extend your right leg and left arm, arch your back, and inhale. Exhale as you return to your original position. Repeat several times, then change position and do the same exercise while kneeling on the other knee.

**3.** Sitting in the chair, bend one knee and lift it toward your shoulder. Touch your raised foot with the opposite hand when your knee has come up to shoulder level. Repeat with the other leg and hand. Keep up a moderate pace while repeating 20 or more times for each side. Breathe regularly at a slow tempo. If possible, accelerate the pace as you go.

**4.** Standing behind a chair that has arms, bend your body forward. Place your hands on its arms, then with your midriff resting on the chairback, carefully raise and extend one leg, then the other. If possible, raise both and balance on the chair. With one or both legs in the air, arch your body gently. Lower your legs and repeat slowly, exhaling when bringing your legs up, inhaling when arching your body. Caution: make sure of your chair before starting. It should be well balanced and solid.

**5.** Sitting on the edge of the chair with your body straight and your arms hanging over the side of the chair, try to raise one leg slowly, keeping it straight, while at the same time trying to reach the upraised foot with the opposite hand. Alternate sides. Exhale when you touch; inhale while you change legs and hands.

**6.** Sitting deep in the chair and grasping the sides of the seat tightly, hold your legs together and swing them from side to side. Accelerate the tempo while continuing the swinging motion 20 to 30 times.

## Muscular Strength Exercises

Two final exercises with a chair help build muscular strength.

**1.** Sit straddling an armless chair, facing its back. Place both hands on the chair back and raise both knees while bending forward and exhaling. Slowly extend your legs out and slightly to the sides. Lean back cautiously and inhale. Repeat 10 to 30 times.

**2.** Sitting on the floor in front of the chair, raise your feet and place them on the chair seat. Try to reach up and touch your toes with your fingertips. As a somewhat more difficult alternative, sit in the chair with your hands on the chair arms. Bend and lift your knees, at the same time trying to lift yourself up with your arms. Exhale when you bend and inhale when you relax. Repeat 10 to 30 times.

## Towel Exercises

In six other exercises a towel can, in effect, be a portable gym. The towel serves as a means of providing resistance and also has a massaging effect.

**1.** To build cardiorespiratory endurance, hold a bath towel by the ends behind you and stretch it taut horizontally at hand level. Inhale deeply, then pull the towel ends forward, crossing your arms in front. Push your crossed arms so as to stretch the towel as far as possible. Exhale while pushing. Uncross your arms, go back to the starting position with your hands stretched out from your sides, and inhale. Repeat 15 to 30 times.

**2.** For flexibility and balance, while in a standing position hold the towel taut in front of you at waist level. Your hands should be held apart about the width of your shoulders. Try to pass one leg over the towel and then bring it back. Repeat with the other leg. Exhale when your knee is highest and inhale when your knee is down. Repeat 10 to 20 times with each leg.

**3.** For muscular strength, hold the towel taut behind your head. Bend one arm, then the other, as you maintain tension in the towel and slowly move it back and forth behind your neck. Inhale when both your arms are extended upward; exhale when one arm is down. Overload gradually by increasing the tension. Repeat 20 to 30 times.

**4.** Again for flexibility and balance, hold the towel stretched across the back of your neck. Take a deep breath and swing your right arm downward

**Towel Exercises**

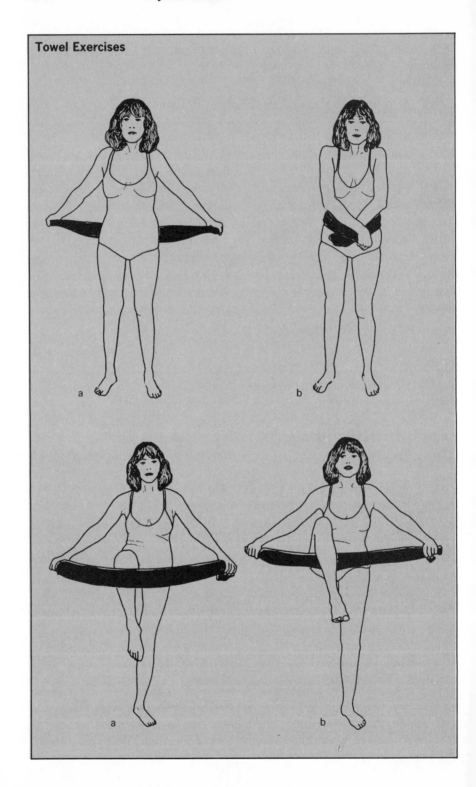

**Towel Exercises**

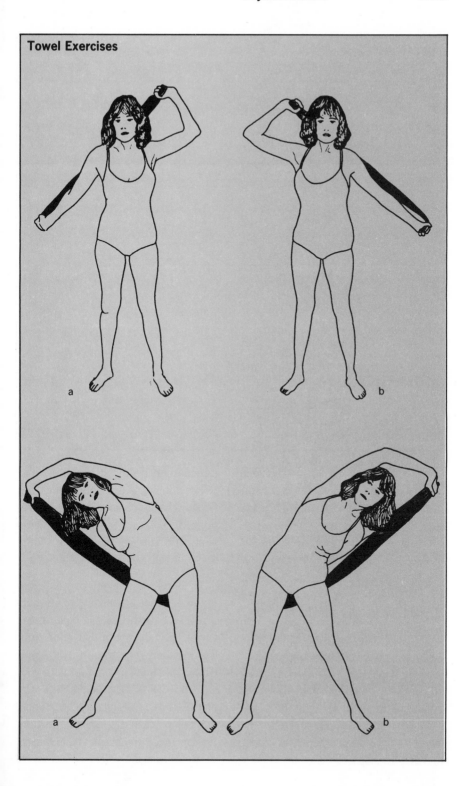

## Towel Exercises

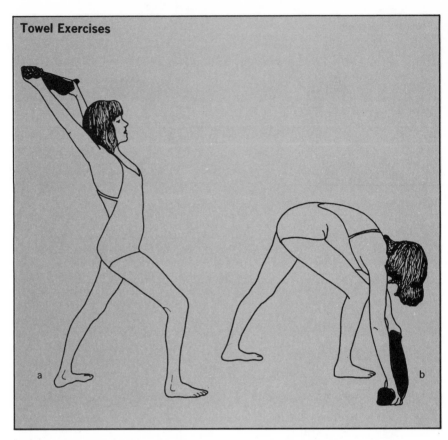

a                                                                    b

behind your back as you bring your left arm up and overhead as far as you can. Bend your body to the right. Exhale while bending over, inhale while straightening up. Repeat 10 to 30 times, then change arm positions and bend to the left, exhaling at the same time. Try to keep your arms as straight as possible at all times.

**5.** For flexibility and agility, assume a lunge position as you would in fencing. One leg should be set well ahead of the other and bent; the other should be straight. Holding the towel with your hands apart, stretch your arms up above your head and back, arching the body slightly. Bring your

arms forcefully down to the floor. The towel should, if possible, touch the floor. The exercise should be repeated 10 to 15 times at a steady pace. Exhale as your arms come down, inhale as they come up.

**6.** For flexibility and coordination, stand upright with your arms outstretched to the sides, holding the towel behind you. Raise your right leg, twisting your trunk to the right. Try to reach your right foot with your left hand while still holding both ends of the towel. Alternate legs. Inhale when you are in the straight position. Exhale at the end of the twist. Repeat 15 to 20 times.

## Shower Routines

Shower shape-ups have two advantages. First, they are simple. Second, they provide the mild movement that in the morning in particular can increase circulation and help the body to wake up.

The shower shape-ups can, of course, be done other places than in a shower. But if you perform them in the shower, be sure the surface on which you are standing and exercising is covered with a nonslip mat—for safety. If you do these exercises while the shower is running, breathe through the mouth, not the nose. Pretend you are swimming.

**1.** For cardiorespiratory endurance, take a deep breath while standing, then slowly bring your arms and shoulders forward. Cross your arms in front of you to squeeze your chest, exhaling at the same time. Slowly move your arms and shoulders back while inhaling. Repeat 10 to 20 or more times.

**2.** For flexibility, while in a standing position take a deep breath and slowly bend your body forward. Move your arms back and up as far as possible while exhaling. Straighten up slowly, inhaling, and repeat 10 to 20 or more times.

**3.** For flexibility and balance, again standing, place your hands on your hips and bend your right knee. Holding your right foot up, try to remain balanced on your left foot for ten seconds. See if you can retain your balance with your eyes closed. Do the same with the other foot. Breathe slowly and deeply. Repeat 10 to 20 or more times with each foot.

**4.** For muscular strength, stand in a slightly crouched position, hands on knees, and slowly bend your knees while keeping your head forward. Press gently on your knees with your hands. Breathe regularly. Exhale when your knees are bent and inhale when they are straight. Repeat 15 to 30 times.

**5.** For flexibility and agility, while standing bend up one arm after the other at the elbow, accelerating gradually. Breathe with every two to six motions of the arms. Repeat as desired.

**6.** For flexibility and coordination, place your left hand behind your neck, inhale deeply, then bend your left knee slowly. Raise your left foot off the floor slowly, bringing it as high as possible. Try to reach your toes with your right hand as you twist your body gently. Exhale as you straighten up. Change arms and do the exercise with the other leg. Repeat with each leg 10 to 30 times.

## The Broom Way

Like the chair and shower routines, the broom exercises are a simple set of movements intended as enjoyable adjuncts to a fitness program. The broom is the only required piece of equipment. But the broom wielder will need a rather large space in which to work out. Otherwise, he or she might find the broom banging on walls, furniture, pictures, and so on.

The half-dozen broom exercises are designed to increase cardiorespiratory endurance (No. 1), build flexibility and agility (Nos. 2, 3, 5, and 6), and develop muscular strength (No. 4).

**1.** Stand with your body bent forward, arms out to the sides, and hands holding the broomstick across the back of your shoulders. Slowly, without touching the broom handle to your head, bring the handle over your head and extend your arms all the way forward. Inhale while your arms are extended in front and exhale as they are bent.

**2.** In a sitting position, with your legs wide apart and arms outstretched to the sides, holding the broom across the back of your shoulders, twist your torso while continuing to hold the broom, trying to reach your right foot with your left hand and then your left foot with your right hand. Maintain a steady pace, exhaling when you reach down and inhaling when you straighten up. Repeat 15 to 20 or more times.

**3.** Again standing, with your arms forward and holding the broomstick horizontal with both hands in front of you, extend one leg behind you as far as it will go. Move that leg forward and up, raising it as high as you can

while maintaining your balance on the other foot. Repeat with the other leg. Inhale while you are bringing your raised leg down; exhale while raising it. Repeat 15 to 25 times.

**4.** In a standing position, with your legs wide apart, hold the broomstick vertically in front of you with both hands. The handle end should rest on the floor. Slowly bend one knee after the other, using the broomstick as support, so that the body shifts from side to side. While bending a knee, exhale. Inhale while straightening up. Repeat 15 to 30 times.

**5.** Standing with your legs wide apart, bend your body forward. The broomstick should be held across the back of your shoulders, hands on either end. Slowly twist your torso until the broom has gone from the horizontal position to a vertical. Accelerate gradually as you repeat the exercise on alternate sides. Breathe in rhythm and repeat 15 to 25 times.

**6.** Kneeling on your left knee, with your right leg extended behind you, hold the broomstick across the back of your shoulders with your outstretched arms. First turn your torso to the left, then slowly twist to the right. Move your right leg sideways and forward and try to reach your right foot with your left hand. Return to the original position and reverse the movement while kneeling on your right knee. Exhale when you are reaching toward your foot, inhale when your body is vertical. Repeat 15 to 25 times.

## Some Movements to Beware of

For varying reasons, controversy surrounds the use of some exercises. Whatever your program, you will want to cast a wary eye on these movements for the reasons indicated:

**1.** *Deep knee bends:* Particularly for the beginner, the deep knee bend, lowering the buttocks until they touch the heels, poses hazards. The deep knee bend stretches the knee's lateral

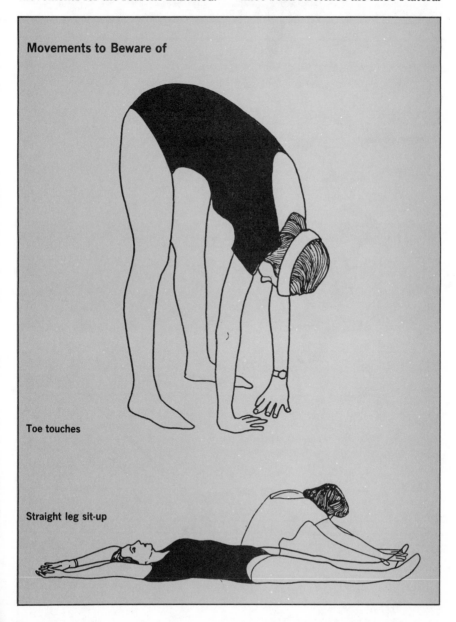

Movements to Beware of

Toe touches

Straight leg sit-up

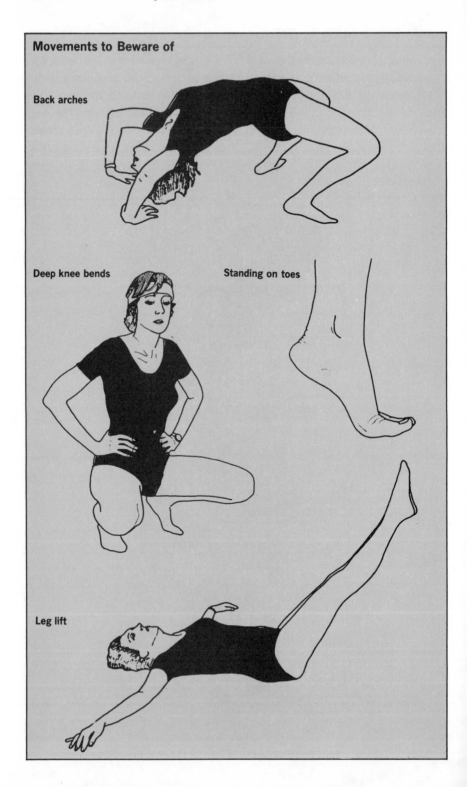

Movements to Beware of

Back arches

Deep knee bends

Standing on toes

Leg lift

ligaments. Stretched too far, the ligaments cease to protect the knee. If the ligaments become overextended, cartilage problems can result.

**2.** *Back arches:* The danger in back arches is that hyperextension may occur. Persons with difficulties such as weak abdominal muscles may find that their conditions become worse if they do this exercise. Physicians maintain that a fitness program should, in the beginning at least, stress abdominal exercises rather than low-back work.

**3.** *Leg lifts:* Performed while the exerciser is lying on his back, leg lifts have been found to help trim the waistline. But they can also lead to problems in persons with a tendency to the low-back ailment called lordosis. The reason is that leg lifts are accomplished through the use of the iliacus and psoas muscles, a set of muscles that can be easily strained when they are not in good condition.

**4.** *Standing on toes:* Recommended in many exercise programs, the repetitive toe stand allegedly strengthens the longitudinal arch. But in reality high toe stands may produce stresses that weaken the arch. Substitutes for high toe stands include heel cord stretches or walking on the heels.

**5.** *Straight-leg sit-ups:* The straight-leg sit-up also requires the use of the iliacus and psoas muscles. But in sitting up the exerciser can hyperextend and strain the back. The effort in sitting up with legs extended in effect tugs at the muscles along the spinal column. Low-back problems in particular can be aggravated.

**6.** *Toe touches:* Toe touching not only forces the knees to overextend; it also exerts heavy pressure on the lower spine. Since the exercise doesn't help to trim the waistline, as it has been alleged to do, toe touching both fails to provide the exercise value claimed for it and presents the risk of back problems.

## Low-Back Pain

Health authorities have estimated that nearly one in every six Americans suffers from low-back pain. Drugs and medications for the relief of such pain earn their manufacturers millions of dollars a year. But low-back pains may often be most effectively attacked with carefully planned and regularly pursued exercise routines.

The causes of low-back pains can vary. Tension can be to blame. A similar result occurs when the lower vertebrae have been compressed or crowded together. In other instances body positions of movements cause direct muscle or ligament strain.

Where such body mechanics have led to low-back pain, the fault usually lies with posture. If the pelvis slants downward, the lower back develops an abnormal curve and presses on the nerves of the spinal column. The pressure becomes so severe sometimes that the disks of cartilage that protect the nerves cannot do their job.

## Muscle Weakness and Tension

Some medical authorities hold that vertebral compression produces only about one-fifth of all the cases of low-back pain that afflict Americans. The other 80 per cent result from simple weakness of the muscles of the back, the abdomen, the hips (the psoas group), the hip extensors (gluteals), and the hamstrings.

Tension also plays a major role. The muscle groups that support and control the movements of the torso tighten up, often because they lack strength and flexibility. And lack of strength and flexibility results from inadequate exercise.

## Relief of Low-Back Syndrome

Is it any wonder that medications that promise to reduce low-back pain sell so well? The search for relief from such pain may occupy many of the waking hours of the sufferer—and cost a substantial amount of money. Yet the best way to relieve low-back syndrome is to avoid it. That means the individual must keep the important muscles involved in trunk support and movement strong and flexible. Such flexibility, once achieved, not only reduces the chances of low-back pain, but also provides the body with greater agility and mobility.

If low-back syndrome cannot be avoided in the first place, it can be relieved through exercise. Physical activities, sports, and games of nearly all kinds that involve movement of the body help eliminate muscle tension. The activities also provide a safe outlet for nervousness and tension which can, as noted, make their own contribution to low-back syndrome.

## The Exercises

Many movements, exercises, and activities that help the fitness beginner to rid himself of low-back pain can be included in a fitness program. They should generally be performed on a firm, flat surface. They require repetition, but the number of repetitions can often be a judgment matter. Each person should gauge his tolerance for such exercises by the ways in which his or her body reacts to them.

The exercises described below are particularly adapted to alleviating the specific conditions for which they are prescribed. But many others to be mentioned later will also help to improve these conditions, if less directly, while also serving one or more

# Good-bye Backache Exercises

## Alternate hamstring stretch

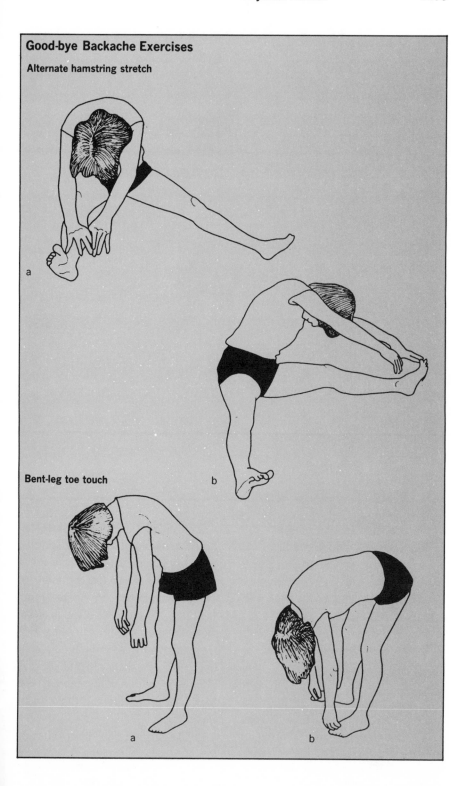

## Bent-leg toe touch

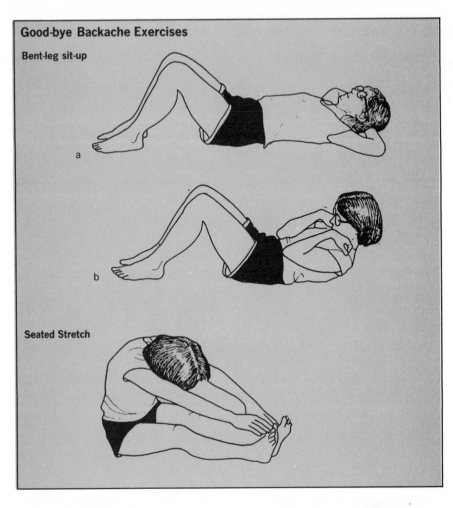

**Good-bye Backache Exercises**

**Bent-leg sit-up**

a

b

**Seated Stretch**

of the five basic fitness goals.

Like those in the preceding set, these exercises should be performed slowly and carefully. The subject should begin by lying on his back with his arms at his sides, palms facing down. The knees should be flexed, either by resting them on a pillow or by placing the feet flat on the ground. Breathe slowly and deeply at least five times, inhaling through the nose and exhaling through the mouth. Thus relaxed, you are ready to proceed with these exercises:

**1.** Contract your abdominal and gluteal muscles at the same time so as to bring your back flat against the floor. After holding that position for six seconds, relax. Repeat the process ten to 20 times. You can perform the same movements with your legs straight. You may want to try contracting the abdominals and gluteals from time to time during the day as a means of strengthening these muscles.

**2.** To stretch your back, starting from the same position and with your

# Good-bye Backache Exercises

## Alternate knee pull

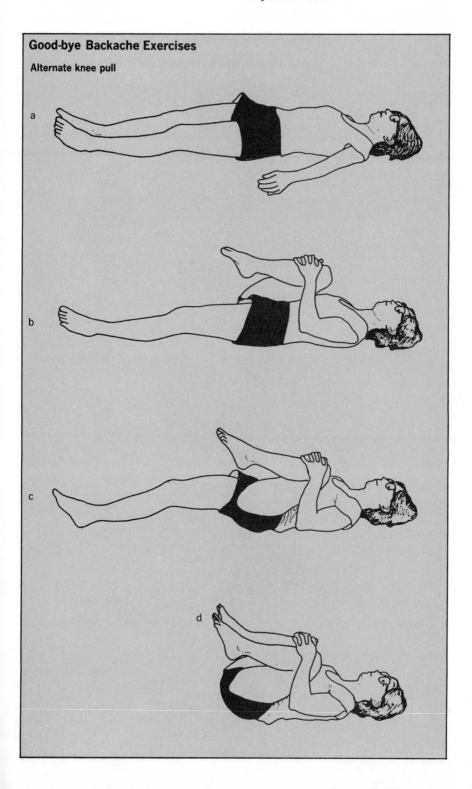

**Good-bye Backache Exercises**

Stand and stretch

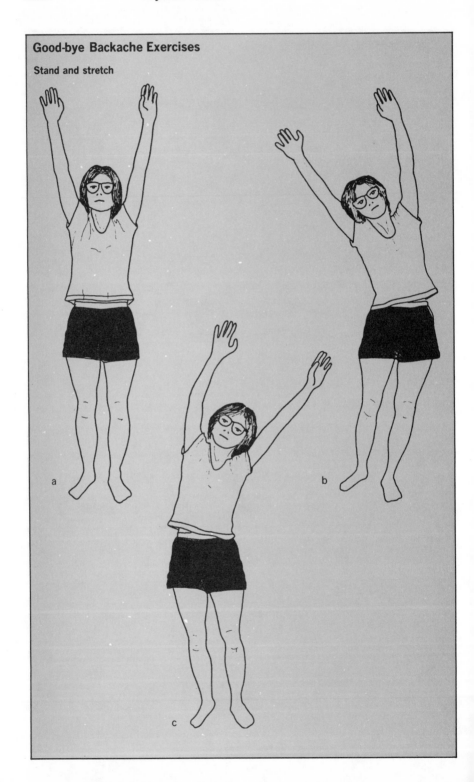

back flat against the floor as above, raise your head. At the same time bring both knees up as far as your chest while clasping your hands around your knees. Exert pulling pressure with your hands for six seconds, then relax and resume your original position. Repeat 10 to 20 times.

**3.** To strengthen the muscles of the hip joint start in the same position, with your arms at your sides. Your knees should be relaxed, your legs stretched out. Simultaneously contract your stomach muscles and flatten your back. Raising your head, bring one knee up to your chest. The other knee should remain relaxed.

Repeat 10 to 20 times, alternating legs.

**4.** Beginning on your hands and knees and keeping your head, neck, and back straight, raise one knee up and back as far as possible. Keep your upraised leg flexed and your back straight. Return to your starting position on hands and knees and repeat 10 to 20 times, alternating legs.

**5.** Stand with your feet together and your hands at your sides. To strengthen your low-back muscles and at the same time stretch your hamstrings, bend over slowly from the hips. Bring your arms back as far as possible. Return slowly to the starting position. Repeat 10 to 20 times.

## Supplementary Back-pain Relievers

Two other exercises help relieve the low-back pains that make life miserable for so many persons. Both exercises contribute to flexibility; both are simple and easy to master.

**1.** In the _head pull-back,_ drop your head until your chin touches your chest. Clasp your hands behind your head. Moving your head upward slowly and then backward as far as possible, keep pressure on the back of your head with your hands. In this isometric movement your head should go back as far as you can move it. Once back, count slowly to five while maintaining the hand pressure. Relax

and repeat half a dozen times. Rest for about five seconds between repetitions.

**2.** In the _monkey slump,_ stand with your feet spread apart and your knees slightly bent. With your hands on your knees, and while breathing in deeply, tense all your body muscles to a moderate degree. Then exhale slowly and let your hands slip from your knees. Your body should slump forward until your hands touch—or almost touch—the floor. Your chin should be level with your thighs. Maintain the slump for three to five seconds. Repeat half a dozen times.

## Yoga

An introduction to yoga can do little      more than sketch some of the main features of this Eastern system of body control and movement. An estimated 300 or more books of relatively recent vintage deal with the subject in greater or less detail. More than 60 authors have written on hatha (physical, or force) yoga alone.

The claims made for yoga cover a broad range. Where one exponent may proclaim yoga's reducing or weight-control merits, another may stress its capacity to restore youth and vitality. A third may emphasize that yoga relieves stress and tension as no other discipline can. A fourth may swear that yoga eliminates low-back pain, straightens shoulders, and cures a multitude of other disorders.

Unquestionably, yoga can do much for the faithful practitioner. But the question for the person seeking total fitness is simple: can yoga help me?

With some qualifications, the answer is Yes.

## Some Background

Yoga began in India some 5,000 years ago. It represents much more than a system of body control. Yoga promises the faithful student that he can, in time, achieve union with the source of all knowledge. The student will thus be awakened to the farthest reaches of his intellectual and spiritual potential.

Yoga means union. It has been described as one of the six main schools of Hindu philosophy. At least 16 systems of yoga have come into currency in Western countries. The 16 promote different paths to similar goals. But of them all, hatha yoga stands out as the form most concerned with revitalizing the body, improving physical health, and providing relaxation. Hatha yoga promises to do these things by teaching a variety of asanas, or postures. The student also learns breathing control. He achieves mental control as well by concentrating on the postures and on their effects.

A brief listing of some of the purposes of yogic postures suggest how broad is the possible range of objectives. Included are postures especially for weight control, sagging abdominal muscles, or back trouble, exercises for women, for relaxation, and for general self-help. Persons over 60 can benefit from specially adapted routines.

## Yoga Can Help

The logic of many asanas is readily apparent. They call, for example, for progressive flexing of the curving segments of the spine from the neck on down through the upper back, lower back, and spinal base. Flexing is accompanied by strengthening. Every joint and ligament undergoes the systematic stretching process. Pressure may also be applied to specific areas of the body to promote improved circulation of the blood. By degrees, the body becomes conditioned to increased demands.

While in various postures, the yoga student learns to practice deep breathing. Deep breathing, properly done from the diaphragm, can encourage relaxation. If it is correctly performed, both the stomach and the chest expand during inhalation and recede during exhalation. A session may close with a final extended relaxation period. Meditation makes it possible to replenish inner resources while absorbing the full benefit of the asanas.

The asanas promote correct deep breathing and thus provide a means of relaxing that can be important to a fitness program. For the fitness worker who wants to learn deep breathing as a road to relaxation, here are two multistep exercises derived from yoga.

## The First Breathing Exercise

**1.** While lying on your back, draw up your knees. Your feet should be placed slightly apart. Inhaling deeply, allow the stomach to relax, then expand. Exhale, at the same time pulling the stomach in so that the diaphragm rises to the point where it presses against the rib cage.

**2.** Continue to breathe diaphragmatically. First slowly fill the lower portions of the lungs, then try to fill the middle and upper parts.

**3.** Exhale. Try to picture the air slowly leaving the upper, then the lower, parts of the chest cavity.

**4.** Continue to breathe in this fashion. Breathe slowly and deeply. Let your breathing become very slow. Your body should relax completely.

## The Second Breathing Exercise

**1.** Start by sitting on a chair with your hands on your thighs and your elbows at your sides. Straighten your spine. Do not lean back against the back of your chair—or touch the back at all.

**2.** Breathe in and out rapidly through your nose. Repeat about 12 times, keeping a wood-sawing rhythm.

**3.** Exhale slowly through your nose until you have emptied your lungs.

**4.** Inhale to the count of seven. Pause for one second, then exhale. Pause again for a second. Repeat until you have completed seven breathing cycles.

## An Overall Assessment

Yoga has been found to be useful in a total fitness program, but it can effect only a limited range of improvements. While it cannot substantially benefit muscular endurance, it does build flexibility and grace. The postures and breathing exercises help to induce relaxation, and may in that process reduce high blood pressure. But evidence indicating that it helps to improve blood circulation is minimal. Yoga does not build muscular strength, but it can help to firm up specific muscle groups. It does not produce a smooth, taut skin despite claims to that effect. Finally, its value in weight control has been questioned. The beginner should take those factors into consideration when deciding whether to schedule yoga sessions into the basic fitness program.

## Calisthenics

Calisthenics have gone out of style to a degree because of the limited effect that they have on circulorespiratory fitness. But they still have many valuable uses. For example, many older people can take part in calisthenic exercises without danger.

Calisthenics have other advantages. They are easy to perform. They require little or no special equipment. They can be used in a fitness program to enhance circulorespiratory benefits. Contrary to the traditional approach, which calls for constantly starting and stopping activity, some calisthenics programs require continuous performance. In these programs the cardiorespiratory benefits can be considerable.

Calisthenics programs for individuals alone or for groups can include vigorous workout patterns that begin producing positive effects, such as increased strength or greater flexibility, in a very short time in nearly all the body's muscle groups. However, calisthenics programs have been found to be of limited value for "spot reducing." In fact, the spot-reducing concept has been attacked as deceptive. Different parts of the body that are burdened with excess fat can be strengthened through exercise: the protruding abdomen will benefit, for example, from sit-ups, V-seats, and curl-ups. But the benefit comes from stronger muscles. The stomach may also become flatter, but the exercise will not remove the fat.

To remove abdominal—or other—fat, the individual should probably choose some other program format, not calisthenics. These persons should, rather, take part in activities that require large-muscle motion, such as walking, swimming, cycling, and jogging.

### Adult Physical Fitness

The Adult Physical Fitness program developed by the President's Council on Physical Fitness is generally acknowledged to be very good. Essentially a calisthenics program, it includes a jog-walk sequence that is

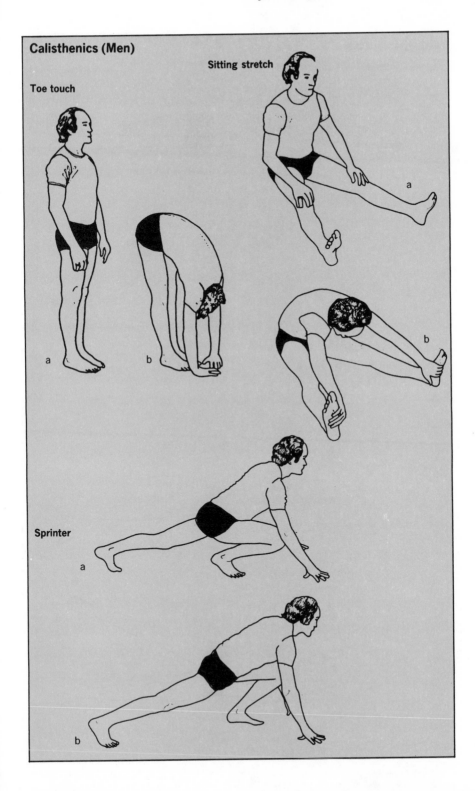

### Calisthenics (Men)

**Toe touch**

**Sitting stretch**

**Sprinter**

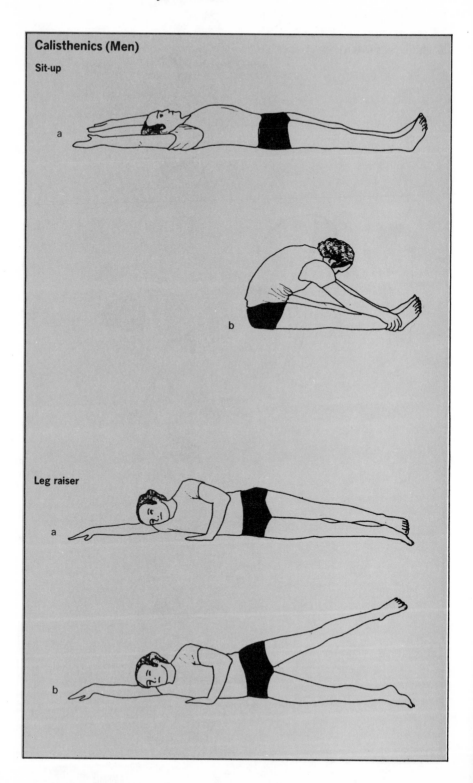

**Calisthenics (Men)**

Sit-up

a

b

Leg raiser

a

b

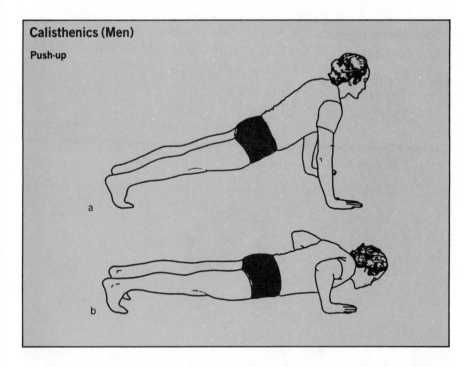

**Calisthenics (Men)**

**Push-up**

a

b

vital to the program's effectiveness. If that sequence is omitted the program fails to measure up to the standards set for basic fitness programs that seek to produce the five basic body improvements.

The program contains separate exercise regimens for men and women. The exercises are basically sound, and participants are led through progressively more difficult levels of activity. In all, five levels are included following an orientation program that introduces the regimen to the beginner. Exercises are described and illustrated for clarity, and charts are provided for those who want to keep records.

## Calisthenics Programs

Calisthenics programs, like most others, fall into discernible patterns. They stress different types of exercise depending on how they were originally conceptualized and drawn up. They can be completely adequate as individualized fitness programs for home use if the exerciser pays attention to certain basics.

Before adapting a calisthenics program to his or her own needs, the individual should make sure that the program has the following characteristics:

The program should include exercises that develop circulorespiratory fitness. These can be added to the basic calisthenics program if they are not integral parts of it from the beginning. For example, a walking or walk-

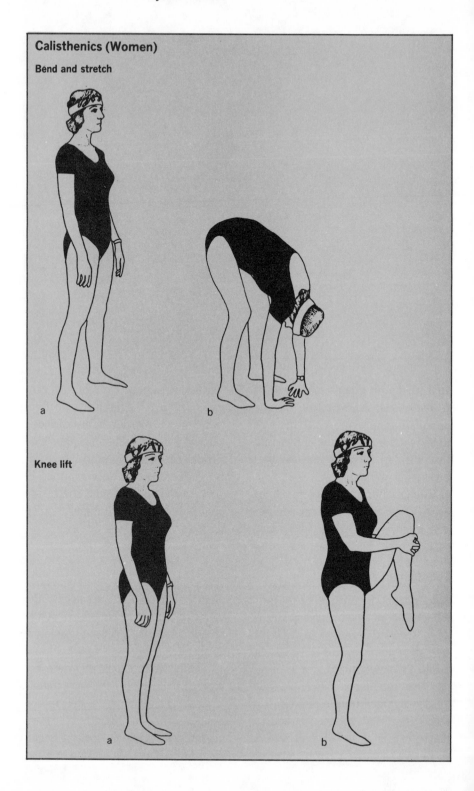

**Calisthenics (Women)**

**Bend and stretch**

a

b

**Knee lift**

a

b

# Calisthenics (Women)

**Wing stretcher**

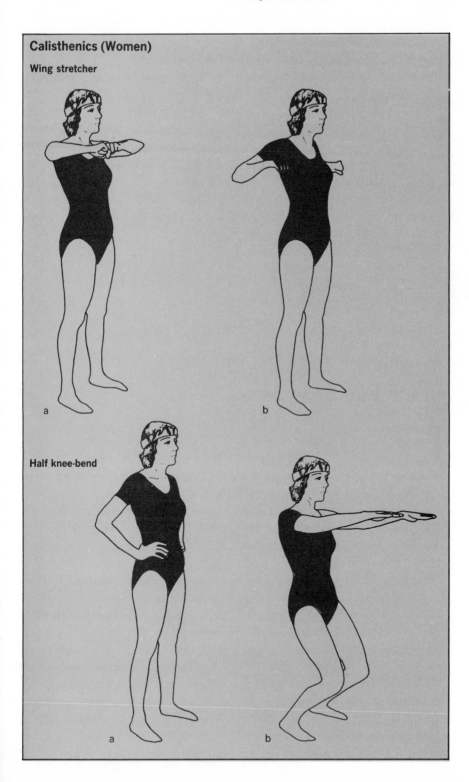

a       b

**Half knee-bend**

a       b

jog section can be added to the basic program. Running in place between calisthenics routines is sometimes a desirable approach.

The program should include exercises that provide work for all the body's major muscle systems.

The program should allow for challenging rates of progression for the out-of-shape beginner as well as the person in very good condition. Progress in the areas of muscular strength and endurance and cardi-orespiratory efficiency are particularly important.

Each session should include a warm-up and a cool-down.

As with other fitness programs, the calisthenics program should include at least three sessions weekly, and each session should last at least 30 minutes.

Questionable exercises should be approached with caution or eliminated.

# Other Fun Exercises

In a period of weeks after starting a fitness program—usually 12 to 24—the dedicated person will probably be ready to branch out into a wide variety of more strenuous activities. More diverse types of exercises are likely to seem attractive. A good fitness program should be preparing the beginner for locomotor sports—those that require the whole body to be in motion—and for brachiation activities, which require movement of the upper body, mainly the arms.

The program, after all, has the goal of maximizing body peformance in all areas of life. In branching out, consideration should be given to those activities that provide enjoyment and at the same time meet physical, social, recreational, and other needs. The activities should not be purely seasonal or participation will be part-time. It may be necessary to mix types of activities so as to ensure year-round participation.

Special training programs in calisthenics may provide the answer, as may a daily walking hour, or dancing. Other people may want to keep it simple—and turn to ancillary exercises that can be performed alone. Still others might opt for yoga or some advanced strength builder exercises. There are several factors to bear in mind as you plan the best way to expand your fitness horizons:

# Model Exercise Circuit Chart

### Station 1: Neck

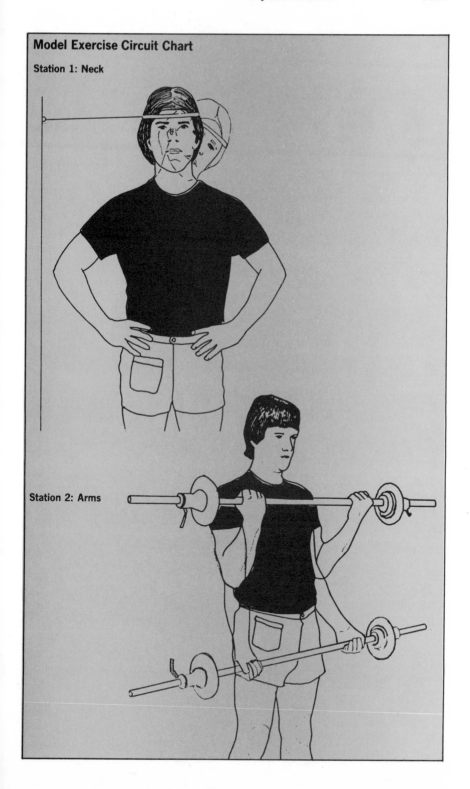

### Station 2: Arms

## Model Exercise Circuit Chart

Station 3: Hands

Station 4: Shoulders

Station 5: Abdomen

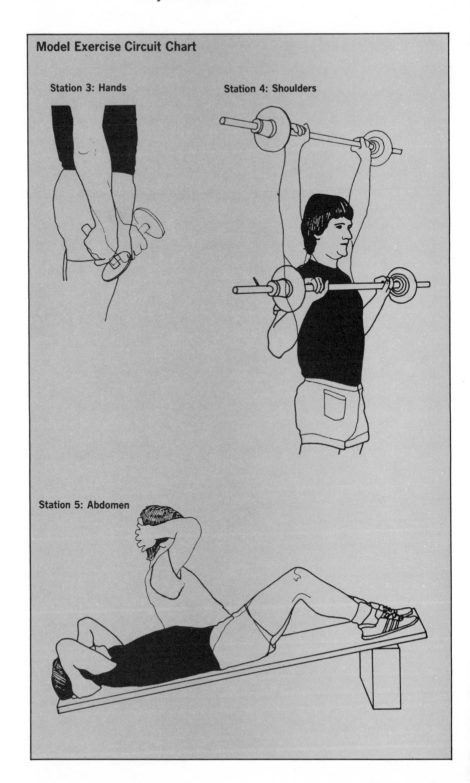

# Model Exercise Circuit Chart

**Station 6: Back**

**Station 7: Chest**

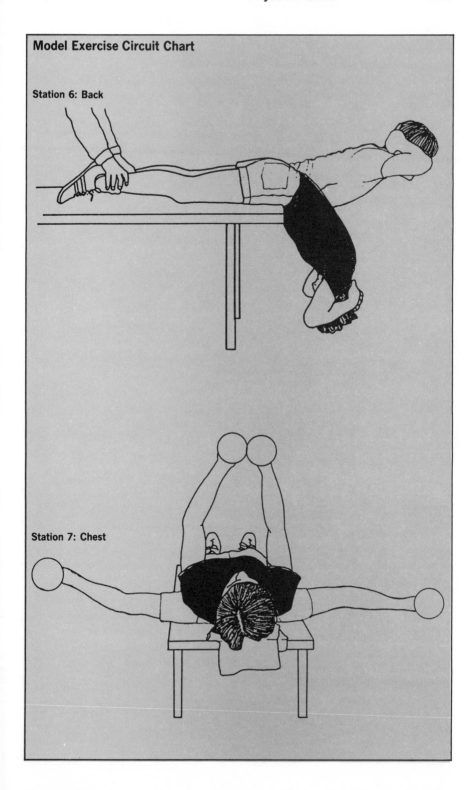

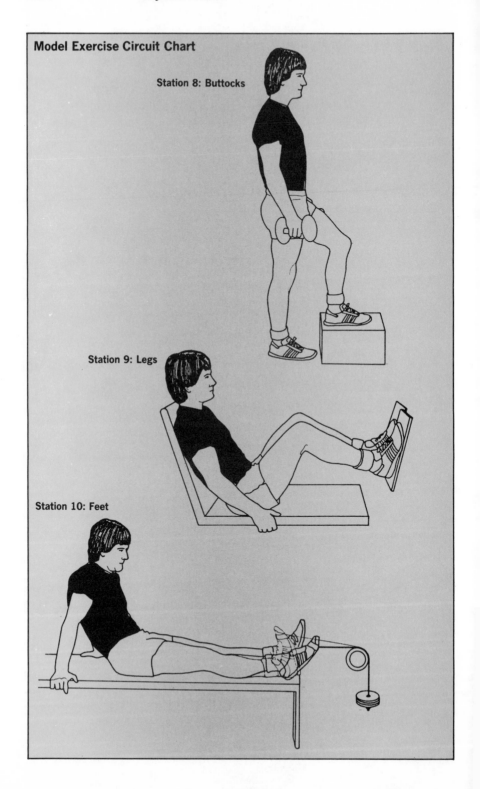

**Model Exercise Circuit Chart**

Station 8: Buttocks

Station 9: Legs

Station 10: Feet

# Group One: Muscle Builders

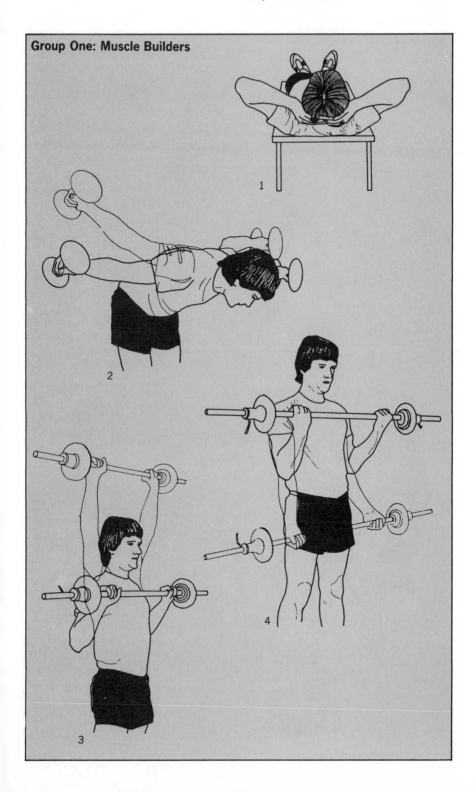

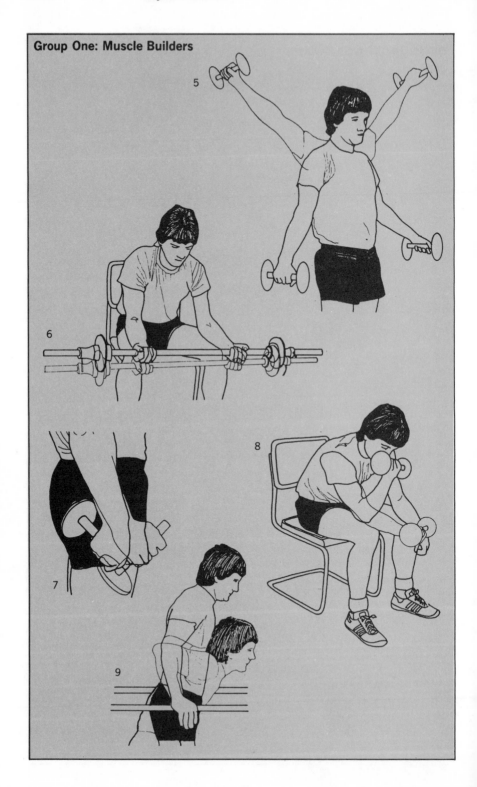

**Group One: Muscle Builders**

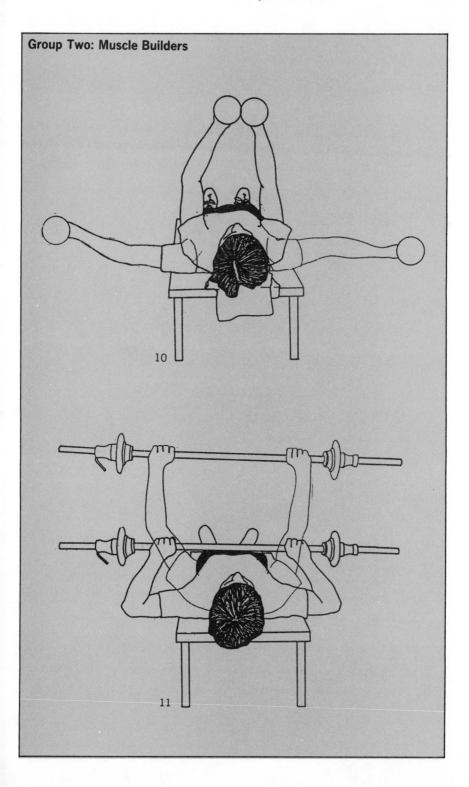

**Group Two: Muscle Builders**

10

11

**Group Two: Muscle Builders**

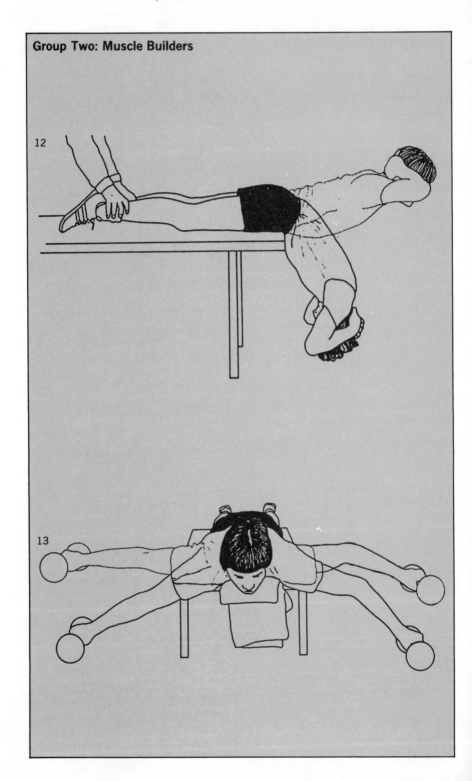

**Group Two: Muscle Builders**

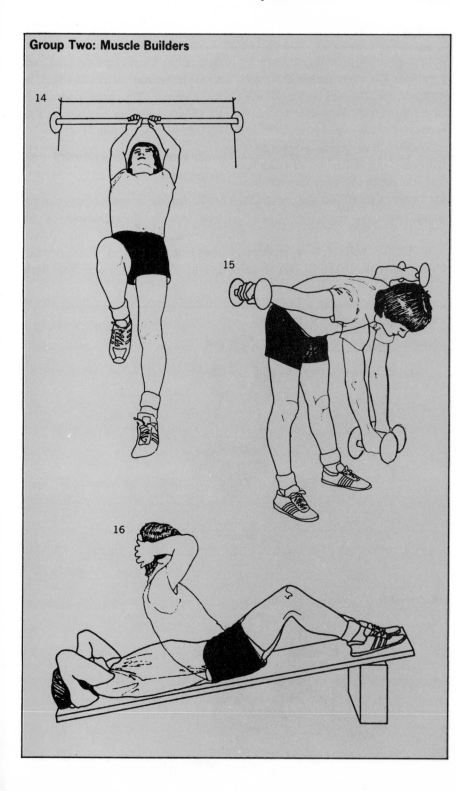

## Walking

Americans love to walk, fitness experts say. But many people don't get the most from the walking they do because they don't approach it as exercise.

Walking does qualify as exercise, however—one of the best. To ensure that you get the benefits that walking can bring, a seven-part procedure is suggested.

**1.** Picture walking as a separate fitness activity. Learn to take your own pulse. Then calculate what your target pulse rate per minute should be for your age. That usually means 70 to 85 percent of your maximum rate (220 minus your age in years).

**2.** Buy a pair of comfortable running shoes.

**3.** Design a starter program for your own use. Promise yourself, for example, that you will walk 20 minutes four days a week. Raise that target to 25 minutes a day, four days,

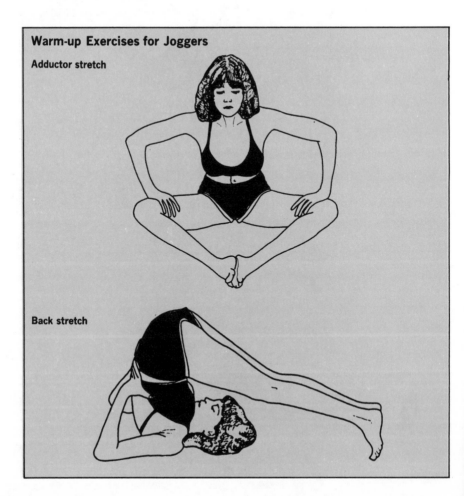

**Warm-up Exercises for Joggers**

Adductor stretch

Back stretch

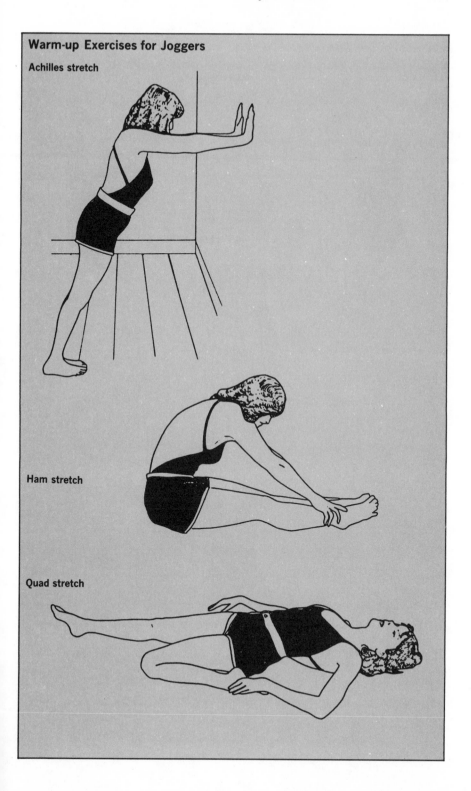

**Warm-up Exercises for Joggers**

Achilles stretch

Ham stretch

Quad stretch

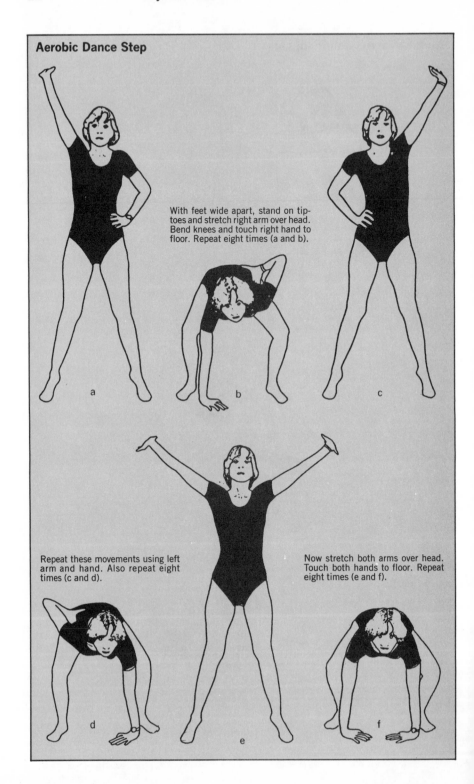

**Aerobic Dance Step**

With feet wide apart, stand on tiptoes and stretch right arm over head. Bend knees and touch right hand to floor. Repeat eight times (a and b).

a

b

c

Repeat these movements using left arm and hand. Also repeat eight times (c and d).

Now stretch both arms over head. Touch both hands to floor. Repeat eight times (e and f).

d

e

f

and then increase the level by increments of five minutes. A good final target might be 45 minutes four days a week.

**4.** Take your own pulse every day and keep a record of your findings. Watch your pulse rate decline as your body becomes more efficient.

**5.** In walking, breathe rhythmically. Let your arms swing by your sides.

**6.** Use your walk as recreation even though you've planned it as a kind of independent fitness program. As you walk, notice colors, trees, buildings, people. Try not to think of work.

**7.** Schedule mini-walks in the mid-afternoon, when your body may be starting to drag. Walk, if possible, instead of taking the usual coffee break. You should obtain a fresh charge of energy and a clearer head.

Everybody walks, it seems. Why regard walking as exercise, then? Because walking can do almost as much for individual fitness as jogging.

There are other reasons for making walking a part of a fitness program, or for walking at every opportunity apart from the program. Walking burns up calories. Walking does not strain joints and muscles as some other exercises do. Walking can be enjoyable, as dedicated walkers have testified down through history.

Conceivably, the typical modern American could go through an entire day without taking more than 15, 20, or 50 long strides. To do so, it would only be necessary to utilize the elevators, autos, escalators, and other devices that make walking unnecessary. But for those who consider walking both fun and a learnable art, walking as exercise puts those devices into the shade.

Let's consider some of the types of walking that the individual can incorporate into his or her life.

## Speedwalking

A technique of walking as fast as possible while swinging the arms back and forth, speedwalking or racewalking is rapidly gaining in popularity. The arms are used to provide rhythm and momentum. The elbows remain bent at 90-degree angles. The speedwalker, like other walkers, needs only comfortable exercise clothes and shoes. Many speedwalkers wear runners' shoes.

Speedwalking burns up 620 to 870 calories an hour. As an exercise, it puts every muscle to work in an aerobic and circulorespiratory way. The exaggerated hip movements help firm up buttocks, thighs, and hips. The beginner should aim for three half-hour speedwalking tours a week, over that period maintaining a rate of three or four miles per hour. Leg-stretching warm-ups before starting and cool-downs at the end of the walk will help in the same ways as warm-ups and cool-downs before and after other exercise sessions.

As the speedwalker progresses, he or she can step up the walking pace to five or more miles per hour. If possible, keep records of the date, the distance walked, and the time consumed.

## Interval Walking

Other approaches to walking are less strenuous, but they offer many of the advantages of speedwalking if performed regularly. Interval walking, for example, involves walking briskly for 30 seconds, then slowly for 30 more seconds. That process is continued until the walker is reasonably tired. Ideally, again, records are kept in interval and other approaches to walking.

## Continuous Walking

In continuous walking the exerciser sets himself an objective and walks until he achieves it. The first time out, wisdom dictates an easy pace. On subsequent walks, perhaps every two or three days, the pace is stepped up.

## Tempo Walking

In the walking format known as tempo walking, the walker moves easily for five minutes. Then he walks at top speed for one minute. The relaxed-then-rapid repetitions are continued over a set distance. Every few workouts, the rapid phase of the tempo walk should be lengthened by five seconds. The cool-down is accomplished by walking easily for five final minutes.

## Long-Stride Walk

A variation on tempo, continuous, and interval walking, the long-stride walk involves what the name indicates: a period of long-stride walking that is inserted into the basic continuous, interval, or tempo walk. Walking with the longest possible strides helps in particular to condition the hips and buttocks. As a variation on the variation, the walker can insert into his walk periods of walking with short strides while the body inclines well forward.

## Hill Walking

After a warm-up of five minutes of easy walking in a flat area, the hill walker sets off to mount a low hill. For best body conditioning, the uphill pace is rapid, the downhill pace moderate. Hill walking calls for discretion; the walker should not attempt too much too soon—as in every other area of fitness conditioning. Steep hills may have to be avoided at first.

## Stationary Walking

Walking in place, or stationary walking, involves little more than simulated walking in which the exerciser lifts his knees as high as possible. Starting at an easy pace, he gradually "walks" faster. Stationary walking can be done according to the continuous, interval, or tempo methods.

## Variety Walking

Excepting the speedwalk, the several approaches to walking can be combined and recombined to taste. One approach can be used one day, another approach the next. In this way, the exerciser injects variety into the walking phase of his fitness program.

# Hopping, Jumping, and Stepping

Various hopping, jumping, and stepping activities can add spice and enjoyment to the fitness program and can prepare the individual for sports and games involving similar movements. All three exercises should be approached with the same respect that is paid to other parts of the fitness program. That means heart rates should be monitored as necessary, the exercises should become regular features of the fitness program, and, if possible, records of performance should be kept.

## Jumping

In the jump, or side-to-side jump, the legs remain relatively straight and are flexed only slightly while the body is in the air.

A small object may be placed on the floor to serve as a guide in side-to-side jumping. A stripe on the floor or carpeting will accomplish the same purpose. Make sure that you clear the stripe or object in a lateral direction. In jumping again, clear it in the other direction. You should maintain a continuous side-to-side motion, with both feet leaving the floor and touching down again at the same time. Jumping, like hopping, should be continued for a minute or more.

## Hopping

If done properly, the kangaroo hop, or plain hop, can build agility as well as circulorespiratory capacity. To hop, place both feet together, bend over with hands reaching backward, crouch slightly, and jump upward. Your knees should be brought up toward your chest while your body is in the air.

Hopping should be continued for one minute or more. Persons in good physical condition, can, of course, continue the exercise for longer periods. It then becomes a genuine aerobic activity.

## Stepping

An exercise routine including hopping and jumping may also include the step exercise. The step involves stepping up onto a bench or other raised, firm object in repetitive movements that are continued for a minute or more.

The jump, hop, and step have been combined in a training circuit that was specifically designed as preparation for participating in high-movement sports. The circuit includes six stations or stages covering up to six minutes each:

1. Side-to-side jumping

2. Quad sitting, in which the seated exerciser tightens his quadriceps or front thigh muscles for 40 to 50 seconds

3. The kangaroo hop

4. Heel and toe raises, in which the exerciser stands with feet apart, rises on his toes, returns to the floor, turns his toes outward, straight ahead, and inward, then rolls back on his heels

5. The bench step

6. Half squats

# Exercise for the Heart Patient, for Postop Patients, and for the Hospitalized

Exercise has been portrayed as a means by which the healthy person can build more health, strength, and fitness. The weight of medical opinion today holds that exercise can and should have an important place in the life of the sick, disabled, or seriously handicapped person.

In each individual case the exercise has not only to be approved and recommended by a physician; the exercises or sports should also be specifically designed to correct problems or help the person regain physical health. At the least, exercises should make it possible for the ailing person to maintain some level of fitness.

Each exercise should be geared to fulfilling a particular purpose. Following breast surgery, a doctor may prescribe arm and shoulder exercises designed to restore strength in the woman's upper body. Following a coronary attack, a graduated program of walking or swimming may be prescribed. Before a heart attack, a person showing signs of severe tension may be told that he should engage in any of dozens of kinds of relaxing activities. These can range from yoga to golf to simple stretching exercises. Or they can include many other activities discussed in this chapter. In each instance, the exercises are chosen with the patient's problems and condition in mind.

## After the Heart Attack

Through regular exercise the heart attack victim earns a second chance in life. But he faces a difficult challenge. He has to devote constant effort to his exercise regimen. If he backslides, or drops out of the program, he usually finds that deterioration sets in within days or weeks.

The training program that the heart attack victim undertakes should be geared to his personal physical situation. He should start it only with the approval of his physician, and should progress at the prescribed rate. In most cases the post-heart attack exerciser will be asked to keep track of his rate of progression. In all cases he will be asked to see his physician at prescribed intervals.

Postcoronary exercise has, like all exercise, specific goals. It can be very effective in increasing cardiac efficiency by decreasing the heart rate and the consumption of oxygen at a given workload. The training, taken initially in small doses, makes it possible for the muscles to extract more oxygen from the blood. The heart can then pump less blood for a given task. In time, the heart becomes less susceptible to the ill effects of stress hormones, or catecholamines, that circulate in the blood. The patient usually learns to respond better to stress-filled situations. He can control his weight more easily.

With improved physical condition may come other benefits. The patient may experience little or none of the depression that is so common following a heart attack. Chest pains may dwindle or disappear entirely. Many patients experience relief from angina—a cramp-like chest pain—as their fitness levels improve.

### Problems and Preparations

The postcoronary exercise regimen calls for advance consideration of a number of problems. A practical problem is that the patient may find that the program cuts into his work, family, and social life. If he lives in a large city, he may have difficulty commuting to and from the clinic, YMCA, or other institution offering the program.

In consultation with his physician, the patient can in most cases develop an exercise program that eliminates many such problems. In so doing, he increases the likelihood that he can continue to exercise consistently. Typically, he reduces the number of medically supervised sessions to a minimal weekly number compatible with training effectiveness and safety. The "minimal number" may be once or twice weekly. Some physicians give their patients specific instructions and then trust the individual to continue on his own.

Authorities believe that a heart attack victim's assumption of responsibility for all or part of his own fitness program teaches the patient to cope with the stresses, strains, and difficulties that he inevitably faces as he moves toward complete rehabilitation. Also, he grows accustomed to normal living more quickly. In a sense, he becomes by degrees independent of physician, clinic, or other medical advisor without neglecting basic precautions or the prescribed periodic checkups.

A stress test should precede the start of the fitness program. The patient can determine his own sustained maximum heart rate by subtracting his age from the figure 220. Thus a man of 40 would have a maximum sus-

tained rate of 180.

In later stress retesting, usually carried out at four to eight week intervals, the patient may be asked to exercise until his heart rate approaches the maximum. Initially, in each of the four to six exercise sessions each week, he works his heart for half an hour at a rate equal to about 70 or 75 percent of the maximum. The man of 40, mentioned earlier, is thus able to bring his exercising heart rate to about 126.

In a second phase, again undertaken with his physician's approval, the patient may be allowed to bring his exercising heart rate as high as 85 per cent of the maximum. A third and even a fourth phase might follow if necessary.

The stress test may be administered with a bicycle ergometer or a treadmill. During the test, the electrocardiogram is monitored continuously. Breath analyses may be taken as a means of estimating the patient's actual maximum oxygen consumption. Afterward, depending on the program, the patient may be placed in a "complicated" or "uncomplicated" category. In the uncomplicated group are those who have worked their hearts to 70 to 75 percent of the maximum heart rate without developing abnormalities in the electrocardiogram. In the complicated group are those who cannot finish the tests because evidence of cardiac ischemia, or lack of oxygen for the heart muscle, has appeared.

As a final preparatory step, the patient may receive a personal exercise prescription. After later stress tests, he learns, he will receive new prescriptions as he progresses. He may, if needed, receive instructions in the methods of taking a pulse count.

### Exercises of Choice

Recommended exercises of postcoronary patients include walking, jogging, swimming, and others. But the exercises cannot be taken randomly. The patient should walk or jog a specific distance, or swim a specified number of laps, while timing himself with a stopwatch. He will probably be told that he cannot use a regular watch in timing his sessions because such a method of measurement lacks accuracy.

A typical clinic session for a postcoronary group might start with a talk or discussion. Patients learn that they can discuss problems relating to their physical situation or their home exercise prescriptions. They also find out about the "do's" and "don't's" that apply to them, about medications and their uses, and about the meanings of various cardiac signs. Sexual problems may come up for discussion; so may fad diets and the values of "cures" for heart disease that have been reported in the media.

The beginner's session may continue with a 10- to 20-minute warm-up. While music provides a rhythmic accompaniment, the patient may go through simple flexibility exercises interspersed with light walking and jogging. In a class session, the group may halt all activity at specified intervals to take a pulse count. If any individual indicates that he is having chest pains or other problems, he may be asked to stop and undergo a further medical assessment, including electrocardiograms. Instruction for all participants will usually cover proper jogging techniques. Following the warm-up, participants go into their prescribed exercise series. They conclude with a cool-down period lasting 10 to 15 minutes.

As postcoronary exercise sessions continue, the patient may be asked to keep a detailed log. Entries cover current prescriptions, the time and distance data on each workout, and pre- and postworkout heart rates. Periodically—usually once a month—the patient takes his resting heart rate, preferably before he gets out of bed in the morning. He may be asked to ascertain the average of three consecutive morning heart counts. In all cases, the distance, speeds, and heart rates are carefully charted for each patient.

Using such information, a physician can easily gauge a patient's progress. In most cases a patient will show improvement within weeks. But doctors believe that an exercise regimen should be continued for at least a year if substantial benefits are to be achieved. Two years may be necessary in many cases.

# When Not to Exercise

Many heart attack patients cannot wait to get started on an exercise program. They may not understand that when a physician advises against exercise of any kind, or prescribes very light exercise at the beginning of a program, he usually has reasons that relate to the condition of the patient's heart.

In myocardial infarction, for instance, a scar forms on the heart. The scar may take as long as six weeks to heal. Exercise taken before the healing process has been completed may cause the heart wall to bulge, forming an aneurysm. The bulging can occur with each heartbeat and can lead to additional serious heart problems.

If a patient has experienced an acute myocardial infarction, a relatively rare occurrence, either the right or the left sides of the heart may be seriously affected. Exercise may not become permissible until complete recovery of pump efficiency has taken place. The period may last for two or three months or more.

An aneurysm in one of the large blood vessels, such as the aorta, may preclude vigorous training for a period of weeks or months.

A patient who senses rapidly progressing anginal pain while exercising may be receiving warnings of another heart attack. Normally, he should stop exercising at once and not resume until he has medical clearance.

A generalized infection of the heart area can accompany such major diseases as rheumatic fever or diphtheria. Infection may also occur with viral problems such as poliomyelitis, influenza, or infectious mononucleosis. The heart involvement, known as myocarditis, makes exercise hazardous, especially where the patient is feverish. A doctor may suggest that the patient wait a week after his temperature returns to normal before resuming his exercise regimen.

Irregular heart action may lead to serious and even fatal ventricular fibrillation, or rapid, irregular contractions of the heart muscle. Fibrillation always precludes additional exercising until the normal heart action can be restored through use of medication. Mild rhythm irregularities may not, however, be considered serious enough to terminate a training program.

Other types of heart problems that may necessitate cessation or modification of an exercise program include some types of valvular heart disease, blood clots in the lungs or peripheral arteries, repetitive heart failure that leads to enlarged heart, and complete heart block. Hypertension that cannot be controlled by medication may indicate that exercise will drive the blood pressure up higher, possibly to dangerous levels. Some forms of congenital heart disease make exercise inadvisable.

In still other cases a physician who recommends that a patient avoid exercise may be basing his judgment on noncardiac conditions. Heavy exercise may, for example, be contraindicated where the patient has severe uncontrolled diabetes. The same may be true of patients with epilepsy or narcolepsy, a tendency to experience sudden, uncontrollable attacks of sleepiness. Because exercise increases the demands made on the lungs, kidneys, and liver, exercise may be ruled out if the patient has kidney or lung diseases, tuberculosis, or other conditions affecting these vital organs.

Inappropriate exercise can aggravate other diseases and physical problems. Those falling in this category include some types of arthritis; chronic low-back trouble, a complaint that may be exacerbated by jogging; anemia; and some relatively rare kinds of neurological, muscular, or glandular diseases.

## Basic Program

While every postcoronary exercise program must be tailored to the needs and capabilities of the individual patient, some generalizations can be made. An outline of a typical walking-jogging program includes, for example, four basic phases. In each, the regimen includes five weekly sessions, with two days of rest taken at any time during the week.

**1.** *Adjustment phase:* In this phase, the patient works into the program by gradual stages. For two weeks he may be asked to walk a mile in 30 minutes. In each of three follow-up two-week periods, he walks 1.5 miles in 42 minutes, 2 miles in 50 minutes, and 2.5 miles in 57.5 minutes.

**2.** *Action phase 1:* In action phase 1, beginning with the conclusion of the adjustment phase, the patient walks a mile in 20 minutes, continuing that routine for two weeks. For two additional weeks he walks two miles in 40 minutes; then for a final two weeks he covers a three-mile course five times weekly in 60 minutes. The time allotted for each walk is slightly higher for the patient who is over 45 years of age.

It should be noted that patients with higher levels of maximum oxygen consumption may be allowed to pass through the three stages with shorter time prescriptions. The patient with a very good level of consumption would probably be allowed to complete the three-mile course in as little as 42 minutes. In approaching the target, he would be moving through a walking-jogging phase of training. The point at which full-time jogging becomes part of the regimen is usually reached where the patient faces the task of covering a mile in 14 or 15 minutes.

**3.** *Action phase 2:* In this phase, the patient graduates to jogging exclusively. The transition may take many months. The exercising patient should always watch for adverse heart symptoms. He may have to make adjustments in his program on the basis of what he observes.

In action phase 2, the patient again

increases the intensity of the workout while simultaneously decreasing the distance covered. Starting out, for example, the patient might walk-jog over a one-mile course in 18 minutes. After two weeks he might allow himself 16 minutes to walk-jog a mile, then continue that program for two weeks. By such easy stages he increases the pace to one mile in ten minutes. He then goes back to the 18-minute mile, but covers a two-mile course. In the end, having gradually reduced the number of minutes per mile, he is covering a three-mile course in 30 minutes, jogging all the way.

4. *Action phase 3:* Using the same gradual approach, the patient progresses to the point where he is jogging five miles in 50 or 60 minutes. The process requires, normally, one year. The ability to undertake such long-distance jogging represents a major accomplishment. In most cases it pays off in terms of high levels of cardiorespiratory fitness. Some heart attack patients have progressed to the point where they have entered marathons.

## Caveats

Even after he has reached a satisfactory fitness level the heart attack victim may have to be careful. He may, for example, avoid exercising at higher altitudes. At elevations over 4,000 or 5,000 feet, the oxygen pressure in the air sacs of the lungs decreases. The oxygen content in the circulating blood is correspondingly reduced.

The postcoronary patient should also watch for signs of overtraining, or staleness. This condition is characterized by chronic fatigue, irritability, susceptibility to minor infections including colds, insomnia, loss of appetite, and loss of concentration. The answer in such cases is to rest for a week or two. The body can then recuperate and adjust.

In many other situations the postcoronary program may have to be modified or suspended temporarily.

Exercise types, times, and places may have to be chosen carefully. No recuperating patient should exercise heavily after a heavy meal; a wait of two hours is usually suggested. Outdoor exercise in very cold weather may have to be ruled out. The cold air may act as an irritant on the large air passages in the lungs—or exposure to cold may cause a sharp rise in blood pressure. Many physicians believe that a heart attack victim should never do isometric exercises.

Finally, patients on medication should consider the effects of exercise-plus-medicine on their heart rates. Small doses of some medications may not affect the heart rate, but larger doses may do so. Medication may also affect the individual's endurance levels; fatigue may set in more quickly where a patient is taking medication.

# All Men (and Women) Were Created Equal

If men and women are essentially equal, can they take up the same sports? Can they participate in the same exercise regimens? Can they fill in their leisure hours with the same recreational activities?

They can, and they should. Women are taking up weight training, to name one example. Women are learning that bodily strength need not necessarily mean bulging biceps and triceps, and that they can be strong and healthy as a result of exercise and athletic endeavor—while also looking—and feeling—more graceful and attractive.

Increasingly, women are taking up exercise programs; indeed, many more women than men of comparable ages are going into sports activities. And, they are developing the exercise and sports-recreation programs that best suit their temperament and tastes. Jogging is only one of many possible answers.

There are some physiological differences between men and women that are of special relevance in a recreational or fitness program. For example, women are more flexible than men at all ages. Also, women normally carry a somewhat greater percentage of fat than men. For that reason, among others, women do not so readily develop the muscle bulges that male weight lifters have.

Women have heart rates that are five to ten beats per minute faster than those for men. This finding is interesting in view of the fact that before puberty girls and boys do not differ substantially in terms of maximum oxygen consumption. It prompts the question of whether or not women's heart rates are culturally conditioned. Are they more rapid than those of men because of the traditions that have long forced different patterns of exercise and other behavior for girls and women? That question has not yet been answered.

Some other differences may be mentioned. The working capacity of the average woman in the postpuberty years has been found to be about 85 percent of that of the average man of comparable age. That effect comes about because of the woman's smaller heart muscle size and strength capacity. Thus women generally find that while exercising their pulse rates rise more rapidly and to higher levels than those of men.

## Some Misconceptions about Competition

It follows that if men and women can take part in the same exercises and sports, they can also take part in the same competitive activities, whether athletic or of some other kind. However, consideration should be given to the physiological differences between the sexes, including the different heart rates. Testing conducted in a physician's office, laboratory, or clinic should follow the same procedures as for men. Training effects should be sought by the same means. And the same precompetition protocols that apply to men apply to women.

Some authorities maintain that women are assuming unnecessary and perhaps serious risks when they take part in competitive activities or sports that involve heavy body contact. The risks center in the breast area, where bruises and contusions can do permanent, painful damage.

But physicians see little difference between the sexes with respect to the desirability of engaging in noncontact activities. Girls and boys, men and women, have nearly equal capacity for competitive sports and games—aside from the limitations noted—and can enjoy such activities equally.

## Some Gynecological Facts

On the basis of extensive evidence, gynecologists agree that:

- Neither premenstrual changes in the body nor menstruation itself need interfere with a fitness program or ancillary activities. A woman should not assume that menstruation and its accompanying inconvenience need necessarily determine her participation or nonparticipation at any given time. That decision should, rather, be made with overall considerations of health and attitude in mind. Bear in mind that female Olympic athletes compete without regard to whether they are menstruating or not.

- Physically fit women appear to avoid many of the leg, back, hormonal, and other problems that seem to afflict women in general more than they do men. The problems thus need not be considered inevitable. They may be outgrowths of the state of "unfitness."

- Menopause need not involve a decrease in fitness activities. On the contrary, keeping fit means keeping normal, "doing your thing," and living and enjoying life. If menopause interferes seriously with the effort to keep fit, something may be complicating the situation, and a doctor should be consulted.

## Exercise during Pregnancy and Postpartum

A fitness program can be continued with modifications during pregnancy. After pregnancy, the new mother can gradually resume—or start—a fitness program. In both cases the physician's advice should control both the

# Expecting the Yoga Way

**The cat/bidalasana**

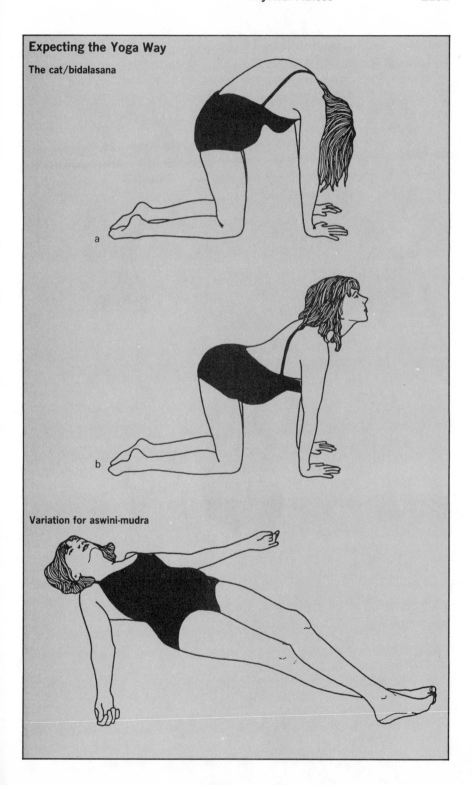

**Variation for aswini-mudra**

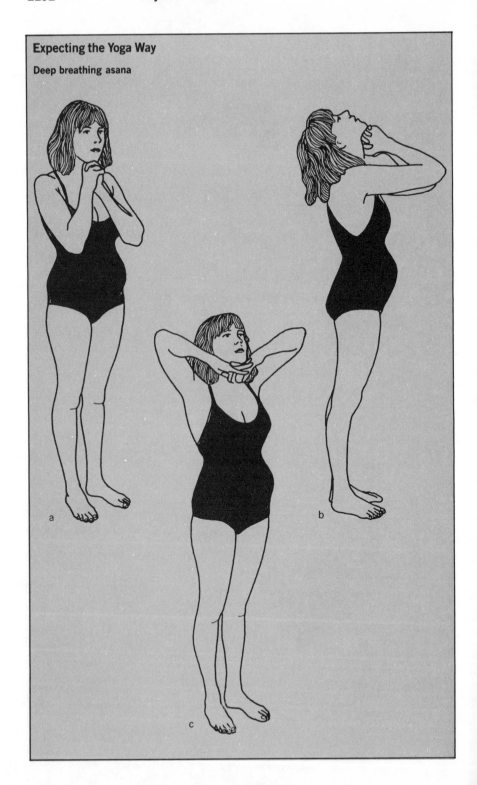

**Expecting the Yoga Way**

Deep breathing asana

intensity of participation and the types of activities.

Clearly, the growing fetus interferes increasingly with strenuous activity. Activity of any kind may become difficult and tiring. After delivery, the problem may become one of "getting your figure back." *The Complete Book of Good Health,* by Phoebe Phillips and Pamela Hatch, contains exercises that your physician may approve for pregnancy and postpartum.

## During Pregnancy

**1.** Start by sitting on the floor with legs spread wide. Placing your hands on your knees, lean forward gently. Let your head sink forward as far as you comfortably can. Let your hands slide toward your toes, stretching down; then bounce two or three times, gently.

**2.** While lying flat on your back with your feet anchored under a bed or chair, extend your arms straight up. Then pull yourself up to a sitting position, moving slowly.

**3.** This one is designed to relieve the backaches commonly encountered in pregnancy. Lying on your back with your knees bent, your soles flat on the floor, arms resting on the floor, press the small of your back against the floor. Hold that position for a slow four-count and release. Breathe deeply. Repeat four or five times.

## Postpartum Exercises

The postpartum exercises can start the day after you deliver if your physician approves. Care should be taken to avoid overexertion or strain, but on the other hand, delaying too long can make it more difficult to get back in shape.

As a separate relaxer, try the back bend. Standing erect, feet slightly apart, let your head fall forward, dragging your upper body with it. Let your hands hang free. Take a deep breath and hold it while straightening up slowly. Once back in the erect position, exhale slowly. Breathe normally. Remember that as you straighten up your lower back muscles should do the work.

## After-the-Baby

Here are eleven more after-the-baby exercises for slimming. The first four can start almost immediately after delivery. Three or four days later, try Nos. 5, 6, and 7. Leave the remaining exercises until about two weeks after delivery.

**1.** Lie on your back, knees bent and feet flat, and breathe in as deeply

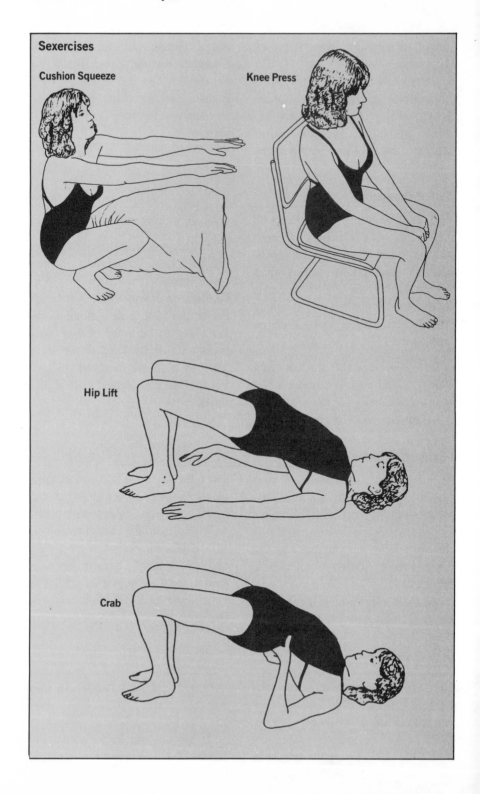

**Sexercises**

Cushion Squeeze

Knee Press

Hip Lift

Crab

as you can. Let your stomach inflate. As you breathe out, draw your stomach in as far as possible. Repeat four times, three times a day.

**2.** Lying on your back still, with legs straight out, bend and stretch your ankles. Point your feet upward. Keeping your ankles as still as possible, wiggle your toes, then rotate your feet at the ankles. Repeat as in No. 1 above.

**3.** Again lying down with your legs straight, press your knees and thighs down as hard as you can. Relax between presses. Repeat as above.

**4.** To strengthen the pelvic muscles, lie on your back with your knees bent and slightly apart. Tighten the pelvic muscles slowly, with the pressure centering at mid-pelvis. Relax, then repeat as before.

**5.** While lying on your back with one leg bent, keep that leg still while trying to shorten the other leg. To "shorten," draw that straight leg up at the hips and waist. Then stretch it down in the same way. Repeat four times once a day.

**6.** While lying on your back with knees bent and feet flat, tighten your stomach muscles and draw them in. Press your waist down with your hands. While keeping your lower back flat, lift your hips slightly. Repeat four times, relaxing between exercises.

**7.** Again lying on your back with your knees bent and arms stretched out at your sides, twist from the waist only. Swing both knees over to the left, then repeat toward the right. Your feet and shoulders should remain in position. Repeat four times, once a day.

**8.** Lie on your back with your arms at your sides and lift your head slightly. Let your shoulders follow your head up. While raised, bend over to one side and reach down with your arm. Repeat on the other side.

**9.** Lying on your back, place your hands on the top part of your chest. Keeping your waist and back on the floor, raise your head and shoulders. Keep your eyes on your knees. Lower and relax.

**10.** Start as you do No. 9, but your hands should be at your sides. Lift your head and shoulders slightly. Bring your right arm up and over and touch the floor on the left side. All movement should come from the upper body.

**11.** In a final exercise, fold your arms under your head. Relax your neck muscles. Lift the right leg and bring it down. Relax and repeat with the left leg.

# Exercises for Early Ages

The wise parent finds out about his child's physical needs and capabilities and tries to provide activity opportunities that match them. The unwise parent tries to force the child into an activity mold in which the child feels uncomfortable or downright embarrassed.

The wise parent understands that maturation refers to both physical and mental aspects of the child's makeup. Maturation in both areas may determine the child's ability to perform well in sports or games that demand a high level of coordination or skill. Maturation may in fact be more important than experience.

## Do's and Don'ts

In regard to this maturation process here are a few "do's" and "don't's" for the parent:

- DO encourage your child to develop good activity habits.

- DO encourage your child to develop good posture habits as a way to be kind to his body.

- DO instruct your child in the rules of safety, good sportsmanship, and other aspects of exercise, sports, and athletic activity.

- DO make sure that your child has adequate medical and dental care.

- DON'T compare your child's performance unfavorably with the performances of others.

- DON'T force your child to take part in any game, exercise, or sport against his will or at too rapid a pace.

- DO take part in exercises or other activities with your child to teach techniques and attitudes in the most personal of all ways—by sharing time.

- Without forcing it, DO encourage your child to become fitness conscious.

## Warning Signs

Children become sick just as adults do. As with adults, a sickness can be primarily physical or primarily emotional. In either case the sensation of weakness or incapacity will be completely real.

A physician should be consulted when a child, during play or exercise, displays any of the following symptoms:

- Blue lips or nails. Blueness should not occur unless the child is playing in cold, damp air—and that in itself might be unhealthful.

- Unusual fatigue. Excessive fatigue does not mean the child is reacting with laziness; it can mean that he needs rest, or a respite from the game.

- Excessive loss of breath. Breathlessness is normal after vigorous activity, but where it persists more than three to five minutes after termination of the activity, a medical examination may be in order.

- Shakiness. Shakiness that lasts more than ten minutes after strenuous activity may be abnormal.

- Cold sweat. The young person who breaks out in a cold sweat is rarely showing a normal reaction.

- Muscle twitching. Muscle twitches may or may not be normal, and should be watched.

In addition, children may exhibit other symptoms after taking part in exercise, games, or sports. These may require a physician's attention, especially if they continue. Among such symptoms are digestive upsets, fainting, headache, dizziness, pain not associated with an injury, disorientation, personality changes, uneven heartbeat, and interrupted sleep.

## Fun Exercises for Preteens

The following exercises, adapted from Pat Stewart's *U.S. Fitness Book,* comprise a simple, easy-to-learn method of introducing a preteen child to a fitness program. The exercises have been designed for children six years old and older. Adult participation or supervision is appropriate if the young exercisers are six to ten years old. For those older than ten, supervision should not be necessary.

**1.** *The wheelbarrow:* Performed with two children, develops arm, shoulder, and abdominal strength. One participant kneels on the floor and places his hands down flat, directly under the shoulders. The fingers should point forward. The other child grasps the kneeling child's ankles and raises the legs. The first

child "walks" forward on his hands while the partner keeps his feet suspended in the air at waist height. The walker should travel only three or four feet at the beginning.

**2.** *The tortoise and hare:* An aerobic exercise, the participants stand at attention. On the count of 1, the youngsters start to jog slowly in place. On the count of 2, the command "Hare" is given and the children double the tempo, lifting their knees high while their arms pump vigorously. On the count of 3, the command "Tortoise" brings the tempo back to an easy jog. The commands can be repeated every minute for four minutes.

**3.** *Trees in the wind:* Helps to develop trunk flexibility. The children

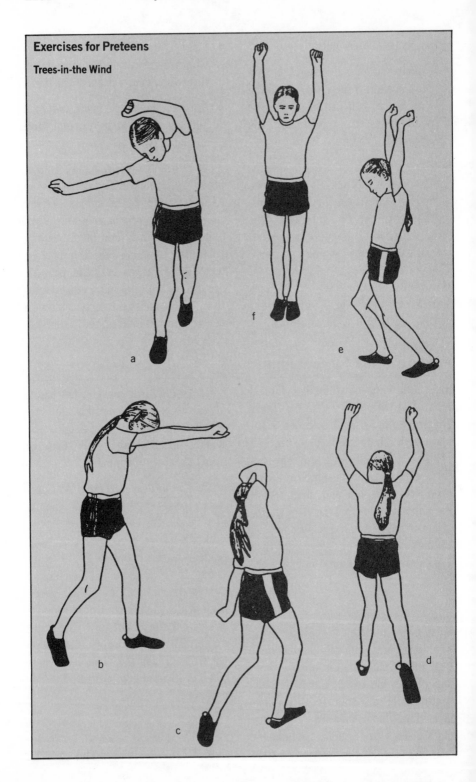

**Exercises for Preteens**

**Trees-in-the Wind**

## Exercises for Preteens

**Bear Walk**

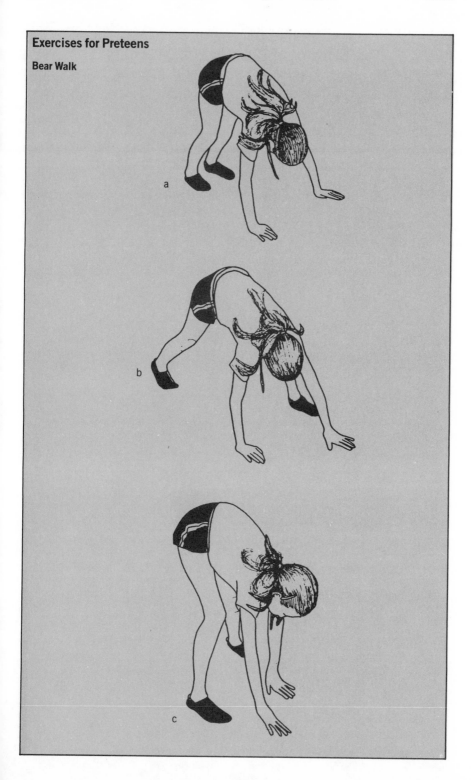

## Exercises for Preteens

**Measuring Worm**

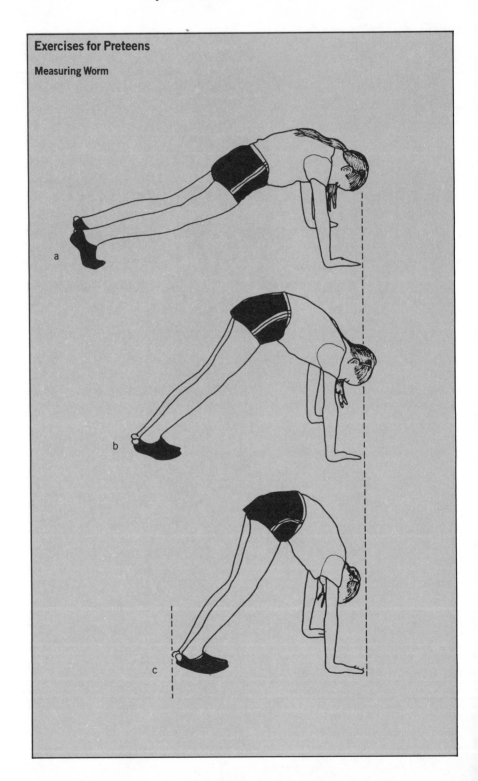

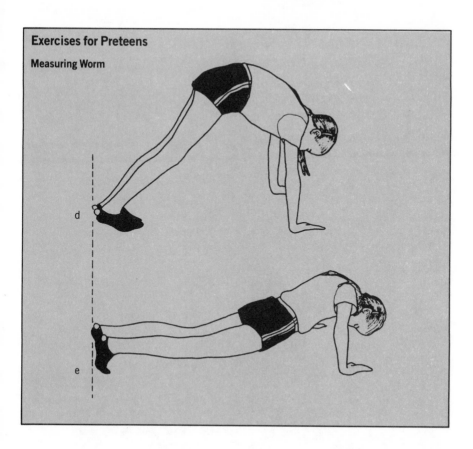

**Exercises for Preteens**

**Measuring Worm**

stand in a circle, arms extended overhead. As the children run slowly in a circle, they bend left, forward, and right, then forward and back like trees swaying in a wind. The exercise can be continued for three or four minutes.

**4.** *The gorilla walk:* For flexibility and coordination, begins with the children standing and spreading their feet to shoulder width. They then bend at the waist and grasp their ankles. The knees should be kept straight. The participants walk forward while holding their ankles. A walk of three or four feet should be a good starting distance.

**5.** *The hop:* A leg-muscle builder, starts with the child standing straight. The child hops forward on the left foot only, taking long steps. Then he repeats on the right foot. A forward trip of three or four feet on each foot is enough.

**6.** *The bear walk:* For leg flexibility requires that the child bend forward from the waist. He places his hands on the floor. Moving around in a circle, the child moves his right arm and right leg at the same time as one step. Then he moves the left arm and left leg. Four circles will do.

**7.** *The rabbit race:* Another exer-

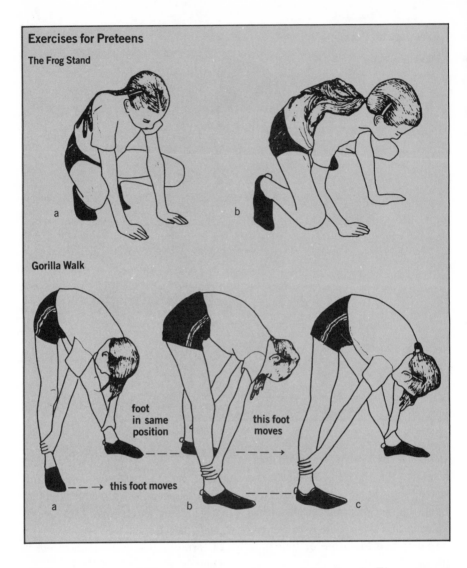

**Exercises for Preteens**

**The Frog Stand**

a    b

**Gorilla Walk**

foot
in same
position

this foot
moves

– – –→ this foot moves

a    b    c

cise for two or more children, the rabbit race promotes circulorespiratory fitness. The participants line up exactly as if they were taking part in a foot race; but they stand three feet apart, side by side, facing a marked finish line 60 feet away. The children race by hopping. They hold their feet together over the entire course, hopping with their toes pointed first toward the left, then toward the right, then straight ahead. They repeat these movements until they reach the finish line. Variations may be introduced. The children may hop on one leg, for example.

**8.** *The frog stand:* Strengthens the arms and enhances balance. The participant squats and places his hands on the floor. The fingers point forward

**Exercises for Preteens**

**The Wheel Barrel**

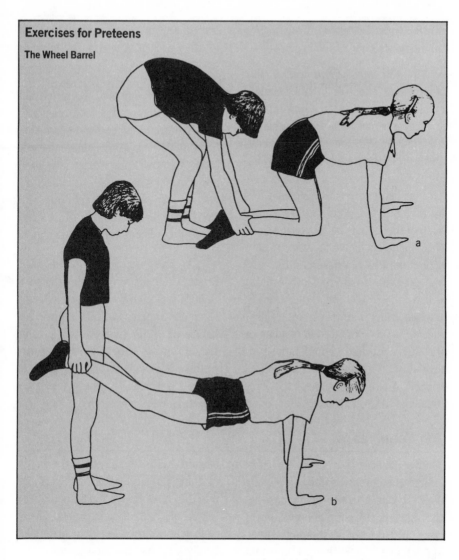

a

b

and the elbows press against the inside of the knees. Leaning forward slowly, the child transfers his weight to his hands, going up on his toes and, if possible, raising his toes off the floor. He balances on his hands, keeping his head up. After several seconds in that position, he returns to the starting position. In repetitions the child tries to maintain his balance for increasingly longer periods.

**9.** *The coffee grinder:* An upper-body strength builder, the coffee grinder requires that the child support his extended body on the right hand and his feet. The body is kept straight. The right arm and both legs are fully extended. The feet are slightly apart. In that position, the child "walks" his feet in a circle around the right arm, which serves as a pivot. The exercise should be repeated with the left arm supporting the body weight.

**10.** *The measuring worm:* Has been found effective in the development of strength in the lower back and hamstrings. The child assumes the push-up position with both hands on the floor and arms straight. Holding his hands in one place, the child "walks" his feet toward his hands. His back arches up. When he has walked his feet forward as far as possible, the child walks his hands forward by slow stages until he has assumed the original push-up position. Both walking actions should be repeated five times.

Two other exercises for children may be used or omitted depending on the child's strength, coordination, and flexibility. Both present a significant hazard of overextension of the knee muscles. Also, in the second exercise, a soft mat may have to be used for the child to kneel on to prevent bruises.

**11.** *The bunny hop:* Requires that the child assume a full squat position. His hands are placed alongside his head behind his ears, palms forward, to represent rabbit ears. The child hops in a circle with both feet together. Completing each hop, he lands again in the squat position. The hopping continues for two minutes.

**12.** *The knee down:* In the knee down, the child stands with the toes of both feet on a line. The child drops to both knees without taking his hands from his sides or moving his toes from the line. Then he returns to the standing position, again without using his hands or other aids. Five repetitions are prescribed.

## The Teen Years

The teenager is approaching maturity in both the physical and the emotional senses. During these years between the ages of 13 and 19, most teens develop an interest in team sports and games. Growth may continue throughout the entire period. Activities requiring stamina become part of the teen's life. If no total or maintenance fitness program has been introduced into the young person's schedule in the earlier years, the time for such a program may have arrived.

Various factors suggest that con-clusion. Many teens reduce the range of their physical activities to make time for school work, social activities, television, and other interests. Many walk less as they learn to drive the family car. As the teen years move on, bicycling comes to be regarded as demeaning or "too much work."

It may help for the parents to take part in fitness activities with their teenagers. But many teens have the maturity to start and continue a total fitness program on their own.

### The Goals

The overall goal remains fitness—fit-ness for school; for homework; for the part-time job, if any; for dancing; for anything else requiring alertness, bodily movement, and endurance. But more limited goals may be set if the teen does not appear to be ready for an ambitious, graduated program.

Parental eagerness may have to be tempered with moderation in this regard. Remember, if the program seems overly ambitious, the young person will be less likely to stick with it. And if the teen does not stay with the program, the overall goals will never be met.

Goals of a more specific nature range across the basic spectrum established for this book. The teen should work—as the adult does—toward circulorespiratory endurance, good body composition, muscular strength and endurance, and flexibility. Training for specific sports and games can be included if that is desired. A 30-minute exercise session three times a week should constitute minimal exposure.

The teen's needs and preferences should always be respected. Few persons, teen or adult, can continue a fitness program if they feel no personal involvement or interest.

## Caveats

The precautions already noted with reference to preteens apply equally to teens. Where a teen has encountered special problems in earlier years, a doctor should be consulted before a program is launched.

Just as adults should be tested, so should teens. The stress test may be accompanied by physical strength and endurance tests similar to those prescribed for adults.

Some teens will want to practice exercises before starting a total program or when adding new movements to an initially limited program. If so, they should be allowed to take as much time as necessary to learn the various movements. A week or two usually suffices.

## The Exercises

The exercises that are adapted particularly to teen use echo some of those that have already been introduced. But many of them add or subtract an element to ensure that they are actually suited to the teenage group. The first three of the teen exercises described below may be regarded as warm-ups.

**1.** *The deep breather:* To perform this circulorespiratory warm-up, you simply stand at attention. On the count of 1, moving slowly and rhythmically, rise on your toes and simultaneously circle your arms inward and upward so that they cross in front of you. Move slowly. Inhale deeply. Completing the 1-count, raise your arms overhead. On the count of 2, circle your arms backward and downward. Lower your heels to the floor and exhale. Repeat for one to two minutes.

**2.** *The wing stretcher:* To increase your flexibility, try the wing stretcher. Standing straight with your elbows at shoulder height, fists clenched, hold your palms in front of your chest. Throw your elbows back vigorously. Then bring them back forward just as vigorously. Keep your head erect. Your elbows should remain at shoulder height. Repeat for one to two minutes.

**3.** *The one-foot balance:* In this balancing exercise, first stand at attention. On count 1, stretch your left leg backward. Bend your trunk forward, extending your arms sideward until you are "flying." Your head is up, your upper body parallel to the floor, and your left leg is extended back and up, toes pointed. Try to hold this position for five to ten seconds, then return. On count 2, switch to the other leg and repeat. Continue the repetitions for one to two minutes.

**4.** *The jumping jack:* In this coordination exercise, first stand at attention. On the count of 1, swing your arms sideward and up. Touch your hands above your head with your arms straight. At the same time move your feet apart toward the sides in a single jumping motion. On count 2, bring your feet back together and your hands to your sides. Repeat for two minutes.

**5.** *The body bender:* This flexibility exercise has four counts or separate movements. To prepare, simply stand

erect with your hands against the back of your head. On count 1, bend sideways to the left as far as you can, moving only from the hips. While keeping your feet stationary and your toes pointed forward, return to the starting position on count 2. On count 3, repeat, but bend to the right. At count 4, return to the starting position. Continue for 15 to 30 repetitions.

**6.** *The windmill:* Another four-count exercise, the windmill promotes flexibility in the middle body. Stand with your knees flexed and apart and your feet spread to shoulder width. Your arms should be extended outward to the sides at shoulder level. On count 1, twist and bend your trunk while bringing your right hand to the left toe. Keep your arms straight and your knees flexed. The other three counts bring you (2) back to the starting position, (3) twisting and bending while bringing your left hand to your right toe, and (4) returning to the starting position. Repeat 10 to 20 times.

**7.** *Back stretcher:* In this exercise for the lower back and thighs, while standing with your feet apart extend your arms overhead. On the count of 1, bend forward from your hips, bending your knees, and touch the floor by extending your arms between your legs and behind them. On count 2, return to the starting position.

**8.** *The jump and touch:* In this leg exercise, go into a half crouch. Pretend you are going to start a broad jump. Your arms should be extended backward. Springing upward, bring your knees toward your chest and your heels toward your buttocks. While in the air swing your arms down and around your legs and attempt to bring your hands together. Come down in the starting position and repeat 5 to 15 times.

**9.** *The squat thrust:* A circulorespiratory exercise, the *squat thrust* was described earlier. The teen version exactly parallels the adult version. Repeat 10 to 20 times.

**10.** *The bear hug:* In the bear hug, a thigh thinner, stand with your feet spread comfortably and your hands on your hips. On the count of 1, step out diagonally to the right. Keep your left foot anchored. Circle your arms around your right thigh, "tackling" your right leg. On count 2, return to the starting position. On counts 3 and 4, perform the exercise on the left side. Repeat 15 to 30 times.

**11.** *The Coordinator:* Stand at attention to start this cardiorespiratory conditioner. On count 1, hop on your left foot. Swing your right leg forward and touch your right toe to the floor in front of your left foot. At the same time raise both arms in front of your body until they reach shoulder level. On count 2, hop again on the left foot. Swing your right foot out to the right and touch the toe to the floor. At the same time bring your arms sideward at shoulder level.

**12.** *Squat jump:* A leg strengthener, the *squat jump* begins as you assume a semisquat position. Clasp your hands on top of your head with feet apart and the heel of your left foot on a line with the toes of the right foot. On count 1, spring upward in a ballet-like movement, reversing the positions of your feet while in the air. Come down to the semisquat position with your hands still on your head. The same movement is repeated on count 2, but the feet are reversed. Continue, reversing your feet on each jump, until you have jumped 10 to 20 times.

**13.** *Knee raise (single and double):* This hip and abdominal-muscle flexor requires that you first lie on your back. Your knees should be slightly bent, with your feet flat on the floor and your arms at your sides. On count 1, raise one knee as high as possible, bringing it close to your chest. On count 2, extend the leg fully so that it is perpendicular to the floor. Count 3: bend your knee and return it to your chest area. Count 4: straighten the leg and return to the starting position.

During this exercise, you should alternate legs. Repeat 15 to 30 times. For variety and even better exercise, move both of your legs simultaneously.

**14.** *Head and shoulder curl:* The curl has also been described earlier. The head should be held up for a 4-count, then returned to the starting position. Repeat 15 to 30 times.

**15.** *Leg extension:* To start this hip and abdominal flexor, you should sit on the edge of a table and extend your legs. Keep your body erect and your hands on your hips. On count 1, flex your knees quickly and swing your feet backward toward your buttocks. Your toes should drag on the floor. With count 2, extend your legs back to the starting position. Keep your head and shoulders high throughout the exercise. Repeat 15 to 30 times.

**16.** *The up oars:* Begin this exercise, another hip and abdominal exercise, by lying on your back. Extend your arms above your head. On the count of 1, sit up and reach forward with the extended arms. Pull your knees up against your chest. Your arms should remain outside your knees. On count 2, return to the starting position. Remember that you are simulating rowing, and keep your movements rhythmic. Repeat 10 to 20 times.

**17.** *Snap and twist:* Still another exercise that helps the muscles of the hips and abdomen, the snap and twist has a count of 4. Lie on your back with your arms stretched out above your head. On the count of 1, sit up quickly and bring the left knee up to your chest. At the same time extend your right arm forward and your left elbow backward. The movements should be vigorous.

On count 2, return to the starting position. Repeat on the opposite side on count 3, and on count 4 return to the starting position. Keep it as rhythmic as possible. Repeat 10 to 20 times.

**18.** *The back twist:* One more for the hip and abdominal muscles, this exercise requires that you lie on your back with your arms extended to the sides and your palms on the floor. Your legs should be pointed straight up. On count 1, keeping your feet together, swing your legs slowly to the left. They should almost touch the floor. Your arms, shoulders, and head should remain on the floor. On the count of 2 return to the starting position; on count 3, repeat to the right, and on count 4 return again to the starting position. Repeat 10 to 20 times.

**19.** *Side leg raise:* Designed to strengthen the lateral muscles of the leg, the side leg raise has a two-count. Lie on your side with your arms extended overhead. Rest your head on your lower arm. Your legs should be extended fully, one on top of the other. On the count of 1, raise your upper leg vertically. On count 2, bring the leg back down. Repeat 10 to 20 times and then turn to the other side and repeat an identical number of times.

**20.** *The sprinter:* In this circulorespiratory exercise, assume the sprinter's squatting position. Your hands are on the floor, your fingers pointed forward, your left leg extended far back. On the count of 1, reverse the positions of your feet. Bring the left foot forward to your hands and move the right leg back in a single motion. On count 2, reverse again and return. Repeat 15 to 30 times.

**21.** *Push-ups:* The push-up strengthens the arm, shoulder, and chest muscles. For boys, the standard push-up is recommended—with the entire body straight and supported on hands and toes. For girls the modified push-up is often preferable. The body is kept straight, but the knees rest on the floor. With practice, both boys and girls should be able to repeat the push-up 10 or 20 times.

**22.** *Bouncing ball:* Another arm-shoulder-chest exercise, the bouncing ball challenges the physically very fit person. From the regular push-up position, push yourself off the floor with your hands. Your hands should actually leave the floor. With practice, you may be able to clap your hands while you are in the air. Repeat as possible.

## Alternatives

Other exercises, or variations of those already described, may tempt the teen fitness enthusiast. At the least, these alternatives inject some variety into the program. The following exercises, as well as those already described, can be overloaded in the three standard ways: by working out with weights, by speeding up the tempo, or by increasing the number of repetitions. (Note: these exercises require somewhat more space than the earlier ones.)

**1.** *All fours:* Get down on your hands and feet (note feet, not knees). "Walk" for two to four minutes.

**2.** *Bear walk:* From the same position, "walk" forward by moving the right arm and right leg simultaneously. Then take another step by moving the left arm and left leg in unison. Continue for two to four minutes.

**3.** *Leap frog:* This old familiar game requires at least two persons, but it can be done with virtually any number. Participants should count off by twos and, on command, the "evens" leap over the "odds." Then the odds leap over the evens. Repeat for two to four minutes.

**4.** *Indian walk:* With your knees bent slightly and your trunk bent far forward, let your arms hang down until the backs of your hands touch the floor. Holding this position, walk forward. Continue for two to four minutes.

**5.** *Crouch run:* Leaning forward at the waist, and keeping your upper body parallel to the ground, run slowly. Continue for two to four minutes.

**6.** *Straddle run:* While running forward, leap off to the right at an angle as you put down your right foot. Leap to the left as your left foot advances. Continue for two to four minutes.

**7.** *Knee-raised run:* Run with your knees moving up as high as possible on each step. At the same time pump your arms vigorously. Continue for two to four minutes.

**8.** *One-leg hop:* Hop forward on your left foot, then on your right. Take five to ten hops on each foot in succession and continue for two to four minutes.

## Some Beginner's Weight-Training Exercises for Teenage Girls

Muscle-building exercises for teenage girls should differ from those prescribed for teen boys in at least two ways. First, the girls' exercises should involve more repetitions and less weight—usually no more than two to 12 pounds. Second, the exercises for girls should be designed to lengthen or stretch muscles—not to build bulging biceps.

Depending on their conditioning levels, some adult women may want to follow the girls' somewhat lighter weight-training regimen. Here are four basic routines recommended for teens:

**1.** *The pullover:* To firm up and tone the chest muscles, and thus build a more attractive bust, lie down on a bench with a two-pound dumbbell or other weight in each hand. Extend your arms straight up and hold for a count of four to six. Lowering the weights to your bent knees, raise them until your arms are extended straight up again. Repeat 10 to 15 times.

**2.** *Thigh high:* For the muscles in the front of your thighs, sit on the floor with your legs straight out and your hands on the floor behind you for support. With a 2½ pound leg weight strapped to each ankle, raise your right leg slowly. Hold for a count of four to six. Lower to the floor and repeat 10 to 15 times. Go through the same routine with the other leg.

**3.** *A leg up:* To give shape to the backs of your legs, try the leg up. Lying on your stomach on the floor with a weight strapped to each ankle, bend your right knee. Your right foot should point up straight. Raise and lower that leg five times, flexing the foot each time, then push your right leg up so that it comes entirely off the floor. Straighten that leg. Repeat 10 to 15 times with that leg, then do the routine with the other leg the same number of times.

**4.** *Leg lifts:* A stomach strengthener, the leg lift requires that you strap one five-pound weight to both feet. Sitting on a chair or bench, hold your feet about two inches off the floor, then raise your legs, keeping them straight, until they are level with your hips. Slowly lower your legs to the two-inches-off-the-floor position. Repeat 10 to 15 times.

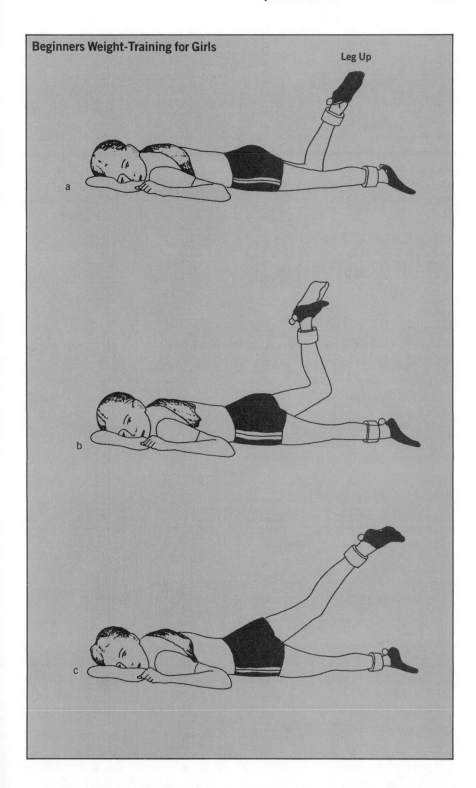

Beginners Weight-Training for Girls

Leg Up

a

b

c

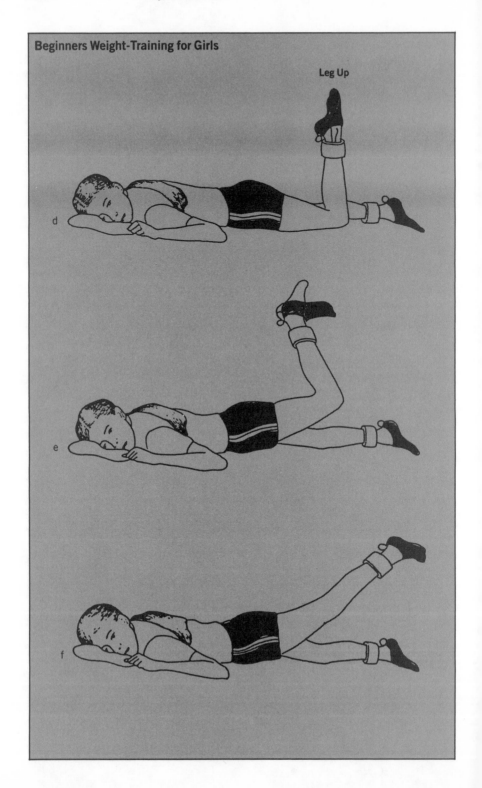

Beginners Weight-Training for Girls

Leg Up

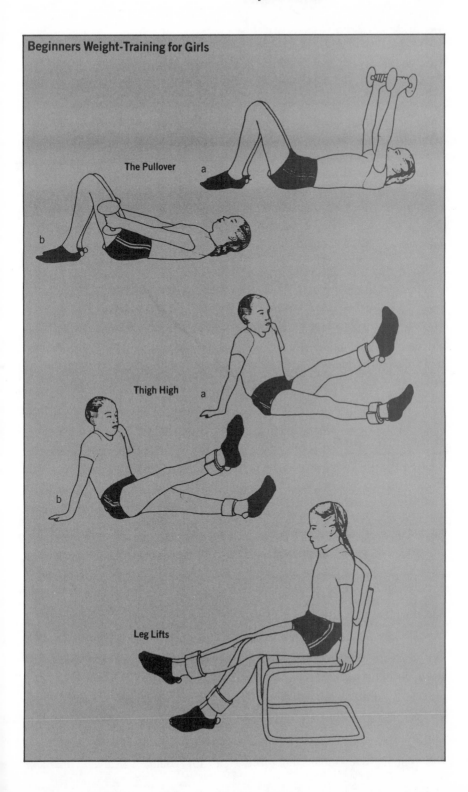

Beginners Weight-Training for Girls

The Pullover

Thigh High

Leg Lifts

# Exercises for Later Life

Young muscles that are not used come to resemble the muscles of the aged. To a very considerable extent, the reverse of that statement is also true: symptoms of aging may in fact be symptoms of disuse. Many senior citizens who exercise can hold off these symptoms and succeed in preserving a youthful appearance, psyche, and level of fitness.

The mention of "psyche" is important. Upon entering his 60s, or the retirement period, or any significant stage of later life, a person may feel that he is dying a small death. He may find it difficult to face the changes that later life brings: reduced involvement, more time to think about himself, a sense of diminishment and decreased importance, and so on.

He may find it less difficult if he has remained physically active, or if he can become physically active. By retaining some vigor, he may also retain a positive feeling about himself. He may have greater courage, and thus be able to try out new and stimulating experiences. He may move with greater ease and grace, presenting a trim and attractive figure. And the fit older person has a degree of independence that his less fit neighbor does not have. He need not call on friends, relatives, or others for help. He retains a large measure of personal freedom.

## Basic Principles

The principles behind a golden-age fitness program are essentially the same as those already specified for younger and mature adults. But the older person, perhaps even more than the younger one, has to move in easy stages. Even after testing and medical clearance, he should not undertake too much too fast. He will probably want to increase repetitions as his program progresses, and gradually add more difficult exercises. The main alternative, to overload by increasing intensity, might cause undue strain.

Physiologically, the older person faces a slightly different problem from the younger. He cannot reach the same high heart rates that the younger one achieves. Thus the older person has a correspondingly lower target heart rate.

The older person may be exercising just as hard as his younger counterpart. But the older person's pulse rate response will be lower. He will have reached the same percentage of his maximum as the younger person, only sooner. Those realities apply to women as well as to men. Women can achieve approximately the same maximum heart rates as men of comparable ages.

Warm-up and cool-down are as important or more so for older people as for younger. Running in place warms up the body effectively; so do easy stretching, pulling, and rotating exercises. In the main part of the workout, vigorous exercise should be alternated with periods of less strenuous activity.

## A Warm-up Routine

The older person planning his or her own fitness program may want to invent a warm-up series of exercises. Alternatively, he may want to try the plan devised as part of the Senior Citizen's Exercise Program. Sponsored

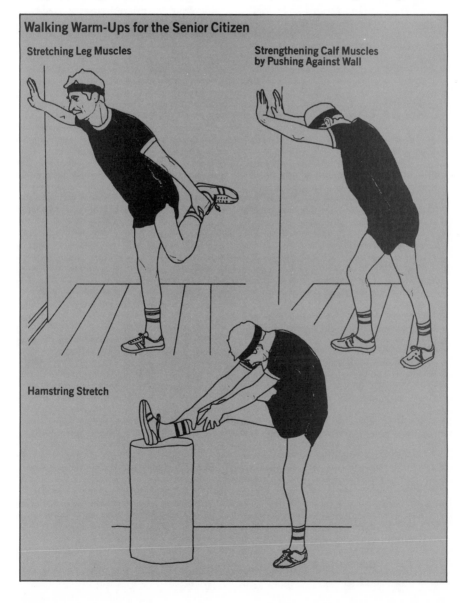

**Walking Warm-Ups for the Senior Citizen**

Stretching Leg Muscles

Strengthening Calf Muscles by Pushing Against Wall

Hamstring Stretch

by the Travelers PEP (Physical Exercise Pays) program, the senior citizen's routine has been recognized by the President's Council on Physical Fitness and Sports. The routine is performed over a five- or six-minute period:

**1.** Take a deep breath while rising on your toes with arms extended over your head. Exhale slowly. Repeat three times, then lift your left and right knees in succession. Repeat the knee lifts ten times.

**2.** Start walking. You will want to increase the amount of walking you do by small increments. Walk erect, keeping your head up and remaining comfortable. Concentrate on walking heel to toe. That means that as you put your foot down, rock forward to your toes, thus strengthening your leg muscles. Gradually pick up the pace of your stride.

## A Ten-part Set for Seniors

The normally mobile older person has many options. He or she can, obviously, create a routine for thrice-weekly or more frequent use. A ready-made program, such as the following program presented by Linda Webb in the Good Housekeeping Institute Exercise and Diet Program, may also do the trick.

The first three movements in the ten-part program can be used by nearly anyone, including persons who are confined to wheelchairs. But such persons are advised to keep the number of repetitions to three in all cases.

**1.** *Arm swing:* One of the simplest of all exercises, the arm swing involves rotating the right arm forward five times, then reversing the motion and rotating backward an equal number of times. Repeat with the left arm. Place both arms together, windmill fashion, and swing five times.

**2.** *Finger squeeze:* Extending your arms forward at shoulder height, with palms down, squeeze the fingers together slowly into a fist, then release. After repeating five times, turn your palms up and squeeze again five times. With your arms extended toward the front, shake your fingers five times.

**3.** *Arm turn:* Extend your arms straight out to the sides. With palms up, cup your hands and rotate your arms so the palms face down. Return to the starting position. Repeat five times. Starting with your palms down, cup hands, and move your arms in the opposite direction. Repeat five more times.

**4.** *Shoulder roll:* Beginning with arms at your sides, roll your shoulders forward slowly. Your shoulders should describe a full circle. After five repetitions, reverse the direction of the roll and repeat five more times. End with a shrug.

**5.** *Body stretch:* Keeping your left foot firmly planted, extend your right

## Ten Exercises for the Senior Citizen
### Arm Swings

### Finger Squeeze

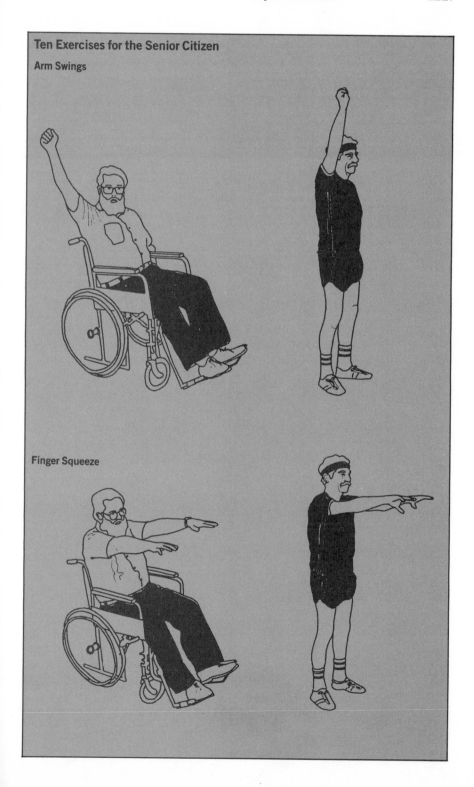

## Ten Exercises for the Senior Citizen

### Arm Turns

### Shoulder Rolls

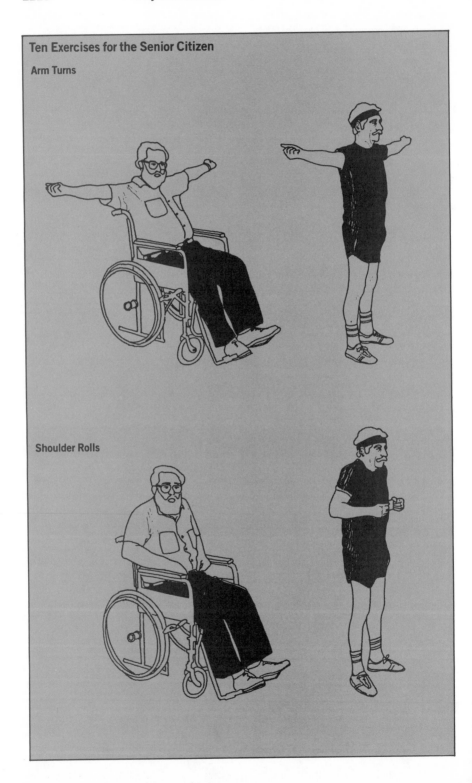

## Ten Exercises for the Senior Citizen

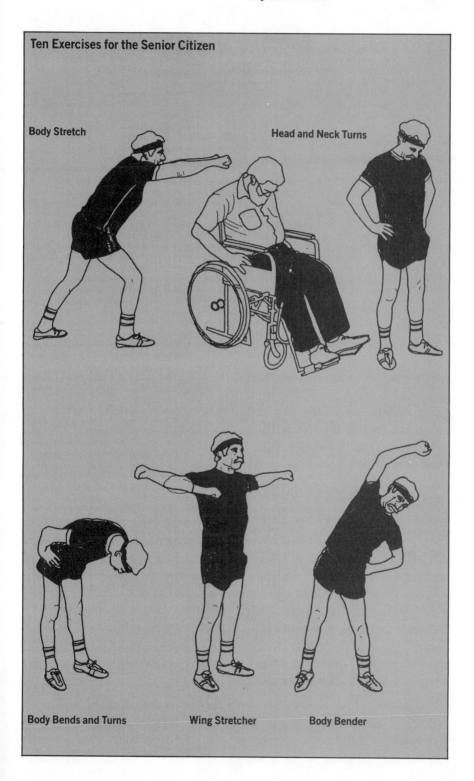

Body Stretch

Head and Neck Turns

Body Bends and Turns

Wing Stretcher

Body Bender

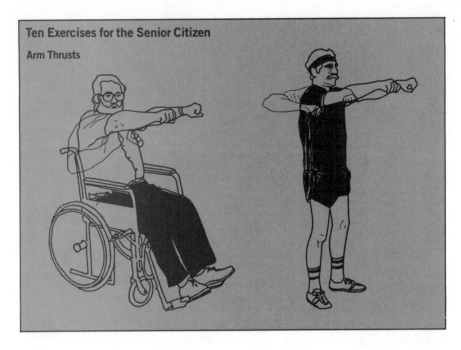

**Ten Exercises for the Senior Citizen**

**Arm Thrusts**

foot forward as far as possible. Bend your body forward at the same time, arms extended out in front, in a kind of lunge. Count to five, stretching a little more on each count. Switch, extending the left foot and keeping the right planted. With each stretch, while holding for the five-count, lift up on the toes of your back foot. Repeat five times with each foot.

**6.** *Head and neck exercise:* Hands on hips, bring your head down and forward so that your chin touches your chest. Then bend your head backward as far as you comfortably can. Bring your head back to the starting position, erect, then turn it slowly to the left, then to the right. Repeat the entire cycle five times.

**7.** *Body bend and turn:* Again with your hands on your hips, bend slowly forward from the waist until you can

bend no farther. Stand straight and lean back from the hips. Return to the starting position, bend slowly to the left, then to the right, and come back to the erect position. Repeat five times.

**8.** *Body bender:* Place your left hand on your left hip. Raise your right hand straight overhead. To a count of two, bend toward the left. Returning to the starting position, change hands, raising the left and putting the right on your right hip. Bend toward the right. Each bend should be done to a count of two. Repeat five times on both sides.

**9.** *Wing stretcher:* Standing with your feet about six inches apart, tighten your leg muscles and draw in your stomach while extending your chest. Bring your arms up, fists clenched, so that both elbows and fists are at shoulder level and your fists are in front of your chest. In this position, with muscles taut, take a deep breath and release it slowly. Vibrate your arms toward the back for a count of three. Repeat three times and work up to five.

**10.** *Arm thrust:* From the same starting position, clenched fists again in front of your chest, thrust your arms forward at shoulder height. Bring your fist back toward your chest and swing your arms out to the sides. Bring your arms back to the chest and thrust them vigorously up and down. Repeat three times.

## Progressing through Fitness Levels

The exercises described above take the fitness-aware senior citizen into a program in the simplest possible way. They should cause little pain or strain. But for optimal results, any program for any participant at any age should provide for progression.

A three-level program may be the perfect answer. The program is self-contained: it offers the older person a long-term alternative that need never be abandoned because it can be overloaded almost limitlessly. On the other hand, the man or woman who wants to utilize the program as a springboard to a more ambitious schedule of physical activities can use it in that way too.

The three-level program that follows is adapted from Pat Stewart's *U.S. Fitness Book.* It has a relatively simple level 1, a more difficult level 2, and a most challenging level 3. At each level the exerciser achieves a balanced workout, using all the muscle groups and giving primary emphasis to circulorespiratory fitness. Before starting, the older person should make sure that he or she is entering the program at the proper level. Standard walking or walk-jog tests along with others noted earlier can provide guidance in determining where to begin.

## The Who and the How

Both men and women can take part in the exercises recommended below. Couples may find mutual encouragement if they can take part together—and may be more inclined to continue the program for that reason. But in the experience of fitness authorities, men usually start at a somewhat higher level than women of comparable ages.

For both men and women, the watchword should be, "Take it easy!" The tempo of the exercise session and the numbers of repetitions should be increased very gradually. In this way, stiffness and soreness can be minimized. But some stiffness and soreness may be expected. If that occurs, it means only that the exerciser needed the workouts.

To encourage consistency and to provide a means of checking

progress, records should be kept—as always. The records should include the date, the exercises performed, the number of repetitions, and so on. Without such records, it may prove difficult to overload sensibly, with an eye to past accomplishments. Without gradual overloading, much of the potential benefit of the program may be lost.

## The Exercises

The older person should follow the instructions given with each exercise. If two repetitions are called for, the exerciser should repeat only twice. The reason is that the exercises have been arranged in such a way that a

Music that suits the tempo of the various exercises may make the exercise session more enjoyable. Comfortable clothing such as slacks or shorts, plus short-sleeved blouses or T-shirts, makes free, rhythmic movement easier. Wear comfortable, properly fitted shoes with nonskid soles and low or no heels.

warm-up, or preparation for a succeeding exercise, is built into each set or station. Thus the exercises should be performed as prescribed if they are to give optimal results.

### Level 1

As much as possible, the exercises at level 1 should be performed in a continuous sequence, with only brief rests between sets. But a rest is always called for if the exerciser feels that he is straining or pushing himself too hard.

It is important to remember that the ability to go through the level 1 exercise routines in continually shorter spans of time indicates progress. But no one should overdo it, or try to set any records. The person should maintain an even pace, avoiding jerkiness. If, after a week of performing the exercises as prescribed, he or she feels that the pace is too strenuous, the pace should be slowed, or some exercises should be eliminated for the time being. Wherever possible the exerciser ought to stick with the set routines for another

week, making such adjustments as are necessary.

Where a range of repetitions is indicated, gradual overloading calls for the addition of one repetition in the second week. But the senior exerciser should proceed with overloading only if he feels ready for it. After the second week, two or more repetitions can be added where allowed—again depending on the way in which he is taking to the program. Many persons will reach the highest number of repetitions on level 1 in three or four weeks.

Once at the level 1 maximum, the exerciser should continue at the same level until he or she can complete the entire series without resting between exercises. Having done that for three successive days, he can move on to level 2.

## Level 2

At level 2, the person follows generally the same procedure as at level 1. Initially, he performs the minimum number of suggested repetitions. In three to five weeks he should have completed the level 2 conditioning phases and be prepared for level 3.

As at the preceding level, the exerciser should move on to level 3 only when, in three consecutive sessions, he is able to perform all the repetitions of the level 2 exercises without stopping to rest between sets.

## Level 3

The same general approach should govern at level 3 as at levels 1 and 2. The exerciser starts slowly and progresses gradually. When the exerciser is able to perform without strain all the prescribed repetitions of the level 3 exercises in three consecutive sessions, he is ready to face the maintenance phase. At this point, several alternatives lie open:

- Go back to the exercise routines indicated earlier for mature adults and devise a completely new program.

- Get into walking and jogging on a more advanced or demanding level.

- Consider a program of relatively easy sports, to be dealt with in the next three chapters, and recreational activities, already covered.

- Take up yoga or calisthenics.

- Construct an augmented program out of the activities in levels 1, 2, and 3.

Whatever the choice, remember that muscles that aren't used deteriorate.

## Beyond the Daily Schedule

Whatever the older exerciser does to extend or supplement the daily schedule, he should keep in mind that he can retain the high level of fitness already achieved only on one condition. The new activities have to include the same basic tasks, and give the same benefits, as those already mastered.

Many persons turn to group activities. YMCAs across the country offer exercise classes for senior citizens, as do local recreation centers. Where a senior exerciser joins a group, he can usually skip his regular level 3 exercises on the days on which classes or meetings are held.

For other persons, sports beckon irresistibly. Swimming is excellent because the exerciser can proceed at his own pace while deriving outstanding physical—in particular circulorespiratory—benefits. But bicycling, tennis, and many other sports are also possibilities. In each of these alternatives, the objective is more movement, and more beneficial movement.

# A-Z Index Reference Guide

## A Note on Using the Index

The pages that follow contain a reference tool that should be very useful for the layman. In using this glossary-index combination the reader will be able to find brief definitions for medical terminology and locate the pages where each major topic is discussed. Where appropriate, cross references to similar or related topics are given. Illustrations and photos are indicated by the page numbers which are in italics.

# Reference Index

**Abdomen:** in human beings, the cavity between the diaphragm and the floor of the pelvis, in which the stomach, intestines, liver, and other organs are located, 17–18

muscles, *11*

*See also* Hernia

Abdominal wounds, 1058

**Abortion:** the expulsion of a nonviable fetus prior to term, either induced or involuntary (miscarriage or spontaneous abortion), 249–50

legal consent, 609

procedure, 249–50

theraputic, 246, 248

*See also* Miscarriage

**Abrasion:** scraped place on the skin, as from a fall, 1058

**Abscess(es):** collection of pus in a body cavity formed by tissue disintegration, and often accompanied by painful inflammation

breast, 802

skin *See* Boils

Abscessed tooth, 725

Absence attacks, 389

**Absorption:** assimilation by means of the digestive process, 54, 55–56

villi, 387

Absorptiometry, 369

Abused children *See* Child abuse

Acanthamoeba keratitis, 528

Accident prevention, 1008

voluntary agencies, 1008

Accidents,

emergency surgery, 603–04

**Accommodation:** the thinning or thickening of the lens of the eye in order to adjust the focus of vision at different distances, 84

**Acetabulum:** the hip socket, 6

Acetaminophen, 1092

Acetophenetidin *See* Phenacetin

Acetylsalicylic acid, 1093

**Achalasia:** failure of a sphincter muscle to relax, causing, in the case of the cardiac sphincter, abnormal dilation of the esophagus, 454

**Achilles tendon:** the thick tendon that connects the muscles at the back of the calf of the leg to the bone of the heel, 14

pains from exercise, 1126

**Acid:** any of various chemical compounds that in water solution are sour in taste, turn blue litmus paper red, and are capable of reacting with another compound (a base) to form a salt

Acid rain, 959

Acid burns, 1058–59

**Acidosis:** chemical imbalance in the blood marked by an excess of acid, sometimes affecting diabetics and leading possibly to diabetic coma, 511, 517

**Acidotic:** having or marked by acidosis

**Acinous cell:** cell in the pancreas that secretes digestive juice, as distinguished from the cells of the islets of Langerhans

**Acne:** common eruptive skin disorder due to clogging or inflammation of the sebaceous glands, 206, 715–16

**Acoustic nerve:** auditory nerve

Acquired immune deficiency syndrome (AIDS)

*See* AIDS

**Acromegaly:** disorder of the pituitary gland characterized by enlarged head, hands, feet, and most body organs, 73, 501

**Acrophobia:** fear of heights, 148, 916

ACTH (adrenocorticotrophic hormone), 72, 73, 75

ACTION, 334

**Acupuncture:** the Oriental art of traditional medicine in which needles are inserted at specific points through the skin to treat disease and induce anesthesia

**Acupuncturist:** one skilled in acupuncture

**Acute:** sudden and severe, as a disease

Acute bronchitis, 492

Acute leukemia *See* Leukemia

Acyclovir, 551, 793

Adam Walsh Resource Center, 189

**Adams-Stokes disease:** temporary loss of consciousness caused by the heart's missing a beat, i.e., its failure to contract and pump blood on schedule

**Addiction:** the compulsive habitual use of a drug for other than medical reasons

*See* Drug abuse; Drug addiction

**Addison's anemia:** anemia, pernicious, 412, 502–03

Additives *See* Food additives

**Adipose:** of or pertaining to fat; fatty

**Addison's disease:** chronic hypofunction (underfunctioning) of the adrenal cortex, characterized by weakness, loss of body hair, and increased skin pigmentation

**Adenocarcinoma:** carcinoma involving epithelial tissue of a gland, 642, 810

**Adenoid(s):** enlarged lymphoid growth behind the pharynx, 654

swollen, 117

**Adenoidectomy:** surgical removal of the adenoids, 654

**Adenoma:** benign tumor which can cause hyperfunction of the parathyroid glands, 508

**Adenopathy:** any glandular disease characterized by swelling of the lymph nodes, 578

**Adenotonsillectomy:** tonsils and adenoids removal

Adhesions, 642

Adipose tissue, 865

**Adolescents:** age groups, teenagers

*See* Teenagers

Adoption, 117–18

**Adrenal cortex:** the outer part of the adrenal gland, which produces several hormones that affect metabolism of foods, secondary sex characteristics, skin pigmentation and resistance to infection, 73

**Adrenalectomy:** surgical removal of an adrenal gland

**Adrenal gland:** either of two small ductless glands situated above each kidney, 73, 74–75, *74,* 498, *502, 503,* 635–36, *635*

   disorders, 502–03

**Adrenaline/epinephrine:**   adrenal hormone which acts to stimulate the heart, dilate the blood vessels, and relax bronchial smooth muscles, 503, 747

**Adrenal medulla:** inner part of the adrenal gland, 502

**Adrenocorticotrophic   hormone/ ACTH:** hormone secreted by the anterior lobe of the pituitary gland which stimulates the growth and function of the adrenal cortex, 394

Adult day care, 1003

**Aerobic:** capable of living only in air or free oxygen, as certain bacteria. Compare *anaerobic,* 728

Aerosol burns, 1059–60

Aerosols, 954

Aedes mosquito, 593

Affective reaction, 919–20

**Afferent:** applied to nerves receiving sensations; sensory. Compare *efferent.*

**Aflatoxin:** toxic substance produced by a fungus that develops typically in stored grains or legumes such as peanuts and that is associated with cancer of the liver, 577

**Afterbirth/the placenta:** so called when expelled from the uterus after the birth of a baby, 258–59

Aggression, 118

Aging, 311–12

   annual check-up, 312–13

   attitudes, 312

   cellular therapy, 338

   fractures healing, 374

   graying of hair, 698

   liver spots, 717

   male menopause, 292–93

   nervous system, 30

   skin, 285–86

   *See also* Elderly; Senility

**Agoraphobia:** fear of open spaces, 916

**Agranulocytosis:** acute disease characterized by almost total disappearance of neutrophils from the blood, and often following the use of certain drugs, 416

**AHF** *See* Antihemophilic factor

**AID** *See* Artificial insemination by donor

**AIDS (acquired immune deficiency syndrome):** a serious condition whose main characteristic is a deficiency in the body's natural immunity against various diseases, 547–49, 584–86

   diarrhea, 456–57

   hepatitis B vaccine, 470

   prevention, 585–86

   symptoms, 548

   thrush, 452

   voluntary   agencies,   1018–19, 1020–21

AIDS-Related Complex (ARC), 586

**Ailurophobia:** fear of cats, 916

Air pollution, 69, 491, 957–61

   allergies, 776

   indoors, 959–60

   lung disease, 491

   *See also* Environment

Air sacs *See* Alveoli

**Airway:**

   1. passageway for air

2. plastic breathing tube for administering artificial respiration from rescuer's mouth to victim's mouth

Al-Anon, 936

Al-Anon Family Group Headquarters, 936, 1020

Alateen, 936

**Albino:** organism with deficient pigmentation. In human beings, skin is usu. milky or translucent, hair is white, and eyes appear pink, 691

**Albumin:** any of a class of protein substances found in the blood, 540

**Albuminuria:** the presence of protein in the urine, 521

**Alcohol:** colorless, flammable liquid distilled from fermented grains, fruit juices, and starches

affect on human body, 929–31

denatured *See* Ethyl alcohol

headaches, 748, 749

impotence, 302

in middle age, 294–96

sexual relations, 264

teenagers, 213, 215–16, 225

types, 927

weight reduction, 871

wood *See* Methyl alcohol

Alcohol abuse,

costs to society, 927

danger signals, 934–35

drinking habits, 928

driving, 295, 639, 933

effect on health, 931–33

possible causes, 933–34

treatment, 935–37

voluntary agencies, 936–37

with other drugs, 933

*See also* Alcoholism

**Alcoholic:** one suffering from alcoholism

Alcoholic beverages

hangover, 930–31

kinds of beverages, 928–29

Alcoholics Anonymous (AA), 936, 1009, 1020

**Alcoholism:** disease characterized by excessive and compulsive use of alcoholic beverages, 927–37

educational materials, 1009

esophagal varices, 452

labor-management programs, 1009

liver cirrhosis, 468–69

malnutrition, 863

tongue cancer, 480

tuberculosis, 480

voluntary agencies, 1009, 1020

**Aldose:** a kind of sugar

**Alexander Graham Bell Association,** 137

**Algophobia:** fear of pain, 916

**Alimentary tract or canal/gastrointestinal tract or canal:** passageway for food utilized in the digestive process, extending from the mouth to the anus, and including the esophagus, stomach, intestines, and rectum

passage of food, 52, *450*

*See also* Gastrointestinal tract

**Alkali:** any of various chemical compounds that neutralize acids and turn litmus paper blue

Alkali burns, 1060

**Alkaloids:** organic substance containing nitrogen and having a powerful toxic effect on animals and man, as morphine or strychnine, 946

**Alkalosis:** chemical imbalance in the blood marked by an excessive alkali content

**Anaerobic:** capable of living without air or free oxygen, as certain bacteria. Compare *aerobic,* 728

**Anal fissure:** crack, split, or ulceration in the area of the two anal sphincters that control the release of feces, 766

**Analgesia:** incapacity to feel pain

**Analgesic:** drug that lessens or eliminates the capacity to feel pain

Analine dyes,

    bladder cancer, 571

Anal pruritus, 708, 766

**Anal sphincter:** the ring of muscle fibers surrounding the anus and controlling the passage of wastes from the body, 59

**Anaphylactic shock:** allergic shock, 1030

Anaphylaxis, 747

**Androgen:** any of various hormones found in males which control the appearance and development of masculine characteristics, also present although in smaller amounts in females

osteoporosis, 369

**Androsterone:** an androgen secreted in the urine, 79

**Anemia:** deficiency in the amount or quality of red blood corpuscles or of hemoglobin in the blood, 411–15, 759

blood pressure, 96

hemolytic: form of anemia caused by an abnormally high rate of breakdown of red blood cells, exceeding the capacity of the bone marrow to replace them with new cells, 412

hemophilic: anemia caused by bleeding into joint cavities in advanced hemophilia, 410

hookworms, 466

iron-deficiency: anemic condition caused by insufficient iron in the diet, 413–14

lead poisoning, 163–64, 958

malabsorption syndrome, 126

pale skin, 412

pernicious/Addison's anemia: anemia characterized by the enlarged size and reduced number of red blood cells, caused by the body's inability to absorb vitamin B$^{12}$, 412

purpura, 410

Rh positive blood, 414–15

*See also* Sickle cell anemia

**Anesthesia:** loss of sensation, 612,

surgery, 608

**Anesthesiologist:** physician specializing in the study and administration of anesthetics, 826

**Anesthesiology:** the branch of medical science that deals with the study and administration of anesthetics

**Anesthetics:** drug, gas, or other substance or procedure that produces anesthesia, 608, 612–16, 954

childbirth, 255–58

general anesthetic: usu. in the form of gas, that produces anesthesia by rendering the patient unconscious, 613–14

intravenous, 614

local anesthetic: applied locally, usu. by injection, to produce regional anesthesia, 615

regional anesthetic: applied locally to produce anesthesia in a region of the body, 614–15

spinal local anesthetic: usu. applied by injection to the tissues surrounding the spinal cord and affecting spinal nerves below the point of injection, 615–16

topical, 614

**Anesthetist:** person trained to administer anesthetics, 608, 610–11

**Aneurysm:** localized dilation of the wall of an artery, forming a pulsating sac and usu. accompanied by pain due to abnormal pressure, 421, 435

brain, 677

surgery, 664

syphilis, 554

Anger, 119

**Angina pectoris:** condition causing acute chest pain because of interference with the supply of oxygen to the heart, 414, 424, 427-29, *428,* 1060

drugs, 429

**Angiocardiography:** visualization by X ray of the heart and its major blood vessels after injection of an opaque fluid, 844

**Angioedema:** swelling of the subcutaneous tissues, 777

**Angiogram:** X ray of a blood vessel obtained by the injection of an opaque liquid material into the blood vessels that supply the brain, 382

kidney cancer, 574

**Angiography:** visualization of the blood vessels, 445

**Angiology:** the branch of medical science dealing with the blood vessels and lymph vessels

Angioplasty *See* Balloon angioplasty

Animal bites, 1060–61

*See also* Cat scratch fever; Jellyfish stings; Scorpion stings; Snakebites; Sting ray

Ankles,

problems with exercise, 1126–27

**Ankylosing spondylitis:** spondylitis, rheumatoid, 356

**Ankylosis:** The stiffening or fixation of a joint, as by disease or surgery

Annual check-ups, 276–77, 312–13

Anopheles mosquitos, 592

**Anorexia:** loss of appetite

**Anorexia nervosa:** emotional disturbance, esp. of young women, char-

acterized by aversion to food and resulting emaciation, 210

secondary amenorrhea, 785

**Anovulatory:** without ovulation, 200

**Anoxemia:** deficiency of oxygen in the blood

**Anoxia:** oxygen deficiency of the body tissues

**Antacids:** any alkaline substance that can neutralize stomach acidity caused by gastric juices, often prescribed in ulcer diets, 453, 460, 1093

hiatel hernia, 641

Anterior lobe, 72–74

**Anterior lobe hypophysis:** the anterior part of the pituitary gland that produces growth hormones and hormones that stimulate other glands, 72–74

Anterior pituitary gland

*See* Hypophysis

**Anterior urethra:** the meatus, or external opening, of the urethra in the penis

Anthelmintics, 465

**Anthrax:** malignant, infectious disease of sheep, cattle, and other animals, caused by a bacillus and sometimes transmitted to humans

**Antibiotics:** any of a large class of substances, such as penicillin and streptomycin, produced by various microorganisms and fungi that have the power to destroy or arrest the growth of other microorganisms, including many that cause infectious diseases

control of tuberuclosis, 481–82

leftover medications, 3

livestock feed, 969

Lyme's disease, 181

meningitis, 166

osteomyelitis, 371

rheumatic fever, 442

spinal tuberculosis, 364

**Antibodies:** substance produced by the body to counteract infection and in response to specific antigens, 746

allergies, 773–74

corticoids, 75

Anticholinergics, 386–87

**Anti-clotting compounds:** *See* Anticoagulant

**Anticoagulant:** substance that retards clotting of the blood, 418

**Anticonvulsant:** medicine used to control epileptic seizures

**Antidepressants:** drug that stimulates physiological activity, thereby tending to alleviate depression, 924

Antidiuretic hormones: *See* Vasopressin

**Antidote:** anything that neutralizes or counteracts the effects of a poison

**Antigens:** any of several substances, including toxins, enzymes, and proteins, that cause the development of antibodies when introduced into an organism, 441, 686

Antigen detection testing, 549

**Antihelminthic:** drug or remedy used to destroy intestinal worms, or helminths

**Antihemophilic factor/AHF:** substance that causes clotting and stops bleeding in hemophiliacs, 410

**Antihistamine:** any of a number of drugs that counteract the nasal engorgement and vasoconstrictor action of histamine in the body, often used in the treatment of hay fever, 484, 747, 781

Antileukotrienes, 747

**Antimetabolite:** chemical that interferes with cell metabolism

Antimony medications, 594, 599

**Antiperspirant:** astringent preparation which acts to diminish or prevent perspiration, 694

Antiseptics,

home nursing care, 993–94

Antispasmodics,

ulcers, 460

**Antitoxin:** antibody produced in response to the presence of a specific toxin, which it neutralizes

**Antivenin:** antitoxin to venom or serum prepared to counteract the effects of venom

**Anuria:** inability to urinate, 553, 539

nephritis, 539

**Anus:** the opening at the lower extremity of the alimentary canal, 59

**Anvil/incus:** the middle of the three ossicles of the middle ear, the bone between the hammer and the stirrup, 87

Anxiety *See* Stress

**Anxiety reaction:** neurosis characterized chiefly by anxiety unrelated to any apparent cause, 913

**Aorta:** the large artery originating from the left ventricle of the heart that forms the main arterial trunk from which blood is distributed to all of the body except the lungs, 34

Aortal-pulmonary artery,

Shunt, 664

**Aortic valve:** the membranous valve between the left ventricle of the heart and the aorta, 442

**Apgar system:** system of rating the health of newborn babies, 259

**Aphasia:** partial or total loss of the power of articulate speech due to a disorder in the cerebrum of the brain, 422

**Aplasia:** arrested development or congenital absence of a part or organ of the body

**Aplastic:** marked by aplasia; underdeveloped

**Apnea:** cessation or interruption of breathing

**Apoplexy:** stroke

**Appendectomy:** surgical removal of the vermiform appendix, 59, 464, 638

**Appendicitis:** inflammation of the vermiform appendix characterized by pain in the right lower abdomen, nausea, and vomiting, 59, 464–65, 1061

**Appendicular skeleton:** skeleton

**Appendix vermiformis:** vermiform appendix, 59, 464, 636–38

Appliances, teeth *See* Orthodontics

**Aqueous humor:** the clear, limpid alkaline fluid that fills the anterior chamber of the eye from the cornea to the lens, 86, 659

**Arachnoid:** the middle of the three membranes that envelop the brain and spinal cord

ARC *See* AIDS-Related Complex

Area Agency on Aging, 1004

**Areola:** the dark circular area around the nipple of a breast or around a pustule

Argon laser: *See* Laser surgery, types

**Arrest:** slow or stop the progress of, as a disease

**Arrhythmia:** variation from the normal heartbeat, 432

Arsenic poisoning, 412, 566

**Arterial:** having to do with or carried by the arteries

Arterial bleeding, 1027

**Arteriogram:** X-ray picture of an artery

**Arteriography:** technique of injecting an opaque substance into the coronary arteries and observing the material by X ray as it runs its course through the heart muscle, 430

**Arterioles:** small artery, especially the one that leads to a capillary, 34, 438

**Arteriosclerosis:** thickening and hardening of the walls of an artery, with impairment of blood circulation, 426–27

eyesight, 528

**Arteritis:** inflammation of an artery, 417–18

**Arteries:** any of a large number of muscular, tubular vessels conveying blood away from the heart to all parts of the body, 33–34, *34*

atheroscleroris, 419–21

disorders, 667

pulmonary: artery that delivers oxygen-poor blood from the heart to the lungs

**Arthritis:** inflammation of a joint, characterized by pain, swelling, and tenderness, 101, 326, 348–60, 410

fungal, 359

gonorrheal: complication of gonorrhea affecting the joints, 358, 550

hemophilic: painful swelling and bleeding in joint cavities, 410

new drugs, 359

pyrogenic: form of arthritis characterized by fever, 358

rubella, 358–59

tuberculosis, 358

voluntary agencies, 1009–10

*See also* Osteoarthritis; Rheumatoid arthritis

Arthritis Foundation of the United States, 354, 1007, 1009–10

Arthritis Health Professions Association, 1009–10

**Arthropathy:** any disease of the joints

Arthroplasty, 361–62

**Articulate:** form a joint, as one bone with another

Artificial embryonation (AE), 238

Artificial insemination by donor (AID), 238

**Artificial respiration:** artificial maintenance of respiration in someone who has ceased to breathe, especially mouth-to-mouth resuscitation, 1026–27

drowning, 1073

Asbestos, 957

Asbestosis, 957

Ascaris *See* Roundworms

Ascending colon, 59

Ascorbic acid *See* Vitamin C

**Asepsis:** prevention of infection by the maintenance of sterile conditions

**Aseptic:** free from disease-causing microorganisms

**Asphyxiation:** loss of consciousness caused by too little oxygen in the blood, generally as a result of suffocation by drowning or the breathing in of noxious gases,

*See* Gas poisoning

Aspiration, 816, 846

Aspiration pneumonia, 454

**Aspirin (acetylsalicylic acid):** analgesic drug that has fever-reducing properties, widely used to treat symptoms of the common cold, rheumatoid arthritis and many other conditions, 749, 1093

allergic reactions, 776

osteoarthritis, 351

treating arthritis, 353

**Assimilation:** the process by which digested food is made an integral part of the solid or fluids of an organism, 54

Association for Retarded Citizens of the United States, 1022

Association for Voluntary Surgical Contraception, 1021

**Asthenia:** lack or less of strength; weakness

**asthma:** chronic respiratory disorder characterized by recurrent paroxysmal coughing caused by spasms of the bronchi or diaphragm, and due in many cases to an allergic reaction, 120–21, 484–86, 776, 1062

allergic, 484–86

voluntary agencies, 1020

Asthma and Allergy Foundation of America, 747, 1020

**Astigmatism:** distorted vision caused by an uneven curvature of the cornea, 146, 524

**Asymptomatic:** condition in which antibodies for a disease are present in the blood but no symptoms of the disease can be observed. Compare *symptomatic.*

**Ataxia:** absence or failure of muscular coordination

**Atherosclerosis;** hardening of the inner walls of the arteries, resulting in a loss of elasticity, and accompanied by the deposit of fat and degenerative tissue changes, 417, 419–21, *420*

weight control, 750

**Athetosis;** derangement of the nervous system in which the hands and feet, especially the fingers and toes, keep moving or twitching, 383

**athlete's foot:** ringworm of the foot, caused by a parasitic fungus, 711, 1127

**Atrioventricular block:** disruption of normal transmission of signals between the upper and lower chambers of the heart, as from scar tissue, that may affect blood flow to the brain and cause blackouts or convulsions, 447

**Atrium** *(pl., atria)* **auricle:** one of the two upper chambers of the heart, which receive blood from the veins and transmit it to the ventricles, 41

**Atrophy:** the wasting or withering away of the body or any of its parts, as from disease or lack of use, 18

Atropine, 1093

**Attenuated:** weakened in strength, as a microorganism for use in a vaccine

**Audiologist:** one who specializes in the treatment of those with hearing problems, 323

**Audiometer:** device that measures hearing, 851

**Auditory canal/auditory meatus:** either of two passageways, the *external auditory canal* leading from the outer ear to the tympanic membrane or eardrum, and the *internal auditory canal* passing through the temporal bone to the brain, 87

**Auditory nerve/acoustic nerve:** nerve consisting of the cochlear nerve and the vestibular nerve and connecting the inner ear with the brain, conveying the sense of hearing and of equilibrium, 88, 89

**Aura:** subjective, momentary sensory perception of an unusual nature that occurs just before the onset of an epileptic convulsion, 388

**Auricle:** atrium, 41

**Auscultation:** diagnostic procedure of listening, as to sounds in the chest with a stethoscope, 831–32, *832*

**Autism:** mental disorder of children, marked by lack of response to external activities, 167

**Autistic:** suffering from or pertaining to autism

Auto and travel insurance, 976

**Autograft:** tissue graft taken from one part of a patient's body for transplanting in another part, 685

Automobiles,

accidents/injuries, 372–73, 378–79

alcohol abuse, 933

harmful exhaust, 958–59

**Autonomic nervous system:** network of nerves originating in the spinal column, and including the sympathetic and parasympathetic nervous systems, that control and stimulate the functions of body tissues and organs not subject to voluntary control, such as the heart or stomach, 27, 28–29

respiration, 64

*See also* Nervous system

**Autopsies:** post-mortem examination of a body, as to determine the cause of death, 344

**Avulsion:** a tearing or wrenching away, as a result of an accident or by surgery

**Axillar:** underarm

**Axillary:** pertaining to or in the region of the armpit

**Axon:** cylindrical fiber in neurons carrying impulses away from the cells, 29–30

AZT (zidovudine), 586

Babies: *See* Infants; Newborns

**Babinski reflex:** reflex of the toes, normal in infants, in which the large toe is extended upward and the other toes splayed when the underside of the foot is stroked, an indication in adults of neurological disease

Baby sitters, 121–22

cooperative arrangements, 121–22

**Baby teeth/deciduous teeth/milk teeth:** the first temporary set of human teeth, 20 in all, which begin to appear about the age of six months and are usu. complete by the end of the second year

**Bacillary dysentery:** a usually acute form of dysentery caused by bacilli, 457

**Bacillus *(pl., bacilli):*** any of a class of straight, rod-shaped bacteria having both beneficial and disease-causing effects

Back,

muscles, *12*

Backaches, 5, 365–67, 749–50

endometriosis, 805–06

gynecologic, 806

kidney infections, 541

low-back, 1151–52, 1154, 1157, *1153–56*

lumbago, 365

pregnancy, 242

sciatica, 365

Back blows, 1033, *1033*

Backbone, 2, 3–6

disease, 10

disorders, 328–29

injury, 9–10

*See also* Spinal column; Vertebrae

Back injuries,

emergency treatment, 1062

Back pain *See* Backache; Sciatica

**Bacteria** *(sing., bacterium):* one-celled microorganisms that come in three varieties—bacillus, coccus, and spirillum—and that range from the harmless and beneficial to the virulent and lethal

pneumonia, 478

tooth decay, 728–29

tuberculosis, 479

Bacterial endocarditis, 43

**Bacteriophobia:** fear of germs, 916

**Bag of waters:** amniotic fluid, 254–55

Balance,

exercises to help, 1142–43

function of ear, 89–90

vertigo, 531

**Baldness/alopecia:** common hereditary condition of males marked by a gradual loss of hair on the crown of the head until only a fringe remains around the sides and in the back, often called *male pattern baldness,* 205, 286–88, 700–01, *700,*

hair transplants, 684

patchy/alopecia areata: sudden but usually temporary loss of hair in patches

Balloon angioplasty, 432

**Barber's itch:** *See* Sycosis,

**Barbiturates:** any of a class of drugs derived from barbituric acid that depress the central nervous system, used medically as sedatives and sleeping pills and in the treatment of epilepsy and high blood pressure, and illicitly to counteract the effects of stimulant drugs, 219, 943–46

slang terms, 945

withdrawal, 944

**Barium:** metallic element used in compounds, especially barium sulfate, in radiography of the gastrointestinal tract because it is radiopaque—impervious to X rays

**Barium enema:** enema in which a barium mixture is used to visualize the inner walls of the large intestine by X ray, used to detect cancer and other diseases, 471, 847

**Barium meal:** liquid containing barium taken orally for the visualization of the upper gastrointestinal tract by X ray

**Barium sulfate:** an insoluble barium compound used to facilitate X-ray pictures of the stomach and intestines, 471

**Barium swallow:** X-ray examination of the esophagus as the patient swallows a liquid containing barium

**Baroreceptors/barostats:** sensitive nerve cells that respond to changes in blood pressure and may help to regulate it, 439

**Basal Body Temperature/BBT:** accurate measure of body temperature taken under uniform conditions, used to determine a women's day of ovulation, 234

**Basal ganglia:** group of nerve cells embedded in the cerebral hemisphere, the largest part of the human brain

**Basal metabolism:** the minimum energy, measured in calories, that the body needs to maintain essential vital activities when it is at rest

**Basal thermometer:** thermometer scaled in tenths of degrees instead of fifths, used by women to determine the time of ovulation

Basic food groups, 860

Bathing,

home care patients, 988–89

preschool child, 113

*See also* Hygiene

Battered child syndrome, 128

*See also* Child abuse

Battery burns, 1058–59

BBT *See* Basal body temperature

Becher type muscular dystrophy, 403

Bedtime,

children's, 122–23

Bedwetting *See* Enuresis

Bee stings *See* Insect bites; Insect stings

Behavior,

curiosity, 134–35

delinquency, 137–38

destructiveness, 138–39

discipline, 140–41

dishonesty, 141

disobedience, 141–42

disorders, 159

frustration, 150

independence, 160–61

manners, 164

regulated by brain, 27

*See also* Delinquency

Belching, 453, 455

**Belladonna:** plant with purple-red flowers whose leaves and roots yield a number of poisonous alkaloids used in medicine, 1093

**Bell's palsy:** facial paralysis due to lesion of the facial nerve, 384–85

Bendroflumethiazide, 1093

Benefits *See* Health insurance

**Benign:** mild or nonmalignant, and responding to treatment

**Beriberi:** disease of the peripheral nerves characterized by partial paralysis and swelling of the legs, caused by the absence of B complex vitamins

Beta-blockers, 432

to treat angina, 429

**Bicuspid/premolar:** one of the four upper or four lower cusped teeth located between the cuspids (or canine teeth) and the molars, 271

Bicycling, 318

Bilateral polycystic ovaries, 800

**Bile:** bitter, viscid alkaline fluid used in digestion, especially of fats, that is secreted by the liver and stored in the gallbladder, 54, 57, 58, 450, 470

*See also* Liver

**Biliary Tract:** duct that conveys bile, 647

**Bilirubin:** pigment found in bile, 469

**Biodegradable:** capable of being broken down, as a chemical compound, by microorganisms, 963

**Biodegrade:** break down (a substance) chemically by the action of microorganisms

**Biological death:** death of the brain, following clinical death, 343. Compare *clinical death.*

**Biomicroscope:** slit lamp microscope

Bionic ear *See* Cochlear implant

**Biopsy:** excision of tissue or other material from a living subject for clinical and diagnostic examination, 816

bone marrow, 846

breast cysts, 802

diagnostic, 816, 817

diagnosis of sarcoidosis, 482

kidneys, 574

lymph nodes, 580, 846

muscle, 840

needle, 848, 851

skin, 840

stomach cancer, 568, 643

venereal warts, 553

**Birth abnormalities:** birth defects

**Birth canal:** passageway formed by the cervix and vagina through which a fetus passes in the birth process

**Birth control:** the regulation of conception by employing preventive methods or devices, 264–270, 789

informing teenagers, 227–28

voluntary agencies, 1013–14

*See also* Contraception; Sterilization; Vasectomy

Birth defects, 245–46

noise pollution, 966

PKU, 175

skeletal system, 345–48

voluntary agencies, 1022

**Birthmark:** mark or stain existing on the body from birth, 718

Bite *See* Malocclusion

Bites *See* Animal bites

Black cancer *See* Melanoma

Black eye, 377, 1062–63

Black fever *See* Kola-azar

**Black lung disease:** form of pneumoconiosis common in coal miners and caused by constant exposure to coal dust, 495–496

**Bladder:** elastic membranous sac near the front of the pelvic cavity, used to store urine temporarily, 97, 532

cancer, 569–71

habits, 570

inflammation *See* Cystitis

pubic fracture, 377

tumors, 544, 632–33

Bladder infections, 769–70

*See also* Cystitis

Bland diets, 874

chart, 895

*See also* Soft diets

**Bleb:** blister formed in the epidermis

Bleaching hair, 703

Bleeders *See* Hemophiliacs

Bleeding,

abdominal wounds, 1058

adrenaline, 74–75

low-volume shock, 1030

emergencies, 1027–28

internal, 1063

minor injuries, 1063–64

*See also* Hemophilia; Nosebleed

**Blepharoplasty:** surgical technique to correct congenital defects in the eyelids or to alter their size or shape, 286, 605, 683

Blindness,

glaucoma, 659

newborns, 550

voluntary agencies, 1012–13, 1021

Blind spot, 84

**Blister:** small rounded sac, especially on the skin containing fluid matter, often resulting from injury, friction, or scalding, 1064, 1127

feet, 755–56

Blood, 32–45

cell manufacturing, 38–39

cross-match, 37–38

circulation to kidneys, 95–96, 534

composition, 35–38

contamination and AIDS, 548

diseases, 407–17

functions, 35

Blue Cross/Blue Shield, 972, 974–75

Body chemistry *See* Endocrine glands; Exocrine glands

Body fluids,

role of corticoids, 75

Body lift *See* Suction lipectomy

Body odor, 693–94

Body scanner *See* Computerized tomography

Body temperature,

skin, 689

Body,

structure, 832–33

Body wastes: *See* Feces; Intestines; Urine

Boeck's sarcoid *See* Sarcoidosis

**Boils:** abscess of the skin caused by bacterial infection of a hair follicle or sebaceous gland, 139, 712, 1064–65

**Bolus:** lump or mass of food that has been chewed and softened with saliva, 50

Bone atrophy, 367

Bone marrow, 9, 38, 411

excess red blood cells, 414

transplant, 687–88

transplants for radiation exposure, 971

**Bones:** hard tissue of which the skeleton of a vertebrate animal is largely composed, 1–10

atrophy: decalcification

brittle: osteogenesis imperfecta

broken: fractures

bruises, 1065, 1127

calcium, 9

composition, 8–9

development, 8–9

disorders, 9–10, 369–72

fractures, 9, 372–79

function, 3

growth, 8, 205

inflammation *See* Osteomyelitis

injuries, 372–79

marrow, 9

metabolism, 508

number in body, 3

osteoporosis, 369

softening *See* Paget's disease

tumors, 371–72

*See also* Skeletal System; Specific names of bones, e.g. Vertebrae

Boredom, 123

**Botulism:** poisoning caused by eating spoiled or improperly prepared or canned food and characterized by acute gastrointestinal and nervous disorders, 468, 1065–66

Bottle feeding, 105–06, 259–60

Bowel cancers, 645

Bowel habits, 60, 133

changes, 564

children, 196

constipation, 455

home care patients, 990

surgery, 609

**Bowman's capsule:** dilated structure surrounding a glomerulus as part of the nephron of a kidney, 95

Braces, teeth *See* Orthodontics

**Brain,** *24,* 24–31, 64  "lesser brains" cerebellum and nervous system

birth defects, 346

cerebral injury, 381

degenerative diseases, 398

hemorrhage, 676

organic disorders, 912

skull injuries, 377

**Brain cage:** cranium

Brain cancer, 577–78

Brain cells,

strokes, 422

**Brain damage:** tissue destruction of the brain caused by an injury before, at, or after birth, 124

alcohol use, 931

delayed puberty, 201

epilepsy, 388

mental retardation, 168

**Brain death:** biological death

Brain lesions,

epilepsy, 387, 388, 392

**Brain scan:** procedure of injecting a radioactive substance into the brain tissue or fluid and recording its movement by X rays, 842

*See also* Computerized tomography

**Brain scanning:** *CAT scanning* of the brain

**Brain stem:** all of the brain except the cerebellum, cerebrum, and cerebral cortex; the midbrain, 26

**Brain surgeon:** neurosurgeon

Brain tumors, 31, *674*

laser surgery, 606

surgery, 673–75

Brain waves recording *See* Electroencephalogram

Breakfast, 297

Breastbone *See* Sternum

Breastfeeding, 102–05, 259–60

advice, 105

breast abscesses, 802

schedule, 105

Breast self-examination, 783, 812–13, *814*

Breast cancer,

Reach-to-Recovery, 1010

Breasts,

augmentation, 681

biopsy for cancer, 816

cancer, 812–19

cosmetic surgery, 680–81

cysts, 801–02

diagnosing cancer, 813–16

enlargement *See* Mammoplasty

lumps, 801

mastectomy, 816–18, *817*

reduction *See* Mastoplasty

Breast inflammation *See* Mastitis

Breath,

bad *See* Halitosis

Breathing,

cessation, 1025–26

mechanism, 472

swallowing, *49*

Lamaze childbirth, 257

*See also* Respiration

**Breathalyser:** device for measuring the concentration of alcohol in the bloodstream of drivers of motor vehicles

Breech delivery,

hip dislocation, 347

**Breech presentation:** birth with the baby positioned to present the buttocks first instead of the head first, 253–54

Bribery, 124

**Bridge:** a mounting for holding false teeth, attached to adjoining teeth on each side

*See* Dentures

**Bromidrosis:** perspiration odor, 23

Brompheniramine, 1093

**Bronchi** *(sing., bronchus):* the two forked branches of the trachea, 66, 67–68, 492, 563

diseases, 474

**Bronchial tree:** the bronchi and bronchial tubes

Bronchial asthma

*See* Asthma

**Bronchial tubes:** the subdivisions of the trachea conveying air into the lungs, 67

**Bronchiole:** minute subdivision in a bronchial tube, 66, 68

**Bronchitis:** inflammation of the bronchial tubes, characterized by coughing, chest pain, and fever, 491–93, *492*

acute: short, severe attack of bronchitis, often brought on by exposure to cold or breathing in of irritating substances, including pollutants

chronic: recurring attacks of bronchitis after periods of quiescence, and characterized by a chronic cough and breathlessness

respiratory allergies, 484–85

smoking, 488

Bronchoscope, 850

Bronchoscopy, 850

**Brucellosis/Malta fever/undulant fever:** persistent infectious disease caused by a bacterium *(Brucella)* transmitted to humans from infected animals, as goats, cattle, or swine, and marked by recurrent fever, sweating, weakness, and generalized aches and pains

Bruises, 1066

bones, 1127

*See also* Bones, bruises

**Bruxism:** habit of grinding the teeth during sleep or when otherwise under strain, 735

**Bubo:** inflammatory swelling of a lymph gland, especially in the groin or armpit, 587

**Bubonic plague:** form of plague characterized by buboes, 587–88

**Buccal:** pertaining to the cheek or mouth cavity

**Buerger's disease:** circulatory disorder associated with cigarette smoking, 214–15

**Bulbar:** pertaining to a bulb, esp. the bulb of the medulla oblongata of the brain

**Bulimia:** disorder involving overeating followed by self-induced vomiting, 210

Bullet wounds *See* Gunshot wounds

**Bunion:** painful swelling of the foot, usually at the outer side of the base of the big toe, 284, 329, 756

**Burkitt's lymphoma:** malignant lymphoma affecting the jaw, found especially among children in Africa, 652

Burns,

diet with, 622

long-term treatment, 1068

shock, 1067–68

thermal, 1067–68

*See also* Acid burns; Alkali burns; Chemical burns

**Bursa:** any of the fluid-filled sacs within the body that tend to lessen friction between movable parts, 6, 15, 360, 756

hip joint, *7*

*See also* Joints; Muscles

**Bursitis:** inflammation of a bursa, 360, *361*, 757, 1065

calcific: painful condition characterized by calcium deposits in the shoulder tendon or calcification in a bursa at the shoulder

Butabarbital, 1093

Bypass surgery, 432

**Byssinosis/white lung disease:** lung disorder caused by inhaling cotton dust

**Cadaver:** dead human body, especially one intended for dissection

**Caesarian section:** surgical delivery of a baby by cutting through the abdominal wall into the uterus, 259–60, *259*, 792

**Caffeine:** chemical found in the leaves and berries of coffee, used as a

mouth, 566–67, 652

myelomas, 583

normal cells, *561*

ovaries, 811

pancreas, 575–76

penis, 628

pollution, 957

prostate gland, 329–30, 546, 572–73, 627

radiation treatments, 819

reticulum-cell sarcoma, 582–83

scrotum, 628

seven warning signs, 568

skin, 566–66

smoking, 214

stages, 560–61

stomach, 567–69, 642–44

testicular, 505

THC chemotherapy, 953

thyroid gland, 579

tongue, 652–53

uterine, 248–49, 506, 809–11

voluntary agencies, 1010–11

Wilms' tumor, 633

*See also* Chemotherapy

**Cancer-producing agents:** carcinogens

Candidiasis *See* Moniliasis

**Canine teeth:** the sharp, pointed teeth, two in the upper jaw (called *eye teeth*), and two in the lower jaw, located between the incisors and the molars

*See* Cuspids

**Canker sore:** small ulcerous lesion in the mouth near the molar teeth, inside the lips or in the lining of the mouth, 451–52, 762

Cannabinoids, 939

**Cannabis** *See* Marihuana

**Cannabis sativa:** the Indian hemp plant, from whose flowering tops are derived marihuana and hashish

**Cannula:** narrow tube inserted into a body cavity or vessel, as to extract a substance or introduce a medication

**Capillaries:** minute blood vessel, 34, *34*, 62, 496

blood cell movement, 39˙

**Caput succedaneum:** swelling under a newborn baby's scalp soon after birth, that usually dissolves in a few days, 102

**Carbohydrate(s):** any of a group of compounds, including sugars, starches, and cellulose, that contains carbon combined with the hydrogen and oxygen, essential in the metabolism of plants and animals, 63–64

basic requirements, 857

cellular respiration, 63–64

metabolism by smokers, 249

reduction for diabetics, 513

**Carbolic acid/phenol:** powerful caustic poison distilled from coal tar oil and used as a disinfectant

Carbon dioxide, 62–64

respiration, 62, 63, 64

Carbon dioxide laser *See* Laser surgery, types

**Carbon monoxide:** colorless, odorless gas that is highly poisonous when inhaled since it combines with the hemoglobin in the blood and thus excludes oxygen, 215

**Carbon tetrachloride:** colorless liquid that can be poisonous if inhaled over a long period, and often used as a fire extinguisher or cleaning fluid

**Carbuncle:** painful, extensive inflammation of the skin, marked by hardness and the discharge of pus, 712, 1068

**Carcinogen:** cancer-producing agent, 959

**Carcinogenic:** causing cancer or increasing the incidence of cancer in a population

**Carcinoma:** malignant tumor that arises in the tissue that lines body cavities and ducts (epithelial tissue), 561, 566

**Cardia:** the opening between the esophagus and the stomach

**Cardiac:** of or relating to the heart

**Cardiac sphincter:** ring of muscle at the entrance of the stomach, or cardia, that opens to allow food to enter from the esophagus

**Cardiac arrest:** a stopping of the heartbeat, 1031

**Cardiac catheterization:** the advancing of a catheter, or thin tube, through the veins to the heart chamber, in order to detect abnormalities and obtain blood samples, 445, 844

**Cardiac massage/cardiovascular pulmonary resuscitation/CPR:** emergency procedure consisting of the application of rhythmic pressure on the chest in order to compress the heart and start it beating again, 1031-32

*See also* External cardiopulmonary resuscitation

**Cardiac muscle:** the striated but involuntary muscle of which the heart is composed, 13

Cardiac shock, 1031

Cardiac sphincter, 448, 454

**Cardiac X-ray series:** chest X rays taken after the patient has swallowed an opaque liquid such as barium sulfate, 844

**Cardiogram:**

1. record produced by a cardiograph

2. electrocardiogram

**Cardiograph:** 432

1. instrument for recording the force of the movements of the heart

2. electrocardiograph

**Cardiologist:** physician specializing in the diagnosis and treatment of heart disease, 825, 842

**Cardiology:** the branch of medical science dealing with the heart, its physiology and pathology, 825

Cardiorespiratory endurance, exercises, 1142

**Cardiovascular:** pertaining to the heart and blood vessels

**Cardiovascular disease/heart disease:** disorders affecting the heart and blood vessels

*See* Heart disease

**Cardiovascular specialist:** physician specializing in the diagnosis and treatment of diseases of the heart and blood vessels

**Caries:** decay of a bone or tooth (*dental caries*) *See* Tooth decay

**Cariogenic:** causing caries, or tooth decay, 728

Carisoprodol, 1094

**Carotene:** orange or red crystalline pigment converted to vitamin A in animal metabolism, 691

**Carotid artery:** either of two major arteries of the neck supplying blood to the head

**Carpal(s):** pertaining to the bones of the carpus, or wrist, *8*

**Carpus:** the wrist

**Carrier:** person who is immune from infection of specific disease-causing bacteria that his body carries and that can be transmitted to others who are not immune

**Cartilage:** tough, elastic supporting tissue, 5, 6, 7

torn, 672

**Cartilage plate/epiphysis:** extremity of a long bone, originally separated from it by cartilage but later consolidated with it by ossification

*See* Epiphyses

**Cast(s):** bit of tissue, often microscopic, having taken the shape of a vessel or cavity in which it was formed, that is found in excretions and may indicate the presence of disease, 837

**Catabolism:** the destructive aspect of metabolism, in which living matter breaks down nutrients into simpler substances. Compare *anabolism.*

**Catalepsy:** abnormal condition characterized by lack of response to stimuli and by muscular rigidity, often associated with a psychological disorder

**Catalyst:** substance or agent that causes a chemical reaction while remaining stable, such as an enzyme or hormone in the human body

**Cataract:** the gradual clouding and opacity of the lens of the eye, leading to impaired passage of light and loss of vision, 526, 658

senile: cataract affecting elderly people due to degenerative changes in the lens, 526

laser surgery, 606

myotonic dystrophy, 405

Catatonic schizophrenia, 918

**Cathartic:** medicine for purging the bowels, 328

*See also* Laxatives

**Catheter:** slender tube for drawing off fluid from a body cavity, especially urine from the bladder, 432, 618

**Catheterization:** the introduction of a catheter into the body

**CAT scanner/body scanner:** computerized X-ray machine used in CAT scanning

**CAT (computerized axial tomography) scanning/body scanning:** procedure for producing a cross-sectional, computer-generated, composite X-ray picture of the body or an organ, as the brain, by rotating about a site and taking a series of radiographs directed to it

*See* Computerized tomography

Cat scratch fever, 1068–69

**Caudal:** situated at the tail end or bottom; posterior

**Caudal anesthesia/caudal/caudal block:** form of anesthesia in which the patient is injected in the region of the lower spinal cord (sacral canal) to block pain in the pelvic area, 256

**Caul:** membrane (*amnion*) surrounding the fetus if it is unruptured and intact about the baby's head at delivery, 254

**Cautery, chemical:** chemosurgery

**Cavities:** dental caries *See* tooth decay

**CBC:** complete blood count;

*See* Blood count

**Cecum:** blind pouch or cavity open at one end, esp., the cavity below the ileocecal valve that forms the first section of the large intestine, 55, 59

**Celiac:** pertaining to the abdomen

*See* Malabsorption syndrome

Cellular death, 343–44

Cellular respiration, 63–64

**Cellular therapy:** treatment for the process of aging in which a person is injected with cells from healthy embryonic animal organs with the idea that the animal cells from the particular organ injected will then migrate to the same organ in the aging body and reactivate it, 338

**Cementum:** the layer of body tissue developed over the roots of the teeth, 4, 722

Central incisors, 112

**Central nervous system:** the portion of the nervous system that contains the brain and spinal cord and controls voluntary action and movement, 24, 27–29, *28*

**Centrifuge:**

1. *(n.)* rotary machine employing centrifugal force to separate substances having different densities, as the constituents of blood

2. *(v.)* subject to a whirling motion to separate component parts, as of blood, that have different densities

**Cephalhematoma:** swelling under a newborn baby's scalp, that usu. dissolves within a few weeks

**Cerebellum:** large section of the brain located below and behind the cerebrum, consisting of a central lobe and two lateral lobes, and which coordinates voluntary muscle movements, posture, and equilibrium, 26

hypothalamus, 72

**Cerebral arteriogram:** an X-ray picture of the brain used to investigate brain damage, esp. after a hemorrhage or stroke, and made by injecting opaque dye into the blood vessels serving the brain and X raying them, 842

**Cerebral arteriosclerosis:** degenerative changes in the arteries of the brain

**Cerebral cortex:** the cells and fibers that look like a convoluted layer of gray matter and that cover the cerebral hemisphere of the brain, 26

**Cerebral hemisphere:** one of the two halves into which the brain is divided

**Cerebral hemorrhage:** hemorrhage into the cerebrum of the brain or within the cranium, *421*

**Cerebral palsy:** inability to control movement caused by nonprogressive brain damage resulting from a prenatal defect or birth injury, 126–27, 383–84

voluntary agencies, 1011

**Cerebrospinal fluid/CSF:** the clear, colorless fluid that surrounds the brain and spinal cord, 25, 382

**Cerebrospinal meningitis:** inflammation of the membranes that cover the brain and spinal cord, 25, 31

**Cerebrovascular:** of or relating to the vessels supplying blood to the brain

**Cerebrum:** the upper anterior part of the brain, consisting of two hemispherical masses which constitute the chief bulk of the brain in man and is assumed to be the seat of thought and will, 25–26

**Cervical:**

1. pertaining to the cervix of the uterus

2. pertaining to the neck or any neck-like part

Cervical cancer.

herpes, 551

herpes simplex virus type 2, 792

trichomoniasis, 552

**Cervical cap:** contraceptive device made usu. of soft plastic which fits over the cervix

**Cervical spine** *See* Cervical vertebrae

Cervical caps, 267

Cervical mucus, 236

**Cervical vertebrae/cervical spine:** the top seven vertebrae of the backbone, which are located in the neck and support the head

**Cervicitis:** inflammation of the cervix of the uterus, 805

**Cervix:** neck of the uterus, 228–29

cancer of, 806–09, 810–11

dialated, *251*, 591–92

incompetent, 247

polyps, 803

removal, total hysterectomy, 808

**Cestode:** tapeworm

**Coated tongue:** condition in which the tongue is coated with a whitish substance, consisting of food particles and bacteria, which can indicate fever, illness, or a temporary lack of saliva

**Cocaine:** white, bitter, crystalline alkaloid used as a local anesthetic and a narcotic, 941–42

freebasing, 942

hotline, 955

slang terms, 945

**Co-carcinogen:** substance which is not cancer-producing but reacts with other substances to produce cancers, 562

**Coccidioides fungus:** fungus, the spores of which can cause coccidioidomycosis

**Coccidioidomycosis/desert rheumatism/valley fever:** infectious disease caused by fungus spores and characterized by symptoms resembling pneumonia and tuberculosis and the formation of reddened bumps, 483

**Coccyx:** the tail end of the spinal cord, 5–6

**Cochlea:** spiral-shaped structure of the inner ear containing the essential organs of hearing, including the organ of Corti, 88–89, 966

Cochlear implant, 324

**Cochlear nerve:** the part of the auditory nerve leading from the cochlea of the inner ear to the brain, conveying the sense of hearing

**Codeine:** white, crystalline alkaloid, derived from morphine and used in medicine as an analgesic and to suppress coughing, 947, 1095

Coffee drinking *See* Caffeine

**Coitus** *See* Sexual intercourse

**Coitus interruptus:** contraceptive method whereby the male withdraws before he ejaculates, 269

**Cold, common:** viral infection of the respiratory tract, 132–33, 474–75, 744–45

**Cold sores:** herpes simplex, 1071

*See also* Herpes simplex

Colic, 132

**Colitis:** inflammation of the colon, 463–64

**Collagen:** fibrous protein that forms the chief constituent of the connective tissues of the body, such as cartilage, skin, bone, and hair, 311

**Collapsed lung** *See* Pneumothorax

**Collarbone** *See* Clavicle

**Colon:** the part of the large intestine extending from the cecum to the rectum and divided into the ascending colon, transverse colon, descending colon, and the sigmoid, 59, 450

ascending: the section of the colon extending up from the cecum along the right side of the abdomen

descending: the section of the colon leading from the transverse colon and extending down the left side of the abdomen

Colon cancer, 564–65, 644–45

Colonic fluid,

constipation, 455

**Colonoscope:** speculum used to examine the colon, 645, 847

**Color blindness:** inherited vision defect consisting of the total or partial inability to discriminate between certain colors, usu. red, green, and blue, 132, 524

**Colostomy:** the formation of an artificial opening in the colon through which solid wastes can pass, 565, 646

**Colostrum:** the creamy, yellowish, milklike substance rich in proteins, that is produced by a mother's breasts the first few days after having given birth, 260

Colostrum, 104

**Colposcopy:** microscopic technique for visual examination of the cervix and vagina, 808

**Coma:** prolonged loss of consciousness, 1091

*See also* Diabetic coma

**Comminuted fracture:** fracture in which bone is splintered or crushed, *373*

**Common bile duct:** duct formed by the juncture of the hepatic and cystic ducts, and carrying digestive enzymes from the liver, pancreas, and gallbladder to the duodenum

Common cold *See* Colds

Communication,

need for, 909–10

Community health care facilities, 999–1000

Community hospitals, 1001

**Compound fracture/open fracture:** fracture accompanied by an open wound, often exposing bone that is completely broken, *373,* 1078

Comprehensive major medical *See* Major medical

**Compulsion:** urgent need to perform certain ritualistic acts, often irrational, a symptom of certain neuroses

Computerized tomography (CT), 331, 383, 842, 845–46

brain tumor, 674

congenital heart disease, 445

**Conception:** union of spermatozoon and ovum, first step in the birth process; fertilization, 229–230

**Concussion:** violent shock to the brain, typically caused by a blow to the head, as in a fall, that impairs the functioning of the brain, usu. temporarily, 377

*See also* Head injuries

**Condom:** membranous sheath for the penis which serves as a contraceptive device, 230, 268

Conduction deafness, 323

**Cone:** one of many photosensitive cone-shaped bodies in the retina of the eye, sensitive to color and daylight vision, *82, 83*

Compare *rod.*

Congeners, 931

**Congenital:** acquired prior to or at birth, or during development as a fetus, as fetal abnormality due to the mother's contraction of rubella

Congenital brain damage, 912

mental retardation, 168

Congenital defects,

surgery, 604

urinary tract, 533

*See also* Birth defects

**Congenital heart disease:** deformity of the heart or of major blood vessels existing from birth, 425–26

Congenital heart disease, 382, 425–26, 444–46

**Congestion:** excessive accumulation of blood or fluid in an organ or tissues

Congestive heart failure, 446–47, *446*

**Conjunctiva:** mucous membrane on the inner part of the eyelid and extending over the front of the eyeball, 165

**Conjunctival sac:** the small sac at the inner corner of the eye between the eyeball and the lower lid that serves as a collecting pool for tears, 87

**Conjunctivitis:** inflammation of the conjunctiva (pinkeye), 527

arthritis, 360

*See also* Pinkeye

**Connective tissue:** the fibrous tissue that binds together or supports the parts of the body, as cartilage, tendons, and ligaments

**Conscience:** superego, 490, 1321

**Constipation:** inactivity of the bowels resulting in difficult, infrequent, or incomplete evacuation, 133, 194, 328, 564, 764–65

appendicitis, 1061

hemorrhoids, 651

**Constrict:** to become narrower, as a blood vessel

**Contact lens:** one of a pair of glass or plastic lenses fitted directly over the cornea of each eye to correct vision defects, 527–28

lens insertion, *527*

Contact dermatitis, 179–80, 706, 777

**Contagion:** communication of disease by contact, direct or indirect

**Contagious:** (of a disease) transmitted by direct or indirect contact

Contagious diseases,

rashes, 179–81

Contaminants,

air borne, 958–59

food, 967–70

food grown in sludge, 963

**Continuous positive airway pressure:** procedure in which high-oxygen is forced into the lungs of newborns suffering from respiratory difficulty

**Contraception:** the prevention of conception, 230

voluntary agencies, 1021

Contraceptive jelly, 267

**Contraceptives:** device or substance designed to prevent conception

Oral/the pill: the birth control pill, which is composed of synthetic hormones that suppress ovulation and thus prevent pregnancy

*See* Birth control

Contractions, 254–55

lightening, 252

**Contraindication:** symptom or sign that makes a particular course of treatment inadvisable

Contusions *See* Bruises

**Conversion reaction/conversion hysteria:** neurosis characterized by manifestation of physical symptoms, such as blindness or deafness, without organic cause, as an expression of psychic conflict, 914

**Convulsion/seizure:** spontaneous violent and abnormal muscular contraction or spasm of the body, 1071

due to fever, 148

*See also* Epileptic seizures

**Cooking and fire safety,** 13

**Corium** *See* Dermis

**Corn(s):** horny thickening of the cuticle common on the feet, 710, 756–57

diabetes, 771

**Cornea:** the transparent lens surface of the eye, 84

transplant, 659, 686

**Coronary:** encircling or crowning, such as the two arteries branching from the aorta and encircling the heart

**Coronary arteries and veins:** the network of arteries and veins that nourishes the muscle and tissue of the heart, 382–83

**Coronary artery disease:** fatty obstructions in the coronary vessels that nourish the heart, thus impairing adequate delivery of oxygen to heart, 424, 429–30

Coronary bypass surgery, *663*

Coronary care units, (CCU), 432–33

**Coronary insufficiency:** insufficient blood circulation through the coronary arteries

**Coronary occlusion:** closure of the coronary artery, due to buildup of fatty deposits or coronary thrombosis, 430, 1080

non-surgical treatment, 432

**Coronary thrombosis:** interference with the blood supply to the heart muscle because of a blood clot in the coronary artery

*See* Coronary occlusion; Heart attacks

**Corpus callosum:** fibrous tissue connecting the two hemispheres of the cerebrum of the brain

**Corpuscle:** one of the cells that make up blood, either a red corpuscle (*erythrocyte*) or a white corpuscle (*leukocyte*), 36

**Corpus luteum:** mass in the ovary formed by the rupture of a Graafian follicle that releases an ovum during each menstrual cycle, 74

cyst, 801

**Cortex:** the outer layer or covering of an organ or part, as of the cerebrum or cerebellum of the brain (called *gray matter*), of the adrenal glands, or of the kidneys, 502

**Corticoids:** any of the hormones manufactured in the adrenal cortex, 75

**Corticosteroid:**

1. any of the steroids secreted by the cortex of the adrenal gland

2. any steroid hormone resembling in its effects the steroids secreted by the adrenal gland, 871

**Corticosterone:** steroid hormone of the adrenal cortex associated with blood sugar levels and other metabolic functions

Cortisol, 1097

**Cortisone:** powerful hormone extracted from the adrenal cortex and also made synthetically, 75, 394, 405, 747

hair loss, 287

**Coryza:** inflamed mucous membranes in the nose, with discharge of mucus characteristic of a head cold, 397

**Cosmetic surgeon:** physician specializing in cosmetic surgery

**Cosmetic surgery:** plastic surgery concerned with improving the appearance of parts of the body, 286, 677–84

Cosmetics, 322

skin care, 694–96

**Costal:** pertaining to or near a rib or ribs

**Cough:** to expel air or phlegm from the lungs in a noisy or spasmodic manner

**Cowpox:** live calf lymph virus, used in smallpox vaccinations

**Coxa:** the hip or hip joint

**Coxa vara:** deformity of the hip joint caused by curvature of the femur toward the joint, thus shortening the affected leg and causing a limp, 368

**Coxsackie virus:** any of a group of viruses causing various diseases in humans, including a form of meningitis

Coughing, 766–67

obstructive airway disease, 492–93

*See also* Croup

Counseling,

cancer patients, 1010–11

child abuse, 129

rape victims, 822

*See also* Marriage counseling

Crabs *See* Pubic lice

Crack *See* Cocaine

**Cradle cap:** disease of the scalp, esp. in babies, marked by yellowish crusts, 133

Cramps, 788

*See also* Dysmenorrhea; Muscle cramps; Premenstrual syndrome

**Cranial nerves:** the twelve pairs of nerves that originate within the brain, *25,* 27–28

**Cranioplasty:** surgical correction of the skull, as to repair a congenital defect

**Craniotomy:** any surgery involving an opening in the skull, 675

**Cranium:** the part of the human skull that encloses and protects the brain, 13

Crash diets, 869

Crawling,

infants development, 107

Crestodes *See* Tapeworms

**Cretinism:** stunted or impaired physical and mental development due to deficiency of thryoxin, a secretion of the thyroid gland, in infancy or during the fetal period, 501

Crib death *See* Sudden Infant Death Syndrome

Cromolyn sodium, 781

**Crossed eyes/crosseye:** strabismus characterized by a tendency of the eyes to turn inward, toward the nose, 134.

Compare *walleye.*

**Cross-match:** to intermix constituents of the blood of a prospective donor with that of a prospective recipient to check blood compatibility

*See* Blood, types

**Croup:** spasm of the trachea, esp. the larynx, occurring in children and marked by difficulty in breathing and a barking cough, 134, 1071–72

**Crown:** the part of a tooth exposed beyond the gum and covered with enamel

Crying,

infancy, 107, 109

**Cryosurgery:** type of surgery in which extremely low temperatures are employed either locally or generally to destroy tissue, as in malignant skin lesions, 322, 566, 651

Cryptorchidism, 629

**Cryotherapy:** inducement of peeling by freezing the skin with carbon dioxide to improve appearance of flat acne scars and shallow wrinkles, 286

**Cryptorchidism/cryptorchism:** failure of the testicles to descend normally

*See* Testicles, undescended

CT Scanning *See* Computerized tomography

**Culdoscopy:** technique for examining the female reproductive organs within the abdominal cavity, 237

**Culture:** the development of microorganisms or living cells in a special medium, as gelatin, often as a means of analyzing a body fluid or tissue for the presence of disease

Culture plates, 779–80

**Cupula:** structure within each of the semi-circular canals of the inner ear, communicating changes in motion

**Curettage:** the scraping of a cavity with a curette, as to remove morbid matter or obtain tissue for diagnosis

**Curette:** small instrument, usu. resembling a spoon or scoop with sharpened edges, used in curettage

**Cushing's syndrome:** excess of hormones secreted by the adrenal cortex, characterized by weakness, purple streaks in the skin, and a moon face, 503, 635

**Cusp:**

1. one of the projections or points on the crown of a tooth

2. One of the triangular flaps of a heart valve

**Cuspid/canine tooth/eye tooth:** one of the two upper or two lower sharp, pointed teeth located between the incisors and the biscuspids, 720–21

**Cutaneous:** pertaining to, affecting, or on the skin

**Cuticle:**

1. epidermis

2. crescent of toughened skin around the base of a nail, 20, 22

Cuts *See* Abrasions

**Cyanosis:** disordered circulatory condition due to inadequate oxygen supply in the blood and causing a livid bluish color of the skin

**Cyanotic:** bluish in color due to cyanosis

**Cyclamates:** sodium cyclamate

Cyclophosphamide, 582

Cyclopropane

anesthetia, 613

for labor, 256

Cyclosporine, 687

**Cyclothymic/cycloid:** describing a personality disorder in which the individual is subject to sharply defined moods of elation or depression, 917

**Cynophobia:** fear of dogs

**Cysts:** saclike mass containing liquid or semi-solid material, 248–49, 634–35

breasts, 801–02

chocolate: ovarian cyst formed from misplaced endometrial tissue growing on the ovary, 801

corpus luteum: ovarian cyst formed from the fluid produced by the corpus luteum, 801

defined, 799

follicular/retention cyst: ovarian cyst formed from the contents of a Graafian follicle, 507, 800–01

reproductive/urinary system, 799–801

vaginal, 800

**Cystectomy:**

1. surgical removal of the gall bladder or of the urinary bladder

2. surgical removal of a cyst, 633

**Cystic duct:** duct that carries bile from the gallbladder to the juncture with the hepatic duct, where the common bile duct is formed, 57

**Cystic fibrosis:** hereditary disease of infants and young children marked by cysts, excessive fibrous tissue, and mucous secretion, 135–36, 245

voluntary agencies, 1011

Cystic Fibrosis Foundation, 136, 1011

**Cystitis:** inflammation of the bladder, characterized by a burning sensation when voiding, frequent need to urinate, and sometimes blood in the urine, 98, 541, 769–70, 793–94

**Cystocele:** hernia in which part of the bladder protrudes through the wall of the vagina, *797, 798*

**Cystoscope:** device used to view the interior of the bladder after being inserted in the urethra, 632, 851

**Cystoscopy:** the technique of viewing the interior of the bladder by means of a cystoscope, 570

**Cystostomy:** the making of an artificial outlet from the urinary bladder

D and C *See* Dilation and Curettage

Dalkon Shield, 265

**Dandruff:** condition marked by itching and flaking of the skin, esp. of the scalp, 699

Daydreaming, 146–47

Day hospitals, 1003

**Db** *See* Decibel

**DBI/phenformin:** drug that stimulates the production of insulin in the pancreas

**D.D.S.:** Doctor of Dental Surgery

Deafness, 91, 137, 322–24, 531

Paget's disease, 370

*See also* Hearing aids

Death,

autopsy, 344

**Dental caries/cavities:** ulceration and decay of teeth; *See* Tooth decay

**Dental floss:** strong, silky filament for cleaning between the teeth

Dental hygiene,

hemophiliacs, 410

oral cancer detection, 567

Dental insurance, 975

**Dentin:** the hard calcified substance that forms the body of a tooth, 4, 722

**Dentist:** one who specializes in the diagnosis, prevention, and treatment of disease affecting the teeth and their associated structures, 138, 839

**Dentistry:** the branch of medical science that concerns the study, diagnosis, prevention, and treatment of diseases of the teeth, gums, and associated structures, 839

children, 172–73

**Dentition:** the kind, number, and arrangement of the teeth in the mouth

**Denture(s):** frame of plastic or other material adapted to fit the mouth and containing one, several, or a complete set of artificial teeth to replace natural teeth that have been lost, 314, 736–39

care, 738–39

complete, 738

eating problems, 316

fitting, 736

partial, 737

Deordorants, 693–94

Deoxyribonucleic acid, 513

**Depilatory:** chemical product capable of removing or loosening hair, 205–06, 704

**Depressant:** drug or other substance that reduces or calms the physiological processes of body or mind, 939, 942–43

Compare *stimulant.*

**Depression:**

1. mental state marked by melancholy, pessimism, or dejection

2. psychotic condition characterized by stuporous withdrawal from reality and intense guilt feelings, 913

herpes attacks, 551

*See also* Suicide

**Depressive reaction:**

1. neurosis characterized by persistent feelings of depression and pessimism unrelated to any apparent cause

2. (involutional melancholia) psychosis usu. occurring in women around the time of menopause, and in men during their 50s, characterized by hopeless melancholy, anxiety, weeping, and often delusions, 915, 919, 920

**Dermabrasion:** the removal of layers of skin by planing with an abrasive tool to dispose of wrinkles or skin blemishes, 286, 322

**Dermal:** of or relating to the skin

**Dermatitis:** inflammation of the skin,

contact: dermatitis caused by a hypersensitive reaction to external contact with a substance or material

**Dermatologist:** physician specializing in the diagnosis and treatment of disorders of the skin, 826, 840

**Dermatology:** the branch of medical science dealing with disorders of the skin

**Dermis/corium/true skin:** the inner layer of the skin, which contains blood vessels, nerves, connective tissue, sweat glands, and sebaceous glands, 20, 690

Desensitization *See* Hyposensitization

Desert rheumatism *See* Coccidioidomycosis

Destructiveness, 138–39

**Detached retina/separated retina:** eye disorder in which the membrane at the back of the eye (retina) is separated from its bed, as by being torn, thus impairing vision, 526, 660, 1239

laser surgery, 606

Development *See* Behavior

**Developmental disability:** any condition which interferes with a child's development, esp. one which will constitute a handicap throughout the individual's life, such as mental retardation or cerebral palsy, 139

Dexamethasone, 1095

**Dextroamphetamine (d-amphetamine)/Dexedrine:** isomer of the amphetamine compound, considered to have a more stimulating effect on the central nervous system than amphetamine, 940, 1095

**Dextrose:** form of glucose (a sugar) found normally in animals, used in intravenous feeding because it is readily assimilated by the blood

**Diabetes, chemical/prediabetic condition:** condition indicating predisposition to development of diabetes, when blood sugar level remains abnormally high for too long after taking a glucose tolerance test, 521

**Diabetes insipidus:** production of excessive amount of urine due to deficiency of antidiuretic hormone, 508, 509

**Diabetes mellitus:** disease associated with inadequate production of insulin and characterized by excessive urinary secretion containing abnormal amounts of sugar, accompanied by emaciation, excessive hunger, and thirst, 76–77, 139, 327–28, 509–21

aging, 520–21

bladder infections, 541

blisters, 1064

boils, 1064–65

Caesarian section, 258

carbuncles, 1068

in children, 519–20

control of the disease, 517–19

diagnosis, 512

eyesight, 528

foot care, 771–72

hair loss, 287

impotence, 302

insulin shock, 515

kidney failure, 535

life long adjustments, 518–19

nephrosis, 540

pancreatic cancer, 575

skin disorders, 710

special diets, 674

symptoms, 328

tuberculosis, 480

voluntary agencies, 1012

weight control, 750

weight of newborns, 102

**Diabetic:** one who has diabetes

**Diabetic acidosis:** advanced stage of diabetes treated with insufficient insulin, characterized by increasing buildup of ketone bodies, drowsiness, and, if untreated, coma, 511, 517

Compare *diabetic ketosis.*

**Diabetic coma:** state of unconsciousness in a diabetic resulting from insufficient insulin, characterized by deep, labored breathing and fruity odor to the breath, 517, 1072–73

Diabetic gangrene, 420–21

**Diabetic ketosis:** early stage of diabetes treated with insufficient insulin, characterized by excessive urination, thirst, and hot, dry skin, 577

Compare *diabetic acidosis.*

**Diabetic retinopathy:** disease of the eye associated with diabetes in which new, abnormal blood vessels form on the surface of the retina, sometimes marked by bleeding, 660

**Diacetylmorphine** *See* Heroin

**Diagnosis:** Identification of a disease or disorder by its characteristic symptoms, or the conclusions reached in a particular instance

Diagnostic procedures, 796, 823

    chart of home tests, 854

    home tests, 955

    insurance payment, 977

    patient's rights, 853

    physical examination, 829

    tests, 853

**Dialysis:** the separating of mixed substances by means of wet membranes, as the action of the kidneys, esp. applied to an artificial process to remove waste products and excess fluid from the bloodstream of a patient with defective kidneys, 536–37, *537,* 687

    home-based, 536–37

    Medicare coverage, 537

**Diaper rash:** rash caused by the ammonia produced by the urine in diapers, 179

    *See also* Chafing

Diaphanography, 815

Diphenhydramine, 1096

**Diaphragm:**

    1. dome-shaped layer of muscle between the chest and abdomen whose contraction enlarges the rib cage for inflation of the lungs in breathing, 64–66, *65,* 472

    2. contraceptive device of molded rubber or soft plastic material used to cover the cervix and prevent entry of spermatoza, 267

**Diphragmatic hernia** *See* Hernia, hiatus

**Diarrhea:** frequent and fluid evacuation of feces, 139–40, 456–57, 461, 764, 1073

    colitis, 463–64

    enteritis, 463

    hookworms, 466

**Diastole:** the instant when the heart is relaxed as the ventricles fill with blood prior to contraction and pumping (systole), 44

**Diastolic pressure:** measure of blood pressure taken when the heart is resting, the lower of the two figures in a reading, 438, 833

**Diathermy:** treatment by means of heat generated within the body by high-frequency radiation

**Diacetylmorphine:** heroin

Diazepam, 943, 1095

Dicyclomine, 1095

Diets,

    acne, 206–07, 715–16

    adolescent eating habits, 206, 207–10

    alcohol, 295

    basic food groups, 314–15

    basic nutrition requirements, 859–62

    bland: diet that is not irritating or abrasive, as the diet recommended for peptic ulcer patients, 620–21

    bone disorders, 371

    constipation, 892

    Daily Food Guide, 892

    dental care, 108, 725–26, 739

    disease prevention, 876–77

    diabetic children, 519–20

    diabetics, 512–13

    elimination diet, 780

    gastrointestinal disease, 471

    hair loss, 287

    heart disease, 325, 436–37

    home care patients, 991

**Disinfectants:** germicides, 993–94

Disk,

  slipped/herniating disk: painful displacement (herniation) of one of the fibrous disks of the spinal column between two vertebrae, such that it presses against nerves and may cause sciatica, 365–66, 667–68

**Dislocation(s):** the partial or completed displacement of one or more of the bones at a joint, 372

  hips, 346–48

  jaw, 377–78

**Displacement:** transference of intense anxiety unconsciously felt about a particular conflict to a substitute, which is regarded consciously with the same intensity of anxiety, a manifestation of the phobic reaction

  *See* Phobic reactions

**Dissociative reaction:** neurosis characterized by escape from a part of the personality by means of dream states, amnesia, forgetfulness, etc., 916

**Distal:** relatively remote from the center of the body, or from a point considered as central. Compare *proximal.*

**Distal muscles:** the muscles of the extremities (the hands and the feet)

Distal muscular dystrophy, 403

**Distillation:** separation of the more volatile parts of a substance from the less volatile by boiling and condensing the vapors into separate liquids

**Diuretic(s):** substance stimulating the secretion of urine, 440, 447, 540, 755

**Diuresis:** excessive excretion of urine, 533

**Diverticulitis:** inflammation of diverticula in the digestive tract, esp. in the colon, 461

**Diverticula** *(sing., diverticulum):* pouches or sacs opening off the large intestine, 461

**Diverticulosis:** the presence of diverticula in the digestive tract, 461, *461*

Diverticulosis, 461, *461*

**Diverticulum** *(pl. diverticula):* abnormal pouch or bulge protruding from an organ or part, as from the colon of the intestines

Divorce, 307–09

  adoption of children, 117–18

  early marriage, 261

  runaways, 183–84

  visitation, 147

Dizziness, 1073

DMSO *See* Dimethylsulfoxide

DMT (dimethyltryptamine), 951

**DNA** *(deoxyribonucleic acid):* chemical in the human cell that controls body development

DOM, 952

**Dopamine:** chemical compound found in the brain, needed in the synthesis of norepinephrine and epinephrine

**Dorsal:** toward, near, or in the back.

  Compare *ventral.*

**Double vision/diplopia:** condition in which a single object is perceived as two images due to inability to coordinate focusing of the eyes

**Douching:** flushing of a body part or cavity, esp. the vagina, with water as a means of cleansing, 269

**Down's syndrome/Mongolism:** congenital mental and physical retardation due to a chromosomal anomaly, accompanied by variable signs including a flat face and pronounced epicanthic folds, 168, 245, 912

**Down/downers/goof balls** *(slang):* barbiturates or other drugs that depress the central nervous system

*See also* Peptic ulcer.

**Duodenum:** the first section of the small intestine, leading from the stomach to the jejunum, 54–55, 449

**Dura mater:** the tough, fibrous, outermost membrane of the three membranes covering the brain and spinal cord

Dust,

pneumoconiosis, 495–96

**Dwarfism:** disorder characterized by stunted growth, 73, 501

**Dysentery:** severe inflammation of the mucous membrane of the large intestine, characterized by bloody stools, pain, cramps, and fever, 457

**Dysfunction:** impairment or abnormal functioning, as of an organ

**Dyslexia:**

1. impairment or loss of the ability to read, as from a stroke

2. in children, impairment of ability to acquire language skills due to motor or perceptual disabilities, 143

*See also* Reading

**Dysmenorrhea:** painful menstruation, 786–87, 788

**Dyspareunia:** painful sexual intercourse, 791, 800, 801, 805

**Dyspepsia:** indigestion, characterized by heartburn, nausea, pain in the upper abdomen, and belching, 454, 876

**Dysphagia:** difficulty in swallowing 454

**Dysphasia:** disorder of the cerebral centers characterized by difficulty in understanding or using speech

**Dyspnea:** labored, difficult breathing

**Dystrophy:**

1. defective or faulty nutrition

2. any of various neurological or muscular disorders, as muscular dystrophy

**Dysuria:** difficult, painful, or incomplete urination, 533, 794

Earache, 143–44, 1074–75

diagnosis, 144

**Eardrum/tympanic membrane/tympanum:** drumhead membrane separating the middle ear from the external ear,

*See* Tympanic membrane

Ear infections, 769

adenoidectomy, 654

colds, 475

Ears, 81, 87–91, *88*

blockage, 769

common disorders, 769

diseases, 528–31

disorders, 655–56, 657

draining fluid, 144

examination, 834

foreign body in, 1075

infections, 143–44, 529–30

injury, 530

pressure, 88

reduction in size, 683

ringing, 531

sound perception, *89*

surgery, 655–56

vertigo, 531

**Earwax:** waxy substance secreted by the glands lining the passages of the external ear, 529, 769

Easter Seal Society, 1002

Eating, 46–50, *52*

alimentary canal, *450*

*See also* Digestive system

Eating disorders, 210

Eating habits, 856

childhood, 879–80

elderly, 316–17

exercise program, 1111

home care patients, 991

middle years, 296–98

psychological aspects, 879–81

weight reduction, 870–71

**ECG:** electrocardiogram

**Echocardiogram:** graph recording the pattern of deflection of sound waves by the heart, used in diagnosing heart abnormalities, 842, 844

**Eclampsia:** toxemia of pregnancy involving convulsions, 241. *See also* Toxemia of pregnancy.

**E. coli/Escherichia coli:** common bacillus found normally in the human intestine, usu. harmless but having certain strains that cause urinary tract and other infections

**ECPR/external cardiopulmonary resuscitation:** closed-chest massage, used for those suffering cardiac arrest, 434–35

**Ectoderm:** outermost layer of tissue

**Ectopic/atopic:** out of normal place or position

**Ectopic pregnancy:** abortive pregnancy outside the uterus, as in the Fallopian tubes or abdominal cavity, 248, 265

**Eczema:** noncontagious skin condition characterized by itching and scaling of the skin, 708, 777

children, 179–80

hay fever, 484

**Edema:** swelling of tissues due to abnormal fluid accumulation, 100, 419, 533, 539

congestive heart failure, 446

kala-azar, 594

kidney failure, 536

nephrosis, 540

pregnancy, 241

**Edentulous:** toothless

Education, 185–86

beyond high school, 222

grades, 150–51

mainstreaming, 152

middle aged women, 303–04

EEG *See* Electroencephalogram

**Efferent:** applied to nerves, communicating impulses so that directive action can be taken; motor. Compare *afferent*.

**Egg cell:** ovum

Egg donation, 238

**Ego:** the self, considered as the seat of consciousness, 911

**Ejaculation:** expulsion of semen during orgasm, 228, *235*

EKG *See* Electrocardiogram

Elastic stockings, 243, 289, 419, 497, 760

Elbows, 7

**Elective surgery:** surgery that is not essential for the maintenance of physical health, as cosmetic surgery, 604–05

**Electra complex:** repressed sexual attachment of daughter to father, analogous to the Oedipal complex involving the son and mother,

**Electric shock:** the body's reactions to the passage through it of an electric current, as involuntary muscular contractions, 1075

Electrical safety, 1042–44

**Electrocardiogram/ECG/EKG:** graph recording the pattern of electric impulses produced by the heart, used in the diagnosis of heart disease, 433, 439, 835–36, *835,* 843–44

**Electrocardiograph:** machine used to record the electric current produced by the heart muscle

**Electrocardiography:** technique of producing electrocardiograms and interpreting them, 433

**Electroencephalogram/EEG:** graph recording the pattern of electric impulses produced by the brain, used in the diagnosis of neurological disorders, 331, 382, 391, 842

**Electroencephalograph:** machine used to record the electric current produced by the brain

**Electroencephalography:** technique of producing electroencephalograms and interpreting them

**Electrolysis:** technique for removing unwanted hair by destroying the hair root with an electric current, 205–06, 288, 704–05

**Electromyogram/EMG:** graph recording the electrical activity of a muscle, 402

**Electromyography:** technique of producing electromyograms and interpreting them, 669, 839–40

**Electroshock:** describing a form of treatment for psychological disorders in which a controlled electric current is passed through the patient's head, producing convulsions and unconsciousness, usu. given in series, 924–25

**Electrosurgery/surgical diathermy:** surgical procedure utilizing electricity to destroy tissue, 322

**Elephantiasis:** lymphatic edema, esp. of the legs and scrotum, a symptom of filariasis, 597

ELISA test *See* Blood tests

Elderly,

adult day care, 1003

aging skin, 692

diabetes, 520–21

home nursing care, 982, 1002–03

housing, 339–42

influenza, 476

kidney failure, 536

Medicare insurance, 979–80

nutrition, 862, 1004

pneumonia, 477

prostatic enlargement, 544–45

specialized agencies, 1023

surgery, 623–24

*See also* Aging

**Embolism:** the stopping up of a vein or artery, as by a blood clot, that has been brought to the point of obstruction by the bloodstream, 422–23

phlebitis, 666

pulmonary: embolism in the pulmonary artery or one of its branches,

**Embolus:** object moving within the bloodstream, as a blood clot or air bubble, that is capable of causing an obstruction (embolism) in a smaller vessel, 418, 421

atherosclerosis, *420*

**Embryo:** the rudimentary form of an organism in its development before birth, usu. considered in the human species to be the first two months in utero,

Embryo adoption (EA), 238

Emergencies, 1036–55

babysitters, 122

calling a physician, 1056

guide to common medical emergencies, 1058–91

moving an injured person, 1056–57,

numbers to call for help, 1035, 1036, 1056

respiratory arrest, 1025–26

surgery, 603

Emergency care centers, 999

Emergency medicine, 826

**Emetic:** medicine or substance used to induce vomiting

Emotional development,

aging, 311–12

bedwetting, 546–47

boredom, 123

children, 118, 119, 120, 121

communication needs, 909–10

dishonesty, 141

friendships, 149–50

frustration, 150

guilt, 910

identity, 221–24

middle age, 642–43

negativism in toddlers, 111

sexual compatibility, 262

sexual inadequacy, 302

sexual maturity, 225–28

suicide, 219–20

teenagers, 221–25

Emotionally disturbed *See* Mental illness

Emotional disorders, 909–25

treatment, 920–25

working mothers, 271–73

Emotional effects,

diabetes, 518–19

hospitalization fears, 157–58

joint diseases, 360–61

pituitary gland, 500

Emotional well-being *See* Mental health

**Emphysema:** puffed condition of the alveoli or air sacs of the lung (or other tissues or organs) due to infiltration of air and consequent loss of tissue elasticity, 93, 491–93, *492,* 563–64

enzyme deficiencies, 494–95

smoking, 488

**Enamel:** the layer of hard, glossy material forming the exposed outer covering of the teeth, 4, 721–22

**Encephalitis:** inflammation of the brain, 31, 395–96

**Encephalogram:** X-ray picture of the brain made by encephalography

**Encephalography:** X-ray visualization of the brain following the removal of cerebrospinal fluid and its replacement with air or other gases

**Endarterectomy:** surgical procedure in which carbon dioxide is forced through hardened arteries to ream out fatty blockages, 429–30

**Endemic:** confined to or characteristic of a given locality, as a disease

**Endocarditis:** inflammation of the membrane (endocardium) lining the chambers of the heart, sometimes caused by bacteria, 443–44, *443,* 730

bacterial: bacterial infection of the membrane (endocardium) lining the chambers of the heart

gonorrhea, 550

subacute bacterial: bacterial endocarditis resulting as a complication of rheumatic fever, usu. fatal

**Endocardium:** the delicate membrane that lines the chambers of the heart, 43

**Endocrine gland:** one of several ductless glands that release secretions (hormones) directly into the blood or lymph and that exert powerful influences on growth, sexual development, metabolism, and other vital body processes, 70–80, *70,* 498, 499,

diseases, 498–508

diagnosing diseases, 850–51

function, 71

premature aging, 277

slipped epiphysis, 368

**Endocrinologist:** physician specializing in endocrinology, 825

**Endocrinology:** the branch of medical science dealing with the structure and function of the endocrine glands and their hormones, 71, 825

**Endoderm:** innermost layer of tissue

**Endodontics:** branch of dentistry dealing with root canal work and the dental pulp, 732

**Endodontist:** dentist specializing in root canal work

**Endogenous insulin:** self-produced insulin

**Endolymph:** fluid within the semicircular canals of the inner ear,

**Endometrial:** of or pertaining to the endometrium

Endometrial cancer, 809–11

Endometrial polyps, 803

**Endometrioma:** mass of tumorlike endometrial cells as a result of endometriosis, 804

**Endometriosis:** condition in which tissue that lines the uterus (endometrium) grows outside the uterus in the pelvic cavity, 804–05

**Endometrium:** the lining of the uterus, 246

**Endoscope:** instrument for examining a hollow organ or an internal cavity, as the urinary bladder or the urethra

**Endoscopy:** examination with an endoscope

**Enema:** liquid injected into the rectum as a purgative or for diagnostic purposes, 765

home care patients, 990–91

pre-operative procedures, 609

Energy,

role of adrenaline, 74–75

**ENT:** otolaryngology (ear, nose and throat)

**Enteric:** pertaining to the intestines

Enteric fever *See* Typhoid

**Enteritis:** inflammation of the intestines, esp. of the small intestine, 463

**Enterocele:** hernia in which part of the small intestine protrudes through the wall of the vagina, 797, 798,

**Enuresis/bed-wetting:** involuntary urination during sleep at night, 546–47

Environment,

effect on health, 956–57

Environmental Protection Agency (EPA), 956–57

**Enzymes:** organic substance, usu. a protein, produced by cells and having the power to initiate or accelerate specific chemical reactions in metabolism, such as digestion

digestive system, 53

fibrinolysin, 409

thrombin, 409

**Eosinophil:** any of a type of white blood cell that stains easily when a particular red dye (eosin) is applied, 774

**Ephedrine:** drug that dilates the bronchi, used to reduce nasal congestion and relieve asthma, 747, 1096

**Epicanthic fold/epicanthus:** vertical fold of skin at the inner corner of the eyelid, found chiefly in certain Asian peoples

**Epidemiologist:** physician specializing in epidemiology

**Epidemic:**

1. *(adj.)* affecting many in a community at once, as a disease, 690

2. *(n.)* the temporary prevalence of a disease in a community or throughout a large area

**Epigastrium:** the upper middle (epigastric) part of the abdomen.

**Epigastric:** pertaining to the upper middle part of the abdomen

Epigastric pain, 463

**Epididymis:** portion of the seminal ducts just above the testis,

**Epidermis/cuticle:** the outer, nonvascular layer of the skin, overlying the dermis, 20, 21

**Epidemiology:** the branch of medical science concerned with the study and prevention of epidemic diseases

**Epiglottis:** the leaf-shaped plate of cartilage at the base of the tongue that covers the trachea during the act of swallowing, 50

**Epileptic:**

1. *(adj.)* pertaining to epilepsy

2. *(n.)* person who has epilepsy

Epileptic seizures, 1075–76

   focal, 389–90

   grand mal, 388–89

   petit mal, 389

   psychomotor, 390–91

**Epilepsy:** chronic nervous disorder characterized by sudden loss of consciousness and sometimes by convulsions, 144–45, 387–93

   causes, 387–88

   diagnosed, 392

   stress reduction, 391–92

   treatment, 391–92

   types of seizures, 388–90

   voluntary agencies, 1021

Epilepsy Foundation of America, 388, 393, 1021

Epinephrine, 503

**Epiphysis:** cartilage plate on the extremity of a long bone, 205

   slipped: the slipping or dislocation of the end of a bone (epiphysis), as of the femur at the hip joint,

**Episiotomy:** incision made during labor to enlarge the vaginal area enough to permit passage of the baby, 256

**Epistaxis:** nosebleed

**Epithelial:** pertaining to the epithelium

**Epithelium:** membranous tissue that lines the canals, cavities, and ducts of the body, as well as all free surfaces exposed to the air, 561

Equilin, 1096

**Erection:** enlarged and firm state of the penis when sexually stimulated, 228

Ergotamine, 1096

**Eruption:**

1. emergence of a tooth through the gums

2. a breaking out of a rash on the skin

**Erysipelas:** acute bacterial skin infection characterized by bright red patches, 713

**Erythema:** redness of the skin, a symptom occurring in various forms in different conditions having various causes, as from infection or a burn

**Erythremia:** polycythemia vera,

Erythrityl, 1096

**Erythrocyte/red blood cell/red corpuscle:** cell found in the bloodstream, often lacking a nucleus, the carrier of the hemoglobin, 36, 411, 837

Erthromycin, 549, 550, 1096

**Erythrophobia:** fear of blushing

Erythrophobia, 916

**Eschar:** dry crust or scab left by a burn caused by heat or corrosive chemical action

**Esophagoscope:** device inserted into the esophagus to permit its inspection, 847

**Esophagus (gullet):** the tube through which food passes from the mouth to the stomach, 50, 66, 448, 452–54

Essential hypertension *See* Hypertension, causes

Estrin, 247

**Estrogen:** any of several hormones found in the ovarian fluids of the female which promote growth of secondary sex characteristics and influence cyclical changes in the female reproductive system, 79, 202, 505, 788, 1096

cancer, 810

excess, 506

osteoporosis, 369

replacement therapy, 506

Estrone, 1096

**Ethanol:** ethyl alcohol

Ethchlorrynol, 944

**Ether:** colorless, volatile, flammable chemical compound used as an anesthetic,

Ethinamate, 944

**Ethmoid bone:** sievelike bone at the base of the skull behind the nose, 91

**Ethyl alcohol/grain alcohol/ethanol:** product of the distillation of fermented grains, fruit juices, and starches, used in beverages, and having intoxicating properties, made unfit to drink, used industrially and as a disinfectant, 927

**Etiologist:** physician specializing in studying the causes of disease

**Etiology:**

1. the cause of causes of a disease
2. the branch of medical science dealing with the causes of disease

**Eunuchs:** in males, the failure at puberty to develop secondary sex characteristics due to disorder or removal of testicles, 504

**Eustachian tube:** passage connecting the middle ear to the upper throat which equalizes air pressure on both sides of the eardrum, 88, 531

colds, 475

**Ewing's sarcoma:** malignant tumor of the shafts of the long bones in children, 372

Examination,

gynecological, 782–84

physical, 827–39

**Excision:** act or procedure of cutting out or removing surgically

**Excise:** cut out or remove by surgery

**Excrete:** to eliminate, as waste matter, by normal discharge from the body

**Excretion:**

1. the act of excreting
2. the body's waste matter, as sweat, urine, and feces

Exercise, 278–81

arthritis patients, 354–55

backache, 367

chart, *1167–78*

children, 145, 1196–97

cool-down period, 1118–19

diabetes, 511, 518

dieting, 871

elderly, 317–19

feet, 283–84, 772

five-minute routines, 1129

flexibility and balance, 1142–43

gynecological problems, 1190

heart attack prevention, 437

heart disease, 325, 437

hernia prevention, 18

male vs female abilities, 1189–90

muscular strength, 1143

obesity, 866

osteoarthritis, 351

osteoporosis, 369

pregnancy and postpartum, 1190, 1193

preteens, 1197, *1198–1203*, 1201–04

post-op patients, 1183–88

quitting smoking, 293–94

for specific muscles, *1132–41*

stretching and pulling, 1124–25

stress relief, 1122–25

teenagers, 210–12

to avoid, 1149, 1151, *1149–50*

varicose veins, 760

warm-up period, 1114, *1115–17,* 1118

weight control, 298, 868–69

*See also* Calisthenics

Exercise equipment, 1110

homemade, *1108*

**Exocrine gland;** any of various glands, such as mammary or sebaceous glands, having ducts that carry their secretions to specific locations, 71, 498. Compare *endocrine gland.*

**Exophthalmic goiter:** hyperthyroidism

**Expectorant:** medicine that promotes the discharge of mucus from the respiratory tract

**Expectorate:** discharge from the mouth, as saliva or phlegm

**Exploratory:** performed for the purpose of making a diagnosis: said of a surgical operation

Extended wear lenses *See* Contact lenses

**Extensor:** muscle whose function is to extend or straighten a part of the body,

**Extension:** state of being extended or straightened,

**External cardiac massage:** cardiac massage

External cardiopulmonary resuscitation (ECPR), 434–35

Extracapsular extraction, 658

**Extraction:** surgical removal of a tooth from the mouth

**Extrinsic:** originating or situated outside an organ or part

**Exudate:** substance filtered through the walls of living cellular tissue, sometimes as a result of disease or

injury, as in the case of inflammation

Eye surgery,

cataract, *525*

corneal transplant, *525*

glaucoma, *525*

retinal detachment, *525*

Eyes, 46 47, 81, 82–87, *82, 523*

"black eye" injuries, 1062–63

color, 691

crossed, 134

diagnostic procedures, 850

diseases, 522–31

disorders, 768

drainage, 87

elderly, 327

examination, 834

focusing, *85, 523*

foreign body in, 1076

infections, 526–27

injuries, 526–27

inflammation, 355

light into vision, 82–83

muscles, *86*

strabismus, 657

structure, 85–86

voluntary agencies, 1012–13

Eyeglasses, 146–47, 524

**Eyeground:** the inner side of the back of the eyeball

Eyelids,

cosmetic surgery, 683

Eyesight *See* Vision

**Eyestrain:** disorder caused by excessive or improper use of the eyes and characterized by fatigue, tearing, redness, and a scratchy feeling in the eyelids, 768

headaches, 748, 749

**Eye teeth:** the upper canine teeth; *See* Cuspids

Face,

birth defects, 346

injury, 377–78

Face lifts *See* Cosmetic surgery; Rhytidoplasty

**Facial canal:** Fallopian canal

Facial nerve,

paralysis *See* Bell's palsy

Facial neuralgia *See* Neuralgia

**Facial plasty:** rhytidoplasty, 286

Facio-scapula-humoral muscular dystrophy, 403

**Fainting:** brief loss of consciousness, 761

*See also* Neurogenic shock

Fallen arches, 755

**Fallopian canal/facial canal:** bony canal in the skull

**Fallopian tubes:** the pair of tubes connecting the ovaries and the uterus, through which the egg must pass at the time of ovulation, 229,

sterilization, 269–70

Family planning,

voluntary agencies, 1013–14

*See also* Birth control

Family practice physician, 826

Family relationships, 304–06

fathers, 147

grandparents, 151

working mothers, 271–73

**Family therapy:** form of group therapy in which the patient group are members of the same family, 923

Fantasies, 146–47

**Farsightedness/hypermetropia/hyperopia:** inability to see nearby objects clearly, 84

*See also* Hyperopia

**Fascia:** fibrous tissue in the form of sheets that connect, surround, and support muscles and organs of the body

**Fascitis:** inflammation of the fascia

Fat,

modified diet, 902–04

modified diet, menus, 904

removal of excess, 681–82

restricted diet (chart), 905–06

restricted diet, menus, 902–06

**Fats:** chemical compound forming an important food reserve and a source of hormones, vitamins, and other products essential in metabolism, 857–58

**Fat pad:** mass of fatty tissue

Fathers, 147

participation in childbirth, 257

single, 310

*See also* Parenting

Fatigue, 282

infertility, 232

physical activity, 1112

**FDA:** Food and Drug Administration

Fears,

children, 147, 157–58

infants, 109

toddlers, 112–13

blushing *See* Erythrophobia,

cats *See* Ailurophobia,

dark *See* Nyctophobia,

dirt and contamination *See* Mysophobia,

dogs *See* Cynophobia,

germs *See* Bacteriophobia,

heights *See* Acrophobia,

insanity *See* Lyssophobia,

open spaces *See* Agoraphobia,

pain *See* Algophobia,

strangers *See* Xenophobia,

*See also* Phobias

**Febrile:** feverish

Fecal blood test,

home test, 855

**Feces/stool:** animal waste discharged following a bowel movement, usu. containing indigestible foods, bacteria, bile, and mucus, 45, 60, 450

Feeding new babies *See* Breastfeeding; Bottlefeeding

Feet, 329

ailments, 284–85, 329

blisters, 755–56

bones, *8*

bunions, 756

calluses, 756

care, 149, 282–83

corns, 756–57

exercises, 283–84

fallen arches, 755

flat feet, 755

plantar warts, 714

shoes, 282–83, 284–85

**Femur:** the long bone that supports the thigh; the thigh bone, *7, 15*

Fenoprofen, 353

**Fermentation:** the conversion of glucose into ethyl alcohol, esp. through the action of an enzyme (zymase) found in yeast, 927

Fertility,

Froehlich's syndrome, 504

tests for, 233–37

*See also* Infertility

Fertility cycles, 234

Fertilization, 229, *236*

Fetal development,

diet, 239

Fetal position,

lightening, 252–53

**Fetus:** organism developing in the uterus before birth, sometimes considered in the human species to begin with the third month in utero, prior to which is called an embryo

**Fever/pyrexia:** body temperature above the normal, 1076–77

children, 148

common cold, 474–75

hair loss, 287

home nursing care, 986

kidney infections, 542

nausea, 170

rheumatoid arthritis, 352–53

roseola, 180

stomach aches, 190

tonsillitis, 195

urinary infections, 196

Fever blisters *See* Herpes simplex

**Fiberoptic:** consisting of or making use of fibers of glass or plastic, as in optical instruments designed for viewing the intestines or stomach

Fiberoptic instruments, 847

**Fibrillation:** irregular, uncoordinated contraction (arrhythmia) of muscle fibers of the heart

**Fibrin:** insoluble protein that forms an interlacing network of fibers in clotting blood, 409

**Fibrinogen:** complex protein found in plasma which, in combination with the enzyme thrombin, forms fibrin, 409

**Fibrinolysin:** enzyme present in the blood that liquefies fibrin, thus dissolving blood clots, 409

Fibroid tumors, 237, 247, 289, 803–04

**Fibroma:** benign tumor composed of fibrous connective tissue

**Fibula:** the outer of the two bones of the lower leg,

Daily Food Guide, 892

measurer in metric, *880*

use of insecticides, 969

Food additives, 877, 967–68

Food and Drug Administration, 938

**Food chain:** the relationship of organisms considered as food sources or consumers or both, as the relationship of a flowering plant to a bee to a bird

Food contaminates, 876–77

Food measures,

chart, 880

**Food poisoning:** digestive disorder marked by nausea and vomiting, caused by bacteria found in decaying or rancid food, 467–68, 876–77, 968, 1077–78, 1053–55

*See also* Botulism

Food storage, 877, 1053–55

**Food tube** *See* Esophagus

**Foot doctor:** podiatrist,

**Foot drop:** condition in which the foot drops when extended in stepping forward, as caused by paralysis of a leg muscle

**Foramen:** natural aperture or passage, as in a bone, 723

Foramen, 723

**Forceps:** two-bladed instrument for grasping and compressing or pulling, various types of which are used by dentists and surgeons

**Forensic medicine/forensic pathology:** subspecialty of pathology dealing with the various aspects of medicine and the law

**Forensic pathology:** forensic medicine

Foreplay, 263

**Foreskin:** the loose skin (prepuce) covering the head of the penis

*See also* Prepuce

Formula (baby): *See* Bottlefeeding

**Fossa:** pit or depression in a surface

Foster Grandparent Program, 334

**Fovea:** shallow rounded depression in the retina, directly in the line of vision at a point where vision is most acute, 83

**Fractures:** break in a bone, 9, 1078–79

decompression of spinal injuries, 379

diet with, 622

healing, 374

metal plate, *375*

skull, 676–77

treatment, 374–75

types, 373, *373*

use of internal appliances, 671, *672*

*See* Closed fracture, Complete fracture, Incomplete fracture

**Fraternal twins:** twins who are not identical, derived from separately fertilized ova, 196

**Freckle:** small, brownish or dark-colored spot on the skin, 717

**Free association:** psychoanalytic technique in which the patient talks freely about anything that comes to mind, 923

Freebase, 942

**Freezing of skin:** cryosurgery

**Freud, Sigmund:** Austrian neurologist (1856–1939) who founded psychoanalysis and shaped the course of modern psychiatry, 911, 923

Friends, 149–50

teenagers, 224–25

**Frigidity:** sexual unresponsiveness in women, 264, 301–02

**Froehlich's syndrome:** failure of secondary sex characteristics to develop in males due to anterior pituitary disease, 504

**Frontal lobe:** the front portion of each cerebral hemisphere of the brain, whose functions are uncertain,

**Frontal lobotomy:** rarely performed surgical operation of cutting into the frontal lobes of the brain to alter behavior

**Frostbite:** partial freezing of a part of the body, esp. of the extremities or ears, 709, 753–54, 1079

**Fructose/levulose:** very sweet crystalline sugar, 296

**FSH:** follicle-stimulating hormone, 74

**Fulguration:** destruction of tissue, esp. malignant growths, by electric cautery, 571

**Functional:**

1. able to function, esp. in spite of structural defect

2. affecting performance, as an illness, but lacking any verifiable physical basis

Functional addiction, 939

**Functional hypertension:** hypertension, essential

**Fundus:** the rounded base or bottom of any hollow organ

Fungal arthritis, 359

**Fungi:** any of a group of plants including the mushrooms, molds, yeasts, and various microorganisms, some of which cause diseases in human beings

infections, 710–11

respiratory diseases, 482–83

**Funnel chest/pectus excavatum:** congenital deformity in which the sternum is depressed

Gait, 832–33

**Galactosemia:** hereditary condition affecting infants who lack an enzyme that converts galactose (a sugar) into glucose in the blood

**Gall bladder/cholecyst:** small pear-shaped pouch situated beneath the liver that serves as a reservoir for bile, 56

diet following surgery, 621

digestion, 450

surgery, 646–48

Gall bladder disease, 470–71

attacks, 1079

**Gallstone(s):** solid substance formed in the gall bladder that can obstruct the flow of bile and prevent the digestion of fats, 470–71, 646–47, 648

jaundice, 469

**Gamete:** either of two mature reproductive cells, an ovum or sperm cell

Gamma camera, 432

**Gamma globulin:** component of blood serum which contains various antibodies

**Ganglion** *(pl., ganglia):* 30

1. cluster of nerve cells outside of the central nervous system

2. cyst of a tendon, as on the wrist,

**Gangrene:** death of tissues in a part of the body, caused by lack of adequate blood supply, 373, 410, 771

diabetic, 420, 521

Gardening,

leisure for senior citizens, 332

Gas (indigestion), 455

Gas poisoning, 1079–80

**Gastrectomy:** surgical removal of all or part of the stomach

**Gastric analysis:** extraction and study of gastric juices, 847

**Gastric juices:** the acid fluid secreted by the glands lining the stomach, containing several enzymes, 460

anemia, 412

**Gastric ulcer:** ulcer of the mucous membrane of the stomach, 460, 638–39, 640

*See also* Ulcers

**Gastritis:** inflammation of the stomach, 463, 763–64

acute: sudden, sharp attack of gastritis,

chronic: recurrent and persisting attacks of gastritis, 763–64

toxic: gastritis caused by the swallowing of a poisonous substance, 763

Gastrectomy, 639–40

**Gastrocnemius:** the large muscle at the back of the calf of the leg

Gastroduodenal fiberscope, 847

**Gastroenteritis:** inflammation of the mucous membrane that lines the stomach and intestines, 764

**Gastroenterologist:** physician specializing in the diagnosis and treatment of gastrointestinal disorders, 825, 847

**Gastroenterology:** the branch of medical science dealing with the study of the stomach and intestines and the disorders affecting them, 825

Gastrointestinal disorders, 471, 880

special diets, 874–75

Gastrointestinal series (GI Series), 471, 847

Gastrointestinal tract, 448

small intestine, 53–56

sphincters, 51

*See also* Digestive system

**Gastroscope:** device that allows inspection of the interior of the stomach, 847

**Gastroscopy:** examination of the stomach with a gastroscope, 568

**Genitals/genitalia:** the reproductive organs, 204

**Genitourinary tract** *See* urinogenital tract,

**Genus:** class or category of plants and animals ranking next above the species, as the genus *Homo* in *Homo sapiens*

**Geriatrics:** branch of medicine dealing with diseases and physiological changes associated with aging and old people

German measles *See* Rubella

**Germicide:** disinfectant or other agent capable of killing disease germs

General paresis, 554

**General practitioner/GP:** physician whose training is not specialized and includes some preparation in pediatrics, surgery, and obstetrics and gynecology, thus enabling him to care for an entire family, 824

**Genes:** hereditary unit contained within a chromosome and associated with specific physical characteristics transmitted from parents to offspring, 205

Genetic counseling, 175, 245–46

**Genetic counselor:** specialist, usu. a physician, who counsels couples on the probability of genetic disorders occurring in their offspring,

Genetic defects,

childbirth, 238

Genetic diseases,

hemophilia, 409

sickle-cell anemia, 413

Genetic testing, 246, 824

Genetics,

influence on appearance, 205

mental retardation, 168–69

skeletal system birth defects, 345–48

*See also* Heredity

**Genitalia:** genitals

Genital herpes *See* Herpes, simplex type 2

Genital itch, 312

Genital warts *See* Venereal warts

Gerontologists, 312

**Gerontology:** scientific study of the processes and phenomena of aging

**Helminths:** parasitic worm that invades the intestines, most often via food or water, 465

**Hemal:** of or relating to blood

**Hemangioma:** reddish, usu. raised birthmark consisting of a cluster of small blood vessels near the surface of the skin, 718

Hematological tests, 846–47

**Hematocrit:**

1. instrument for measuring the relative amount of plasma and red corpuscles of the blood by centrifuging it (whirling it around to separate parts having different densities)

2. measurement of relative amount of plasma and red corpuscles by a hematocrit

**Hematologist:** physician specializing in the study of the blood and in the diagnosis and treatment of blood diseases, 825, 842

**Hematology:** the branch of medical science dealing with the blood, including its formation, functions, and diseases, 825

**Hematoma:** blood tumor, 1064

subdural: mass of blood clots or partially clotted blood in the space beneath the outermost (dura mater) and middle (arachnoid) membranes covering the brain,

**Hematuria:** blood in the urine, 533

**Hemiplegia:** paralysis of one side of the body, involving both the arm and leg

**Hemiplegic:** one affected by hemiplegia

Hemodialysis *See* Dialysis

**Hemoglobin:** pigment of red blood corpuscles serving as the carrier of oxygen and carbon dioxide, 36, 62, 411, 691, 838

Hemolytic anemias, 412, 417

**Hemophilia:** inherited disorder characterized by an incapacity of the blood to clot normally, thus resulting in profuse bleeding even from slight cuts, typically affecting males only, 238, 407, 409–11

voluntary agencies, 1015

Hemophilia arthritis, 410

**Hemophiliac/bleeder:** one afflicted with hemophilia, 409–10, 585

**Hemorrhage:** discharge of blood from a ruptured blood vessel, 38

low-volume shock, 1030

Hemorrhagic diseases, 408–11

**Hemorrhoidal:**

1. of or pertaining to the blood vessel in the rectal area

2. of or pertaining to hemorrhoids

**Hemorrhoidectomy:** surgical removal of hemorrhoids

**Hemorrhoids/piles:** swollen varicose veins in the rectal mucous membrane, 461–62, *461*, 564, 650–51, *650*, 765–66

prolapsed: hemorrhoids that protrude from the anus, 651

**Hemotoxic:** (of certain poisonous snakes) transmitting venom that is carried by the bloodstream of the toxified animal, 1087. Compare *neurotoxic.*

**Henle's loop:** U-shaped part of a tubule of the kidney,

*See* Kidneys, tubules

**Heparin:** chemical compound that prevents coagulation of the blood, 409

**Hepatic:** of or relating to the liver

Hepatic duct, 57

**Hepaticologist:** physician specializing in the diagnosis and treatment of liver diseases

**Hepaticology:** branch of medical science concerned with the study, diagnosis, and treatment of diseases of the liver

**Hepatitis:** inflammation of the liver, 469–70

infectious: inflammation of the liver caused by a viral infection usu. transmitted by food and water contaminated by feces from an infected person,

serum: form of infectious hepatitis usu. spread by blood transfusions or by infected hypodermic needles,

Hepatitis B, 469, 470

**Hereditary:** acquired through one's genetic makeup by inheritance, as physical characteristics, diseases, etc. Compare *congenital.*

alcohol abuse, 934

baldness, 205, 286–87

chronic disease, 277

genetic counseling, 245–46

influence on obesity, 866–67

kidney failure, 533

mental retardation, 168

physical traits, 205

skin aging, 285

**Hernia/rupture:** protrusion of an organ or part, as the intestine, through the wall or body cavity that normally contains it, 17–18, 153, 156, *453,* 462

children, 153, 156

femoral, 650, *650*

hiatus/diaphragmatic hernia: hernia in which the lower end of the esophagus or stomach protrudes through the diaphragm, 156, 453–54, *454,* 640–41, *640*

inguinal: protuberance of part of the intestine into the inguinal region (near the groin), 156, 602, 648–49

strangulated: hernia that has become tightly constricted, thus cutting off blood supply, 603, 649

types, 462

umbilical: hernia in which an abdominal part protrudes through the abdominal wall at the navel, 156

vaginal wall, 797–98

ventral: projection of part of the intestine into the abdominal wall,

**Herniate:** slip away from its proper position as an organ or part to form a hernia,

**Herniating disk:** slipped disk, 365–66, 368–69, *368*

**Herniation:** forming of a hernia

**Heroic:** extraordinary or extreme, as measures undertaken when life is in immediate danger

Heroic measures, 603

**Heroin/diacetylmorphine:** addictive narcotic drug derived from morphine, illegal in the U.S., 217, 947–48

slang terms, 945

**Herpes:** any of various acute viral diseases characterized by the eruption of small blisters on the skin and mucous membranes

**Herpes simplex:** virus that causes cold sores and other skin conditions in humans, 586, 713

*See also* Cold sores

Type 1/HSV-1: variety of herpes simplex that causes cold sores, 586, 713

Type 2/HSV-2: variety of herpes simplex that often affects the genital region and can result in congenital damage to the baby of an infected mother, 547, 551, 792–93

Herpes zoster, 714

**Heterograft/xenograft:** tissue graft taken for transplanting from a donor of a different species from that of the patient receiving it

**Hexachlorophene:** antibacterial agent used in some soaps

Hiatus hernia *See* Hernia, hiatus

**Hiccup/hiccough:** involuntary, spasmodic grunt caused by spasms of the diaphragm and the abrupt closure of the glottis, 767, 1081

**Hydronephrosis:** enlargement of the kidneys with urine due to an obstruction of the ureter, 544

**Hydrophilic:** having an affinity for water, as the soft contact lens, 527

**Hydrophilic lenses:** contact lenses, soft plastic

**Hydrophobia:** rabies

**Hydrotherapy:** treatment of disease by the use of water

Hydroxyzine, 1097

Hygiene, 130

acne, 715–16

bathing, 692

bladder infections, 541

children, 113

circumcision, 130

cystitis, 541

hair, 689, 692–93, 698–99

home care patients, 988–90

middle eye, 282

parasitic diseases, 465–66

pre-operative procedures, 609–10

preschool children, 113

skin, 689, 692–93

*See also* Oral Hygiene

**Hymen:** thin membrane usu. partially covering the entrance of the vagina in virgins

Hyoscyamine, 1093

Hyper-, 498

Hyperactive *See* Hyperkinesis

**Hyperacusis:** abnormal and sometimes painful acuteness of hearing, 384

**Hyperaldosteronism:** syndrome of muscle weakness, hypertension, and excessive excretion of urine, due to oversecretion of an adrenal hormone, 635

**Hyperbaric:** of or using pressures in excess of the usual pressure of the atmosphere, as a chamber for treating one suffering from decompression sickness

**Hyperfunction:** disorder of an endocrine gland, characterized by excess secretion of a hormone

**Hyperglycemia:** abnormally high amount of sugar in the blood, 517

**Hyperkinesis:** behavioral disorder of children marked by overactivity, excitability, and inability to concentrate, 159

**Hyperkinetic:** suffering from or pertaining to hyperkinesis

**Hypermetropic:** farsighted

**Hyperopic:** farsighted, 146, 159, 524, 527

**Hyperplasia:** excessive production of cells, resulting in enlargement of tissue or of an organ

**Hyperplastic:** characterized by hyperplasia

**Hypersensitivity:** unusual sensitivity or allergic response to a particular substance

Hypersensitivity pneumonitis, 960

**Hypertension/high blood pressure:** excessively high blood pressure, sometimes caused by a disease (secondary hypertension) and sometimes not (essential hypertension) 45, 96, 241, 424, 426, 438–40, 524–25

adrenal medulla malfunction, 503

causes, 439

diabetes, 521

essential/chronic hypertension/ functional hypertension: hypertension, or high blood pressure, that is not a symptom of disease and has no known cause, 439, 760

eyesight, 528

heart attack prevention, 436–37

impotence, 302

kidney failure, 535, 536

malignant: form of essential hypertension with an acute onset and rapid rise in pressure, 440 secondary: hypertension arising as a consequence of another known disorder, 439–40

sexual activity, 337

stroke, 422

symptoms, 439–40

tinnitus, 769

treatment, 440

weight control, 750

Hypertensive heart disease *See* Heart disease, hypertensive

**Hyperthyroidism:** abnormal and excess activity of the thyroid gland, resulting in oversecretion of thyroxin and an abnormally high metabolism, characterized by fatigue, weight loss, rapid pulse, intolerance to heat, and sometimes by protruding eyes (in which case the disorder is called *exophthalmic goiter*), 77–78, 501–02

**Hypertonic:** characterized by an abnormally high degree of tension , as muscle

**Hypertrophic:** characterized by hypertrophy

Hypertrophic arthritis *See* Osteoarthritis

**Hypertrophy:** excessive development of an organ or tissue due to enlargement of the size of its constituent cells

**Hyperventilation:** abnormally fast or deep breathing, resulting in loss of carbon dioxide from the blood and sometimes causing dizziness and muscle spasms

Hypnosis,

childbirth, 257

**Hypnotic:** tending to produce sleep

Hypo-, 499

**Hypoallergenic:** less likely to produce an allergic reaction

cosmetics, 695

**Hypochondria:** extreme anxiety about one's health, usu. associated with a particular part of the body

and accompanied by imagined symptoms of illness

**Hypochondriac:**

1. *(n.)* one suffering from hypochondria

2. *(adj.)* pertaining to the upper right or left parts of the abdomen

**Hypodermic:** pertaining to the tissue just under the skin or to an injection made under the skin

**Hypofunction:** disorder of an endocrine gland, characterized by too little secretion of a hormone

**Hypogastric:** pertaining to the lower middle part of the abdomen

**Hypogastrium:** the lower middle (hypogastric) part of the abdomen

**Hypoglycemia/low blood sugar:** abnormally small amount of glucose in the blood, which can lead to insulin shock, 515, 516–17, 880

**Hypoglycemic drugs:** drug intended to reduce the amount of glucose in the blood by stimulating the release of insulin from the pancreas, 516–17

Hypoglycemic reactions,

children with diabetes, 520

Hypophysis, 500

**Hypophysis cerebri:** pituitary gland

**Hyposensitization:** program for desensitizing allergy patients by injecting them with progressively larger doses of pollen or other allergens to build tolerance levels, 486

**Hypotension:** excessively low blood pressure, 96

**Hypothalamus:** region of the brain below the thalamus, important in regulating the internal organs and associated with the functioning of the pituitary gland, 72, 210, 500

**Hypothermia:** artificially low body temperature produced by gradually cooling blood, used to slow metabolism and reduce tissue oxygen need so that heart and brain can withstand short periods of interrupted blood flow during surgery,

**Hypothyroidism:** deficient functioning of the thyroid gland, resulting in undersecretion of thyroxin and an abnormally low metabolism, characterized by lack of energy, thick skin, and intolerance to cold, 77, 501

**Hypotonic:** characterized by an abnormally low degree of tension, as muscle, 400

**Hysterectomy:** surgical procedure in which the uterus is completely removed, 289, 506–07, 784, 808, 809, 810, 811

radical: surgical removal of the uterus, cervix, ovaries, and Fallopian tubes, 810

total: surgical removal of the uterus and cervix, 808

**Hysteria:** neurotic condition characterized by impulsive, demonstrative, and attention-getting behavior and sometimes by symptoms of organic disorders

**Hysterogram:** X-ray examination of the uterus and surrounding areas, 237

**Id:** the concealed, inaccessible part of the mind, the seat of impulses that tend to fulfill instinctual needs, 911

**Identical twins:** twins having the same genetic makeup, derived from a single fertilized egg, 195–96

**Identification:** mental process, often unconscious, by which a person associates with himself the attributes of another with whom he has formed an emotional tie

**Idiopathic:** (of diseases) originating spontaneously or of unknown cause

**Ileitis:** inflammation of the ileum of the small intestine

**Ileocecal valve:** the valve between the ileum of the small intestine and the cecum, the first section of the large intestine, 55, 59

**Ileum:** the last section of the small intestine, following the jejunum and leading to the large intestine, 54, 55–56, 59

**Iliac:** pertaining to or near the ilium, 367

**Ilium:** the large upper portion of the hip bone, 6

**Immune:** protected from a communicable or allergic disease by the presence of antibodies in the blood

**Immunity:** resistance to infection or lack of susceptibility of an organism to a disease or poison to which its species is usu. subject, either by means of antibodies produced by the organism itself *(active immunity)* or by another and subsequently introduced into its body *(passive immunity)*, as by injection

alcohol abuse, 932

thymus, 79–80

**Immunization:** act or process of making immune, esp. by inoculation, 159–60

DPT, 193

infants, 106, 108

influenza, 476

measles, 165

mumps, 170

poliomyelitis, 176, 398

pregnancy, 243–44

reactions, 160

recommended schedule (chart), 161

tetanus, 193

**Immunize:** make immune, as by inoculation

**Immunoglobulin:** any of various proteins of the body that are active as antigens or otherwise contribute to the formation of antibodies

Immunoglobulin E, 777

**Infarct:** tissue rendered necrotic (dead) by an obstructed blood supply, as because of a thrombus (clot) or an embolus, 431

**Infarction:** death of tissue due to deprivation of blood caused by an obstruction, as in a coronary thrombosis (heart attack)

**Infections:** communication of disease by entrance into the body of disease-causing organisms

**Infectious:** (of a disease) transmitted by organisms, as bacteria

**Infectious mononucleosis/glandular fever/kissing disease:** acute communicable disease marked by fever, malaise, and swollen lymph nodes, esp. in the throat, 416–17

**Inferior vena cava:** the large vein that brings blood from the lower part of the body to the heart, 41

**Infertility:** inability to conceive or to produce offspring, 231–38

**Inflammation:** localized reaction to infection, injury, etc., characterized by heat, redness, swelling, and pain

of arterial walls *See* Arteritis

of bladder *See* Cystitis

of bone *See* Osteomyelitis

of brain *See* Encephalitis

of brain coverings *See* Meningitis

of bursa *See* Bursitis

of facial nerve *See* Bell's palsy

of femoral head *See* Legg-Perthes' disease

of glomeruli *See* Nephritis

of gums *See* Gingivitis

of joints *See* Arthritis

of larynx *See* Laryngitis

of liver *See* Hepatitis

of mucous membrane *See* Laryngitis

of prostate *See* Prostatitis

of skin *See* Dermatitis

of spinal joints *See* Spondylitis, rheumatoid

of stomach lining *See* Gastritis

of tendons *See* Tendinitis

of tendon sheath *See* Tenosynovitis

of tongue *See* Glossitis

of veins *See* Phlebitis

of vertebrae *See* Osteomyelitis, spinal

See also Arthritis; Rheumatoid arthritis

**Influenza/flu/grippe:** acute, contagious, sometimes epidemic disease caused by a virus and characterized by inflammation of the upper respiratory tract, fever, chills, muscle ache, and fatigue, 475–76, 745

**Ingrown toenail:** toenail that has grown into the surrounding flesh,

**Inguinal:** pertaining to or near the groin

Inguinal area,

undescended testicles, 203

Inguinal hernia, 462, *648*

*See also* Hernia

Inhalants, 939, 953–55

allergies, 746

**Inner ear:** the innermost part of the ear, containing the essential organs of hearing within the cochlea, the auditory nerve, and the semicircular canals that govern equilibrium, 88

damage from noise, 966

**Innervation:** distribution or supply of nerves to a part

**Inoculate:**

1. immunize by administering a serum or vaccine to

2. introduce microorganisms into (a culture medium)

**Inoculation:** act or process of inoculating

common viruses, 745

**Inoperable:** characterized by a condition that excludes surgery as a course of treatment

Inotropic drugs, 432

Insanity,

syphilis, 554–55

Insecticides, 969

Insect bites

allergic reactions, 776–77

tropical diseases, 587–97

*See also* Chigger bites; Spider bites; Tick bites

Insect stings, 161–62, 1082

**Insomnia:** chronic inability to sleep, 754

**Insufficiency:** inability to function adequately, as the heart (cardiac insufficiency)

**Insufflation:** tubal insufflation

**Insulin:** protein hormone secreted by the islets of Langerhans in the pancreas that checks the accumulation of glucose in the blood and promotes the utilization of sugar in the treatment of diabetes, 58, 76–77, 139, 509–10, 513–14, 1097,

dose, 514

endogenous, 1228

sites for injection, *514*

therapy for children, 519

types, 513–14, *513*

Insulin pump, 515–16

**Insulin shock:** condition caused by too low a level of blood sugar, and characterized by sweating, dizziness, palpitation, shallow breathing, confusion, and ultimately loss of consciousness, 515, 1072–73

*See also* Diabetic coma

**Insulin shock therapy:** former method of treating psychotic patients involving large injections of insulin, inducing coma, 924

Insurance *See* Health insurance

**Insult:** injury to tissue caused by stress or trauma

**Integument:** skin, 19

Intelligence,

childs, 162–63, 167–69

**Intelligence quotient/IQ:** a score obtained from standardized tests indicating the level of a person's intelligence, 163

**Intensive care unit (ICU):** section of a hospital specially equipped and staffed to monitor the vital systems of patients and provide close, round-the-clock care for a relatively brief period, as for patients just removed from surgery or for those in an unstable or critical condition, 617

arthritis, 348–60

bleeding, 410

diseases of, 348–61

injury, 9–10

replacement, 350, 361–62, *362*

rheumatic fever, 441

*See also* Bursas; Cartilage; Rheumatology

Joslin, Dr. Elliott, 510

Juvenile Insulin Dependent Diabetes (JIDD), 519

**Kala-azar/black fever/dumdum fever/visceral leishmaniasis:** form of leishmaniasis that is usually fatal if not treated, 593

Karposi's sarcoma, 548, 584, 586

**Keratin:** horny substance that is the main constituent of nails and hair, and in nonhuman animals of claws and horns, 21, 697

**Keratosis:** disease of the skin characterized by an outer layer of horny tissue

Ketamine, 614

Keto-acidosis, 515

**Ketone bodies:** organic compounds that are a by-product of fat metabolism, 511

Ketosis, 515

Kidney disease,

  hypertension, 439

  symptoms, 532–33

  voluntary agencies, 1015–16

Kidney pelvis, 97

**Kidney stones/renal calculus:** mass of hard material, such as crystallized salt, that may collect within the kidney and obstruct the flow of urine, 508, 541, 542–43, *543*

  gout, 357

  symptoms, 630–31

**Kidneys:** a pair of organs located at the rear of the abdomen near the base of the spine, whose function

is to filter the fluid portion of the blood in regulating the composition and volume of body fluids, and to dispose of waste in the form of urine, *93,* 94–96

blood pressure, 96

cancer, 573–75

cysts, 634–35

function, 94

gout, 357

processing fluids, 94–95

removal, 633

transplants, 538, 686–87

tubules, 96

tumors, 633–34

**Kidney failure, acute:** sudden loss of kidney function, characterized by decreased amount of urine, passage of bloody urine, edema, fatigue, and loss of appetite, 533–37

Kidney stones, 1083

Kissing disease *See* Infectious mononucleosis

Knees, 7

  deep bends, 1149

  injuries, 672, 1083

  joints, 7

  problems from jogging, 772

  problems with exercise, 1127

**Kyphosis:** backward curvature of the spine characterized as a humpback or hunchback, 363

**Labia:**

  1. *pl.* of labium

  2. the folds of skin and mucous membrane of the vulva, consisting of the outer folds *(labia majora)* and the inner folds *(labia minora)*

**Labium:**

  1. *sing.* of labia

  2. lip or liplike part or organ

**Latent:** not visible or apparent, as symptoms of a disease at an early stage

**Lateral:**

1. relating to or directed toward the side
2. more distant from the midline of the body, as compared to a nearer (medial) position

**Lavage:** cleansing or washing out of an organ, as the stomach

**Laxative:** substance that has the power to loosen the bowels, as milk of magnesia, 278, 455, 765

*See also* Cathartics

**L-dopa/levodopa:** medicine used in treating the symptoms of Parkinson's disease, 386–87, 1098

Lead poisoning, 163–64, 958, 1050–52

anemia, 412

mental retardation, 169

*See also* Pica

**Leaflet:** flap of a heart valve,

Learning,

reading, 181

**Learning disability:** condition in which a child cannot acquire certain skills or assimilate certain kinds of knowledge at or near the normal rate, 143, 164

LeBoyer childbirth method, 257–58

LeBoyer, Dr. Frederick, 257

Leeches, 1084

Leg cramps, 243

**Legg-Perthes' disease:** inflammation of the bone and cartilage in the head of the femur (thigh bone), 368

Legionnaires disease, 960

**Leiomyoma:** benign tumor consisting of smooth muscle tissue, 569

**Leishmaniasis:** tropical disease resembling malaria in which an animal parasite is transmitted by the sandfly, 593–95

Leisure time,

community resources, 306

later years, 331–35

middle age, 304–07

**Lens:** biconvex transparent body behind the iris of the eye that focuses entering light rays on the retina, 84

Lens implant, 658–59

**Lepromatous:** characterized by nodular skin lesions, as a form of leprosy, 601

**Leprosy/Hansen's disease:** chronic bacterial disease characterized by skin lesions, nerve paralysis, and physical deformity, 600–01

**Lesion:** any abnormal change in an organ or tissue caused by disease or injury

oral cavity, 451–52

**Leukemia:** form of cancer involving the blood and blood-making tissues, characterized by a marked and persistent excess of leukocytes, 414, 415–16, 561, 580–82

Leukemia,

acute, 581

granulocytic: form of leukemia characterized by predominance of granulocytes (or neutrophils), 581

lymphocytic: form of leukemia characterized by uncontrolled over-activity of the lymphoid tissue, 560

multiple sclerosis, 395

new drugs for, 581–82

purpura, 410

voluntary agencies, 1021

Leukemia Society of America, 1021

**Leukemic:** of or characteristic of leukemia

**Leukocyte/white blood cell/white corpuscle:** white or colorless cell found in the bloodstream important in providing protection against infection, 36, 415, 838

Liver scan, 848

**Liver spots/chloasma:** yellowish brown patches that appear on the skin, 717

**lobe(s):** rounded or protruding section or subdivision, as of an organ, 26, 68

Local anesthetics, 615

Lockjaw, 193

**Loiasis:** form of filariasis transmitted by a biting fly from monkey to man or vice versa, 598

**Loins:** the part of the body between the lower rib and the hip bone

Long-term care See Nursing homes

Loniten,

hair loss, 288

**Lordosis:** abnormal inward curvature of the spine, 242, 363

**Lordotic posture:** posture characteristic of some women in late pregnancy, in which the shoulders are slumped, the neck bent, and the lower spine curved forward to bear the weight of the fetus, 242

**"Lou Gehrig's disease":** sclerosis, amyolotrophic lateral,

See Amyotrophic lateral sclerosis

Low blood sugar See Hypoglycemia

Low-volume shock, 1030

Lower back pain See Sciatica

**LSD/lysergic and acid diethylamide:** colorless, odorless, tasteless drug produced synthetically that causes the user to experience hallucinations, 217, 949–51

effects, 950

slang terms, 945

**LTH:** lactogenic hormone, 74

**Lumbago:** pain in the lower back,

See Backaches

**Lumbar:** pertaining to or situated near the loins

Lumbar puncture, 382, 391

epilepsy, 1096

meningitis, 396

**Lumen:** space enclosed by the walls of a blood vessel, duct, etc.

Lumpectomy, 818, 819

Lung capacity, 276, 279

Lung cancer, 293, 562–64

asbestos workers, 563

smoking, 563–64

**Lungs:** either of two porous organs of respiration in the chest cavity of humans, having the function of absorbing oxygen and discharging carbon dioxide, *488*

carbon monoxide, 215

collapse, 67, 378, 497,

disorders, 661

interaction with heart, 60–62, *61, 473*

radon gas, 961

role of blood, 34–35

smoking and cancer, 214

structure, 681

transplants, 688

Lung diseases, 472, 476–78, 478–82, 487–97

voluntary agencies, 1011

See also Respiratory diseases

**Lunula:** the living part of the nail, the pale, half-moon shape at the nail base, 22

**Luteinizing hormone/LH:** a hormone secreted by the anterior lobe of the pituitary gland that stimulates a Graafian follicle to release an ovum during each menstrual cycle and converts the follicle into corpus luteum,

**Luteotrophic hormone:** lactogenic hormone,

**Luteotrophin:** lactogenic hormone,

Lyme disease, 181

**Lymph:** transparent fluid resembling blood plasma that is conveyed through vessels (lymphatic vessels) and lubricates the tissues, 39–40

circulation, 40

**Lymphangiogram:** the visualization by X ray of lymph nodes after injection of an opaque fluid, 847

**Lymphatic:** pertaining to or conveying lymph

Lymphatic system, 39–40, *40*

Hodgkin's disease, 579–80

**Lymph node/lymph gland:** one of the rounded bodies about the size of a pea, found in the course of the lymphatic vessels, that produce lymphocytes, 39–40

bubonic plague, 587

enlargement, 580–81

lymphogranuloma venereum, 556

**Lymphoblast:** young cell that matures into a lymphocyte

**Lymphocyte:** variety of leukocyte formed in the lymphoid tissue, 39, 415

Lymphocytic leukemia,

acute, 125

**Lymphogranuloma venereum/LGV/ lymphogranuloma inguinale:** venereal disease affecting the lymph nodes, 556

**Lymphoid:** pertaining to lymph or to the tissue of lymph nodes

**Lymphoma:** abnormal (neoplastic) growth of lymphoid tissue, symptomatic of various diseases, as lymphocytic leukemia or Hodgkin's disease, 561, 579

drug treatment, 583

**Lymphosarcoma:** malignant growth of the lymphatic system, 582

**Lysergic acid diethylamide** *See* LSD,

**Lysozyme:** enzyme present in tears that is destructive to bacteria, 87

**Lyssophobia:** fear of becoming insane, 916

**Macrobiotic:** of or pertaining to macrobiotics

**Macrobiotics:** the idea, Oriental in origin, that an equilibrium should be maintained between foods that make one active (Yang) and foods that make one relax (Yin), 879

**Macrocephalic:** individual with macrocephaly

**Macrocephaly:** excessive head size, 346

**Macula:** spot or discoloration. *See also* Macula lutea; Senile macula degeneration

**Macula lutea:** yellowish area in the retina related to color perception and marked by most acute vision, 83

Magnesium,

teenage diet, 209

Magnetic resonance imaging, 842

Main lining (drug abuse), 217

Mainstreaming, 152

Major medical insurance, 975

Make-up *See* Cosmetics

**Malabsorption syndrome/celiac disease:** syndrome characterized by bulky, foul-smelling stools and other symptoms due to the inability of the body to absorb certain nutrients from the intestinal tract, 126

**Malaise:** feeling of being run-down, listless, uncomfortable, weary, and generally unwell

**Malaria:** disease caused by certain animal parasites transmitted by the bite of the infected Anopheles mosquito, causing intermittent chills, and fever, 591–93

how transmitted, *591*

immunizations, 244

Male climacteric, 292–93

Male pattern baldness

*See* Baldness

Male reproductive system,

surgery, 625–30

**Malignancy:**

1. malignant tumor

2. state of being malignant

**Malignant:** so aggravated as to threaten life, usu. resistant to treatment, and often having the property of uncontrolled growth, as a cancer

Malignant melanoma

*See* Melanoma

**Malleus** *See* Hammer,

**Malnutrition:** nutritional deficiency, as of essential proteins, vitamins, or minerals, causing impairment of health and certain specific diseases, 164, 863–64

from diseases, 863

from medications, 863

liver cirrhosis, 468

thrush, 452

tuberculosis, 480

*See also* Pica

**Malocclusion:** faulty closure of the upper and lower teeth, 172, 735, 739–40

improper bite, *740*

tinnitus, 769

**Mammogram:** X-ray picture of the breast by the technique of mammography,

**Mammography:** specialized X-ray examination of the breasts, 802, 1030–31

**Mammoplasty:** surgical procedure to augment the size of the breasts, 681

Managed care, 981–82

**Mandible:** the lower jawbone, 720

**Mania:** psychotic condition characterized by excessive activity, elation, extreme talkativeness, and agitation,

**Manic-depressive reaction/affective reaction:** psychosis charac-

terized by mania or depression or by the alternation of both, 912–20

Manners, 164

March of Dimes Birth Defects Foundation, 1022

**Marihuana:** the dried leaves and flowers of the hemp plant *(Cannabis sativa),* which if smoked in cigarettes or otherwise ingested can produce distorted perception and other hallucinogenic effects, 216–17, 952–53

slang terms, 945

THC use for glaucoma, 660

Marriage, 261–62

honeymoon, 262–63

male climacteric, 292

menopause, 291

*See also* Divorce

Marriage counseling, 261–62

*See also* Sex therapy

**Marrow:** either of two types of soft, vascular tissue found in the central cavities of bones—*red marrow,* which produces red blood cells, and yellow marrow, composed mainly of fat cells;

*See* Bone marrow

Massage, 744

**Mastectomy:** surgical removal of the breast, 816–18, *817,* 818–19

modified radical, 818

post-operative therapies, 819–19

pre-surgical staging, 816

radical: surgical removal of the breast, underlying chest muscles, and lymph glands in the armpit, *817,* 818

simple: surgical removal of the breast only, *817,* 818

wedge excision, 818

**Master gland** *See* Pituitary gland

Masters, Dr. William H., 300–01, 336

**Mastitis:** inflammation of the breast, 260

**Mastoiditis:** inflammation of the air cells in the mastoid process

**Mastoid process:** process of the temporal bone behind the ear

**Mastoplasty:** surgical procedure to reduce the size of the breasts, 680

**Masturbation:** the touching or rubbing of the genitals for sexual pleasure and usu. orgasm, 171, 205, 227, 337

**Materia alba:** white, viscous mixture of mucus, molds, tissue cells, and bacteria adhering to teeth or to the spaces between teeth and gums, a potential source of disease, 729

**Maxilla:** the upper jawbone, 720

Meals-on-Wheels, 1004

**M.D.:** Doctor of Medicine

Mealtimes, 1111

**Measles/rubeola:** contagious viral disease, esp. of children, marked by rash, fever, and conjunctivitis, sometimes having severe complications, 164–65

**Meatus:** passage or canal in the human body, esp. one with an external opening, such as the anterior urethra of the penis

Mechanical sperm barriers See Cervical caps; Diaphragms

Meclizine, 1098

**Medial:**

1. middle, or relatively near the middle

2. nearer to the midline of the body, as compared to a more distant (lateral) position

Medic Alert Foundation, 515

**Medical:**

1. of or relating to medicine

2. of or relating to the treatment of disease by nonsurgical means

Medical check-ups,

infertility exam, 235

**Medical history:** the questions asked by a doctor of a patient that are designed to give an outline of the patient's state of health, 606–07, 829

See also Health records

Medical information,

emergencies, 603

Medical day care, 1003

Medical records See

Health records

Medical supply houses, 1003

Medicare, 979–80

dialysis, 537

HMOs, 981

medigap coverage, 979–80

Medications,

administering to children, 165–66

anesthesia, 607, 608, 610

effect on nutrition, 863

home medical supplies, 1036–39

**Medicine:**

1. the profession dealing with the maintenance of health and the treatment of physical and psychological disorders, 823

2. the treatment of disease by nonsurgical means

Medigap insurance, 979–80

**Medulla:**

1. medulla oblongata: the lower part of the brain continuous with the spinal cord that controls certain involuntary processes such as breathing, swallowing, and blood circulation, 64, 74, 502

2. the inner portion of an organ or part, as of the kidneys or the adrenal glands

Medulla oblongata, 26

**Melanin:** dark brown or black pigment of the skin, 21, 691, 718

**Melanoma/black cancer:** malignant tumor formed of cells that produce melanin, 566

**Membranes:**

hyaloid: the delicate membrane that envelops the vitreous humor of the eye

intact: caul

periodontal: the membrane covering the bony tissue (cementum) around the roots of teeth

tympanic: eardrum

**Menarche:** the first menstrual period of a girl, 198–200

**Ménière's disease/Ménière's syndrome:** symptoms including vertigo, ringing or buzzing sensations (tinnitus), nausea, and vomiting, associated with disease of the inner ear and often leading to progressive deafness of one ear, 531

**Meninges:** the membranes that cover the brain and spinal cord, 25, 395

**Meningioma:** uncontrolled new cell growth in one of the membranes (arachnoid) covering the brain and spinal cord, 364

**Meningitis:** inflammation of the membranes that cover the brain and spinal cord, 166, 396, 586

aseptic/viral meningitis: meningitis thought to be caused by a virus instead of a bacterium,

gonorrhea, 550

*See also* Cerebrospinal Menningitis

**Meningococcal:** pertaining to meningococcus, a bacterium

**Meningococcus:** bacterium that causes a form of meningitis, 502

**Menopausal:** of or occurring during the menopause

**Menopause/change of life/climacteric:** the cessation of menstruation and the end of a woman's capacity to bear children, normally occurring between 40-50 years of age and often marked by hot flashes, dizzy spells, and other

physical and emotional symptoms, 289–92, 506, 790

emotional attitude, 291

exercise, 1190

"faulty" eggs, 247

osteoarthritis, 349

post-menopausal bleeding, 790

relations with husband, 291

sexual activity, 336

surgical: abrupt onset of menopause in women due to surgical removal of the uterus and ovaries, 633

urethral caruncle, 795

Menorrhagia, 785–86

**Menses:** menstruation

**Menstrual:** of or relating to menstruation

Menstrual cycles, 199–200, *200, 201,* 229–30

disruption, 801

hormonal control, 505

regularity for adolescence, 199–200

timing ovulation, 232

Menstrual disorders, 506, 784–90

Menstrual molimina, 788

**Menstruation/the menses:** periodic bloody discharge of the unfertilized ovum and tissue from the uterus of a female of child-bearing age, 79, 115, 197–201, 784–86

activities during, 201

anorexia, 210

bloodclots, 789

exercise, 1190

odor, 789

onset, 198–99, 784–85

oral contraceptives, 789

regularity, 784–86

Mental health,

adjustments with a new baby, 102–3

**Methanol** *See* Methyl alcohol

Methacycline, 1099

Methyclothiazide, 1099

**Methotrexate:** drug used in the treatment of psoriasis and leukemia

**Methyl alcohol/wood alcohol/methanol:** flammable liquid obtained through the distillation of wood or made synthetically, poisonous if taken internally, 927

Methyl tertbutyl ether (MTHE), 648

Methylpheniclate, 941, 1099

Methyprylon, 944

Metronidazole, 552

**Metorrhagia:** erratic or unpredictable menstrual bleeding, 786

**Microcephalic:** individual with microcephaly

**Microcephaly:** abnormal smallness of the head, with imperfect development of the cranium, 346

**Micrographia:** very minute handwriting, a symptom of some nervous disorders, 386

**Micron:** 1/1000th of a millimeter (symbol *mu,* Greek letter *mu*)

**Microsurgery:** surgery or dissection of minute parts, as of individual cells, with the aid of a microscope and esp. precise instruments, 656

**Micturate:** urinate

**Micturition:** urination

Middle age *See* Middle years

**Middle ear:** the part of the ear between the eardrum and the inner ear, including the tympanum and the ossicles—hammer, anvil and stirrup, 87–88

Middle years, 275–310

physical fitness and exercise, 275–76, 278–81

teeth care, 724

**Migraine/sick headache:** recurrent severe form of headache, temporarily disabling, usu. affecting one side of the head and often accom-

panied by nausea, dizziness, and sensitivity to light, 748, 966

**Miliaria:** prickly heat

**Milk teeth:** baby teeth

**Minerals:** naturally occurring, homogeneous, inorganic material, some of which, as salt and iron, are required by the body,

food additives, 968

role in diet, 858–59

**Minimal brain dysfunction/minimal brain damage:** condition of children who suffer from a motor or perceptual impairment due to slight brain damage, 124

Minimal residue diet, 621

Minoxidil,

hair loss, 288

**Miscarriage/spontaneous abortion:** the involuntary expulsion of a nonviable fetus after the first three months of pregnancy, 246–48

habitual abortion, 249

sickle-cell anemia, 413

smoking, 239

symptoms, 247–48

trophoblastic disease, 248–49

**Mitral valve:** the membranous valve between the left atrium and left ventricle of the heart that prevents the backflow of blood into the atrium, 442

**Mittelschmerz:** pain during ovulation about midway between menstrual periods,

Mobile coronary care units, 434

**Modality:**

1. method of treatment or its application esp. a physical procedure

2. any form of sensation, as touch or taste

**Molar:** any of the three upper and three lower grinding teeth with flattened crowns at both sides of the rear of the mouth, making 12 in all, 721

Mold spores, 775

Moles: permanent pigmented spot on the skin, usu. brown and often raised, 718

melanoma, 566

Molluscum contagiosum: contagious viral disease marked by raised lesions containing waxy material, 557

Money

children 124, 169

Mongolism: congenital disorder characterized by mental retardation,

See Down's syndrome

Moniliasis/candidiasis: fungus infection involving the skin or mucous membranes of various parts of the body, such as the mouth, esp. in babies (when it is called thrush), or the vagina, 791

Monocyte: relatively large leukocyte,

Mononucleosis: infectious mononucleosis

Monosodium glutamate (MSG), 968

Monovalent: pertaining to a form of the Sabin polio vaccine in which each dose gives protection against a different strain of polio, 176. Compare trivalent.

Morning sickness: nausea and vomiting experienced by some pregnant women in the morning hours, esp. in eary pregnancy, 240–41

Morphine: addictive narcotic drug derived from opium, used medically to relieve pain, 217, 946–47

Morphinism: abnormal condition of the body system caused by an excessive dose or habitual use of morphine,

Morton's toe: painful inflammation of the nerves in the region of the metatarsus of the foot (metatarsalgia) between the third and fourth toes,

See Metatarsalgia

Mosquitos, 162

Burkitts lymphoma, 652

filariasis, 597–98

malaria, 591–93

yellow fever, 593

Mothers,

advice to new mothers, 102–03

single, 310

Motion sickness: nausea and sometimes vomiting caused by the effect of certain complex movements on the organ of balance in the inner ear, typically experienced in a moving vehicle, ship, or airplane, 170, 1084

Motor nerve/efferent nerve: nerve that conveys information from the central nervous system to a muscle with a directive for action,

Mouth

cancer, 566–67, 651–52

examination, 834

Mouth-to-mouth respiration/ mouth-to-mouth resuscitation: form of artificial respiration in which the rescuer places his mouth over the victim's mouth and breathes rhythmically and forcefully to inflate the victim's lungs and start respiration, 1026–27, 1026, 1075

Mouthwash, 451

MS: multiple sclerosis

Mu: micron

Mucosa: mucous membrane, 484

Mucosal: of or pertaining to the mucous membrane

Mucosal test, 780

Mucous: pertaining to, producing, or resembling mucus

Mucous membrane/mucosa: membrane that lines many of the body's inner surfaces, kept moist by glandular secretions

Mucus: viscous substance secreted by the mucous membranes

**Multipara:** woman who has borne more than one child

Multiple births, 195–96

**Multiphasic:** having many phases or aspects: said esp. of testing performed in the course of a comprehensive physical examination

**Multiple myeloma:** malignant tumor of the bone marrow occurring at numerous sites,

**Multiple sclerosis/MS:** chronic disease in which patches of nerve tissue thicken (sclerose), causing failure of coordination and other nervous and mental symptoms, 30, 31, 393–95

demographics, 393

eyesight, 528

symptoms, 393–94

treatment, 394–95

voluntary agencies, 1017

Multiwire gamma camera, 432

**Mumps:** contagious, viral disease marked by fever and swelling of the facial glands, 170, 451

immunization, 244

infertility, 234

meningoencephalitis: inflammation of the brain and of the membranes (meninges) covering the brain, as a result of mumps, 170

Muscle biopsy, 401–02

Muscle control *See also* Cerebral palsy

Muscle cramps, 758, 1085

Muscle disease, 399–406

diagnoses, 401–02

Muscle-relaxing techniques, 1122–25

Muscles, 10–18

abdomen, *399*

atrophy, 18

cardiac, 10

charly horse, 1069

contraction, *16*

cramps, 1128

extensor, 15–16

flexor, 15–16

forearm movement, *17*

skeletal, 11

smooth, 12

soreness, 1128

stress reduction, *17*

structure, 13–14

thorax, *399*

*See also* Ligaments; Tendons

**Muscular dystrophy/MD:** any of various diseases of unknown cause characterized by the progressive wasting away (atrophy) of the muscles, 402–04

Muscular Dystrophy Association, 1022

**Musculoskeletal system:** the human body's network of muscles and bones

**Myasthenia gravis:** chronic disease characterized by muscular weakness and general and progressive exhaustion, 405–06

**Mycobacterium:** kind of rod-shaped, aerobic bacterium

**Myelin:** semisolid fatlike sheath that surrounds the axon of a neuron, 30

**Myelitis:**

1. inflammation of the spinal cord

2. inflammation of the bone marrow

**Myelogram:** X ray of the spinal cord obtained by the injection of a radio-opaque liquid material into the spinal cord area, 383

**Myeloma:** malignant tumor of the bone marrow, 583

**Myocardial infarction:** the process of congestion and tissue death (necrosis) in the heart muscle caused by an interruption of the blood supply to the heart, 43, 44, 430–31, *431*

**Myocardium:** the muscular tissue of the heart, 43, 431

**Myomectomy:** surgical excision of a type of uterine fibroid tumor,

Myoneural junction defect, 406

**Myopathy:** any abnormality or disease of the muscles,

See Muscle diseases

**Myopia:** nearsightedness, 84, 146, 522, 524

correction with contact lenses, 527

Myotonia congenita, 404

**Myopic:** nearsighted

**Myotonia:** disorder characterized by increased rigidity or spasms of muscle, 404–05

congenita: congenital disease characterized by temporary muscle spasms and muscle rigidity,

**Myotonic dystrophy:** chronic, progressive disease characterized by weakness and wasting of muscles, cataracts, and heart abnormality, 404–05

**Myringotomy:** surgical incision of the eardrum, 144, 656

**Mysophobia:** fear of dirt and contamination, 916

Nails, 21–22, 705–06

hangnail, 758

nail antomy, 758

Nail-biting, 171

Naloxone, 955

morphine overdose, 947

**Naprapathy:** the treatment of disease by the manipulative correction of ligaments and connective tissues

**Narcolepsy:** disease in which the patient is overcome by drowsiness or an uncontrollable desire for sleep, 940

**Narcosis:** stupor or unconsciousness produced by a narcotic drug

**Narcotic:**

1. any of various substances, such as morphine, codeine, and opium, that in medicinal doses relieve pain, induce sleep, and in excessive or uncontrolled doses may produce convulsions, coma, and death, 939, 946–49

2. inducing sleep, in anesthesia,

anesthetics, 614

**Nares:** the nasal passages or nostrils

**Nasopharyngeal:** pertaining to the nasopharynx, 530

**Nasopharynx:** the upper part of the pharynx above and behind the soft palate

National Association for Children of Alcoholics, 936

National Association for Mental Health, 1002

National Association for Retarded Citizens, 169

National Center on Child Abuse and Neglect, 128–29

National Center for Missing and Exploited Children, 184, 189

National Clearinghouse for Alcohol Information, 937

National Council on Alcoholism, 937, 1009

National Crime Information Center (F.B.I.), 189

National Easter Seal Society, 1017–18

National Education Association, 335

National Federation of Parents for Drug-Free Use, 955

National Genetics Foundation, 246

National Health Council, 1007

National Hearing Aid Help Line, 323

National Hearing Aid Society, 323

National Hemophilia Foundation, 1015

National Kidney Foundation, 1015–16

National Mental Health Association, 1016–17

hearing loss, 323

Nerves,

  damage, 30, 31, 520, 601

  glossopharyngeal, 91

  lingual: nerve beneath the floor of the mouth that conveys taste sensations to the brain motor,

  motor/efferent, 24

  olfactory: the special nerve of smell,

  optic: the special nerve of vision connecting the retina with the occipital lobe of the brain,

  sensory/afferent nerve: nerve that conveys information and stimuli from the outside world to the central nervous system, 24

  spinal: the thirty-one pairs of nerves that originate in the spinal cord, 27

  *See also* Senses

**Nervous breakdown:** popular, non-technical term for any debilitating or incapacitating emotional disorder

Nervous habits, 171

Nervousness,

  infertility, 232

Nervous system, 27–31, *381, 841*

  and aging, 30, 276

  autonomic, 26–27

  cranial nerves, *28*

  diagnostic procedures, 382–83

  disorders, 30, 31, 381–406

  excessive alcohol, 930–31

  functions, 23–24

  heart beat, 43

**Neural:** of or relating to a nerve,

**Neuralgia:** acute pain along the course of a nerve

  trigeminal/facial neuralgia/tic douloureux: acutely painful neuralgia of a region of the face, with paroxysmal muscular twitchings, associated with branches of the

trigeminal (cranial) nerve in the affected area, 673

**Neuritis:** inflammation of a nerve

**Neuroblastoma:** malignant tumor of the nerve tissue of the adrenal glands, found esp. in children, 125

**Neurofibroma:** tumor on a nerve fiber, 364

**Neurogenic shock:** shock resulting from impairment of the regulatory capacity of the nervous system due to pain, fright, or other stimulus, 1030

Neurological disorders,

  diagnostic techniques, 842

**Neurologist:** physician speciailzing in the care and treatment of the nervous system, 382, 827, 839, 841

**Neurology:** the branch of medical science that deals with the nervous system,

**Neuron:** nerve cell with all its processes and extensions, such as the axon and dendrites, 24, *29,* 29–30,

  motor: horn cells, anterior

**Neuropathologist:** physician specializing in neuropathology,

**Neuropathology:** the branch of medical science that deals with the study, diagnosis, and treatment of diseases of the nervous system,

**Neurosis/psychoneurosis** *(pl., neuroses):* mental disorder having no organic cause and less severe than psychosis, 914

Neuroleptics, 943

**Neurosurgeon:** physician specializing in surgery of the nervous system, 826, 841

**Neurosurgery:** the branch of medical science that deals with the treatment of disease of the nervous system by means of surgery, 673

**Neurosyphilis:** syphilis of the brain and spinal cord,

**Neurotic:**

  1. one who has a neurosis

**Obsessive-compulsive reaction:** neurosis characterized by obsessions that are relieved temporarily by the compulsive performance of certain acts, 914–15

**Obstetrician:** physician specializing in obstetrics, often a gynecologist as well, 98, 826

**Obstetrics:** the branch of medical science dealing with pregnancy and childbirth, 782

**Obstructive-airway disease:** condition characterized by the presence of chronic bronchitis and pulmonary emphysema, and involving damage to lung tissue and the bronchi, 492-95

smoking, 494–95

**Obturator:** special device inserted into a cleft palate to close it against the flow of air, 131

**Occipital:** of or relating to the lower back part of the skull (occiput)

**Occipital lobe:** the rear portion of each cerebral hemisphere which receives messages from the optic nerve, 84

**Occlusion:**

1. the act of closing or shutting off so as to block a passage, as a blood vessel

2. the manner of being shut, as the teeth of the upper and lower jaws, 723

**Occupational disease:** disease resulting from exposure in one's occupation to toxic substances or other hazards to health, 495, 971

Occupational Safety and Health Administration, 971

**Ocular:** of or relating to the eye

Ocular muscular dystrophy, 1108

**Oculist:** ophthalmologist

Oculopharyngeal muscular dystrophy, 404

**Oedipal complex:** repressed sexual attachment of son to mother, analogous to the Electra complex involving the daughter and father

Oil glands *See* Sebaceous glands

Oil spills, 964

**Olfaction:** the act, sense, or process of smelling

**Olfactory:** pertaining to the sense of smell or the capacity to smell

**Olfactory lobe:** the portion of each cerebral hemisphere of the brain on the underside of the frontal lobes, the centers for smelling

Olfactory nerve, 91

**Oliguria:** decreased production of urine, 533

**Onchocerciasis:** form of filariasis transmitted by a blackfly and sometimes leading to blindness, 598

**Oncologist:** physician specializing in the diagnosis and treatment of tumors

**Oncology:** the branch of medical science concerned with the study of tumors, 825–26

**Open bite:** form of malocclusion in which incisors of the upper and lower jaws do not meet when the jaws are together

Open fracture *See* Compound fracture

**Open surgery:** surgery involving an incision and opening of the skin

prostate gland, 627

Operating room,

equipment, 611–12

**Ophthalmic:** of or pertaining to the eye

Ophthalmological Foundation, 1012–13

**Ophthalmologist/oculist:** physician specializing in the care and treatment of the eyes, 826

**Ophthalmology:** the branch of medical science dealing with the structure, function, and diseases of the eye, 826

**Ophthalmoscope:** optical instrument for examining the interior of the eye, 834, 850

**Opiates:** drugs derived from opium, as morphine

synthetics, 948–49

Opioids, 946

**Opium:** narcotic drug obtained from the opium poppy from which morphine, codeine, heroin, and other drugs are derived, 217, 946

Opportunistic diseases, 584

**Optic/optical:** pertaining to the eye or to vision

**Optician:** one who makes or sells eyeglasses and other optical equipment

**Optic nerve:** special nerve of vision, conveying sensations from the retina to the brain, 83–84

**Optometrist:** one who practices optometry

**Optometry:** profession of measuring the power of vision and prescribing corrective lenses

**Oral:** pertaining to or situated near the mouth

Oral cancer *See* Mouth cancer

Oral contraceptives, 264–65, 1100

pulmonary embolism, 497

side effects, 265

*See also* Birth control; Contraceptives

Oral hygiene, 212–13, 762–63

brushing teeth, 726–28, 727

dental floss, 727–28

diet, 725–26

elderly, 313–14

fluoridation, 725

halitosis, 451

middle age, 285

tongue cancer, 652

*See also* Dental care

**Oral surgeon/dental surgeon:** dentist who specializes in oral surgery, 839

**Oral surgery:** the diagnosis and surgical treatment of diseases, injuries, and defects of the mouth and jaw

**Orbit:** either of the bony sockets of the eyes

**Orchidopexy/orchiopexy:** surgical correction of an undescended testicle, 629

**Orchiectomy:** surgical removal of one or both testicles, 573

**Orchitis:** inflammation of the testicles, 170

Organ transplants, 684–88

kidney donor programs, 1015–16

**Organic:**

1. of or pertaining to an organ of the body

2. having a physical basis, as a disorder

3. of or pertaining to animals or plants

4. pertaining to foods grown only with natural fertilizers of animal or plant origin

**Organic foods:** foods grown with the use of organic fertilizers only, such as compost or animal (not human) manure, and without the use of pesticides or herbicides, 878–79

**Organ of Corti:** the true center of hearing within the cochlea of the inner ear, a complex spiral structure of hair cells, 89

**Orgasm:** the climax of the sexual act, normally marked by the male's ejaculation of semen and by relaxation of tension of both male and female

**Orthodontia:** orthodontics

Orthodontic appliances, 741–42

**Orthodontics/orthodontia:** the care and treatment of irregularities and faulty positions of the teeth, including the fitting of braces, 172–73, 213, 739–42

**Orthodontist:** dentist specializing in orthodontics

**Orthopedics:** the branch of surgery dealing with the treatment and correction of deformities, injuries, and diseases of the skeletal system and its associated structures, as muscles and joints

**Orthopedic surgeon:** orthopedist, 374–75, 826, 839

Orthopedic surgery, 667

**Orthopedist/orthopedic surgeon/ orthopod:** surgeon specializing in orthopedics

**Orthopod:** orthopedist

**Orthoptist:** medical technician trained to diagnose defects of the eye muscles and to provide corrective exercises

**Oscilloscope:** instrument for visibly representing electrical activity on a fluorescent screen, 402

**Osseous:** osteal

**Ossicles:** three small connecting bones of the middle ear, the hammer (or malleus), the anvil (or incus), and the stirrup (or stapes), that transmit sound from the eardrum to the cochlea, 1, 88

disorders, 656

hearing loss, 656

**Ossification:** conversion into bone

**Ossify:** to convert or be converted into bone

**Osteal/osseous:** of or relating to bone

**Osteitis:** inflammation of a bone, 731–32

**Osteoarthritis/degenerative joint disease/hypertrophic arthritis:** chronic degenerative disease that affects the joints, 326, 349–51, 351, 368

causes, 349

symptoms, 350

**Osteogenesis:** formation and growth of bones, 370

imperfecta: condition in which bones are abnormally brittle and liable to fracture due to a deficiency of calcium, 370

**Osteogenic:** pertaining to osteogenesis

Osteogenic sarcoma, 372

**Osteomyelitis:** inflammation of the bone tissue or marrow, 10, 370–71, 730

spinal, 364

**Osteopath:** physician trained in osteopathy

**Osteopathy:** system of healing based on a theory that most diseases are caused by structural abnormalities that may best be corrected by manipulation

**Osteophyte(s):** abnormal bony outgrowth, 350

**Osteoporosis:** reduction in bone mass and increase in interior space, porosity, and fragility of bone, 363, 369

demineralization, *369*

**Otitis media:** inflammation of the middle ear, 653, 656

nonsuppurative: inflammation of the middle ear resulting from a blocked Eustachian tube and fluid collection in the middle ear, causing hearing damage

**Otolaryngologist:** physician specializing in the diagnosis and treatment of the ear, nose, and throat, 826–27

**Otolaryngology:** the branch of medicine dealing with the study and diseases of the ear, nose, and throat, 826–27

**Otologist:** one who specializes in the ear and its diseases, 323

**Otology:** the branch of medical science dealing with the functions and diseases of the ear

Pain,

during labor, 255–58

post-operative, 617–18

Pain receptors, 81

Paint,

lead poisoning, 1051–52

**Palate:** the roof of the mouth, 49

hard: the bony part of the roof of the mouth

soft/velum: the soft, muscular tissue at the rear of the roof of the mouth

**Palpation:** diagnostic procedure of feeling, pressing, or manipulating the body, 830–31, *831*

**Palpitation:** rapid or fluttering heartbeat, 436

*See also* Arrthythmia

**Palsy/paralysis:** Bell's palsy, cerebral palsy

**Pancreas:** large gland situated behind the stomach and containing the islets of Langerhans that produce insulin and glucagon, and secreting pancreatic juice via small ducts to the duodenum, 56, 71, *76, 507, 508*

diabetes, 507

pancreatic duct, 58–59

Pancreatic cancer, 575–76

Pancreatic enzymes, 54–55, 450

**Pancreatic juice:** secretion of the pancreas containing digestive enzymes

**Pancreatitis:** inflammation of the pancreas

**Pandemic:** epidemic occurring over a very large area or worldwide, 476

**Papanicolaou, Dr. George N.:** developer of a test, called the *Pap smear* or *Pap test,* for detecting cancer of the cervix, 807

**Papanicolaou smear** *See* Pap smear

Papaverine, 1100

**Papillae** *(sing., papilla):* tiny, nipple-shaped projections that cover the

inner layer (dermis) of the skin and the surface of the tongue, 20

fingerprints, *21*

tongue, 48–49

**Papillary tumor:**

1. papilloma: benign tumor of the papillae of the skin, as a wart or corn, 570

2. malignant tumor of the bladder, so called because it is nipplelike in shape (Latin *papilla* means nipple), 544

**Pap smear/Papanicolaou smear/ Pap test:** method of early detection of cervical cancer consisting of painless removal of cervical cell samples, which are stained and examined, 291, 552, 783–84, 807–8, 829

cervical cancer, 560

venereal warts, 553

**Pap test** *See* Pap smear

**Papule:** pimple

Paraldehyde,

to treat hangovers, 296

Paralysis

nerve damage, 31

poliomyelitis, 397

sickle-cell anemia, 413

spinal injuries, 379

spinal tuberculosis, 364

stroke victims, 422

tumors, 365

*See also* Poliomyelitis

**Paralysis agitans:** Parkinson's disease

**Paranasal sinus:** air cavity in one of the cranial bones communicating with the nostrils, 69

Paranoia, 919

**Paranoid:** describing a personality disorder in which the individual is extraordinarily sensitive to praise or criticism and subject to suspicions and feelings of persecution, 917

**Paranoid reaction/paranoia:** psychosis characterized by invariable delusion, usu. of persecution, sometimes of grandeur

Paranoid schizophrenia, 918–19

**Paraplegia:** paralysis of the lower half of the body

**Paraplegic:** one who is paralyzed in the lower half of the body, including both legs

**Parisites:** animal or plant that lives in or on another organism (called the host), at whose expense it obtains nourishment

intestinal, 465–67

worms, 465–67

Parasitic diseases,

anemia, 412

**Parasiticide:** medication designed to destroy parasites such as body lice

**Parasympathetic nervous system:** the part of the autonomic nervous system that controls such involuntary actions as the constriction of pupils, dilation of blood vessels and salivary glands, and slowing of heartbeat, 28. Compare *sympathetic nervous system.*

**Parathormone/parathyroid hormone:** hormone secreted by the parathyroid glands, important in regulating the amount of calcium in the body, 78

**Parathyroid glands:** four small endocrine glands near or embedded within the thyroid gland, usu. two per side, that regulate blood calcium and phosphorus levels, 78, 500

Paregoric, 1100

Parent-child relationships, 114

boredom, 123

bribery, 124

curiosity, 134–35

disobedience, 141–42

intelligence in children, 163

responsibilities, 274

single parents, 309–10

suicide, 220

teenagers, 222–23

Parents,

drinking habits, 928

relationship with toddlers, 110

Parents Anonymous, 129

Parents United, 129

Parents Without Partners, 129, 310

**Paresis:**

1. partial paralysis

2. general paralysis *(general paresis)* caused by degeneration of the brain as a result of syphilis

**Parkinson's disease/paralysis agitans/parkinsonism:** chronic, progressive nervous disease characterized by muscle tremor when at rest, stiffness, and a rigid facial expression, 31, 385–87

**Parotid gland:** either of two large salivary glands located below and in front of the ear, 47, 451

mumps, 47, 170

**Paroxysm:** sudden onset of acute symptoms, as an attack or convulsions

Paroxysmal tachycardia, 760-61

**Parrot fever:** psittacosis

Partials *See* Dentures

**Particulate matter:** fine particles in smoke that are dispersed by the wind and fall back to earth

**Parturition:** act or process of giving birth

**Passive-dependent:** describing a personality disorder in which the individual needs excessive emotional support from an authority figure, 917

**Patch test:** skin test for determining hypersensitivity by applying small pads of possibly allergy-producing substances to the skin's surface

*See* Prick test

**Patchy baldness:** alopecia areata

**Patella:** the knee cap

**Pathogen:** disease-causing bacterium or microorganism

**Pathogenic:** disease-causing

**Pathologic:** caused by or relating to disease

**Pathologic fracture:** fracture that occurs spontaneously, as because of preexisting disease, without external cause

**Pathologist:** physician or expert specializing in pathology, 827

**Pathology:** the branch of medical science dealing with the causes, nature, and effects of diseases, esp. disease-induced changes in organs, tissues, and body chemistry

Patients,

home care comfort, 987–90

information on diagnosis,853–54

rights, 851–53

**PCBs/polychlorinated biphenyls:** chemicals related to DDT and having many industrial uses, posing a potential threat to health as a water pollutant from industrial wastes, 963

PCP (Phencyclidine hydrochloride), 951

slang terms, 945

Peace Corps, 334

**Pedal:** of or relating to the foot

**Pediatric dentist:** dentist specializing in the care and treatment of the teeth of children, 138, 839

**Pediatrician:** physician specializing in the care and treatment of children, 827

**Pediatrics:** the branch of medicine dealing with the care and treatment of children and their diseases

**Pedodontics:** branch of dentistry specializing in the care of children

**Pedodontist:** dentist specializing in pedodontics, 172–73

**Pellagra:** disease caused by a vitamin deficiency and characterized by gastric disturbance, skin eruptions, and nervous symptoms, 863

Pelvic bone, 7

**Pelvic girdle:** the part of the human skeleton to which the lower limbs are attached, 3, 6

Pelvic inflammatory disease (PID), 266, 547, 555–56

gonorrhea, 550

Pelvic X-ray, 242

**Pelvis:**

1. the part of the skeleton that forms a bony girdle or basin joining the lower limbs to the body, and consisting of the two hip bones and the sacrum

2. the central area of the kidney from which urine drains into the ureter

bones disorders, 367–68

fractures, 375

**Penicillin:** powerful antibacterial substance found in a mold fungus and prepared in several forms for the treatment of a wide variety of infections

allergic reactions, 776

gonorrhea, 550

nephritis, 539

treating pneumonia, 477

syphilis, 555

Penicillin V, 1100

Penicillin g, 1100

Penicillamine, 354

**Penis:** tubular male organ of sexual intercourse and excretion of urine, located at the front of the pelvis, 99, 228

tumors, 622

Pentaerythritol Tetranitrate, 1101

Pentamidine, 596

Pentobarbital, 1101

**Pentothal/sodium    Pentothal/thiopental:** trademark for an ultrashort-acting barbiturate used as an anesthetic, as in dentistry

Pep pills *See* Amphetamines

**Pepsin:** enzyme secreted by the gastric juices of the stomach, 53

**Peptic ulcer:** ulcer of the mucous membrane of the stomach (gastric ulcer) or small intestine (duodenal ulcer) caused by the action of acid juices, 459, 471

diet following surgery, 621

surgery, 639–40

**Percussion:** diagnostic procedure of striking or tapping the body with instruments or with the fingers, 831–32, *832*

**Perianal:** situated around the anus.

**Pericarditis:** inflammation of the pericardium

**Pericardium:** the membrane that surrounds and protects the heart, 43

**Peridental:** periodontal

**Perimeter:** device for determining peripheral vision

**Perineal:** of or pertaining to the perineum

**Perineum:** region of the body at the lower end of the trunk, between the genital organs and the anus

prostate surgery, 627

**Periodontal/peridental:**    situated around a tooth

Periodontal disease, 313–14, 724, 730, 733–36

treatment, 735–36

**Periodontal membrane:** membrane, periodontal, 4

**Periodontia:** periodontics

**Periodontics/periodontia:**    the branch of dentistry dealing with

the diagnosis and treatment of periodontal (gum) diseases

**Periodontist:** dentist who specializes in periodontics, 839

**Periodontitis:** inflammation of the tissues around a tooth, leading to destruction of the alveolar bone, 734

**Periodontium:** the supporting structures of the teeth, comprising the gingiva, alveolar bone, and periodontal ligaments, 723

**Periosteum:** the tough, fibrous membrane that surrounds and nourishes bones, 8

**Peripheral nervous system:** the nerves and ganglia outside the brain and spinal cord, 27

Peripheral smear, 846

**Peristalsis:** wavelike muscular contractions of the alimentary canal that move the contents along in the processes of digestion and excretion, 50–51, 55, 450

**Peristaltic wave:** the alternate contraction and relaxation of muscles in the alimentary canal in peristalsis, 50

**Peritoneoscopy:** technique for examining the female reproductive organs within the abdominal cavity, 237

**Peritoneoscope/laparoscope:**    instrument used for examining the organs within the abdominal cavity, esp. the female reproductive organs, 270

**Peritoneum:** the serous membrane that lines the abdominal cavity enclosing the abdominal organs, 60

**Peritonitis:** inflammation of the lining (peritoneum) of the abdominal cavity, 464, 637

**Peritonsillar abscess/quinsy:** abscess in the tissues adjoining a tonsil as a complication of tonsillitis

**Pernicious:** severe, destructive, and often fatal

**Pernicious anemia:** severe, progressive anemia caused by lack of vitamin B12, formerly fatal but now controllable, 412

**Personality disorder/character disorder:** any of a group of mental illnesses that apparently stem from an arrested development of the personality, 917

Perspiration, 19, 22–23, 689, 693–94

Pertussis, 159–60, 196

**Pessary:**

1. device worn inside the vagina as a contraceptive or to support uterine prolapse, 797

2. medicated suppository for use in the vagina

Pethidine *See* Meperidine

**Petit mal:** minor epileptic seizure, with very brief loss of consciousness, 144, 389

Compare *grand mal.*

Pets,

allergies, 485–86

children, 174–75

**Peyer's patches:** oval areas of lymphoid tissue in the intestine that manufacture lymphocytes, 38

**Peyote:** the mescal cactus of Mexico or the powerful hallucinogenic drug obtained from its dried upper part (called buttons), 951

**Phalanges** *(sing., phalanx):* the bones of the fingers or toes, 1, 8

*See also* Fingers

**Pharmacist:** one skilled in the compounding and dispensing of medicines

**Pharmacologist:** expert in pharmacology

**Pharmacology:** the science of the action of medicines, their nature, preparation, administration, and effects

**Pharyngitis:** inflammation of the pharynx, commonly called a sore throat

**Pharynx:** the part of the alimentary canal between the palate and the esophagus, serving as a passage for air and food, 50, 66

Phenacetin, 1101

Phenazopyridine, 1101

Phencyclidine hydrochloride
*See* PCP

Phenformin, 516

Pheniramine, 1101

Phenmetrazine, 941

Phenobarbital, 391, 943, 1101

Phenobarbitone *See* Phenobarbital

Phenylbutazone, 1101

Phentermine, 1101

Phenylephrine, 1102

**Phenylketonuria/PKU:** inherited metabolic disorder that can cause mental retardation if not treated by a special diet soon after birth, 168, 175, 245, 912

Phenylpropanolamine, 1102

Phenytoin, 1102

**Phlebitis:** inflammation of the inner membrane of a vein, 418, *418,* 666–67, *666*

**Phlebotomy/bloodletting/venesection:** the opening of a vein for letting blood

**Phlegm:** viscid, stringy mucus secreted in abnormally large amounts, as in the air passages

*See* Sputum

**Phobia:** intense anxiety irrationally felt for any of a variety of things or situations, such as closed or open places, animals of a particular kind, heights, etc., a manifestation of the phobic reaction, 913

children, 147–48

types, 915–16

**Phobic reaction:** neurosis characterized by displacement of anxiety of a conflict to a substitute, such as a particular domestic animal, closed places, etc., 915–16

**Phonocardiogram:** graph recording the sounds produced by the heart, used to evaluate heart murmurs and other abnormal sounds, 844

Phosphorus,

teenage diet, 208–09

Physical addiction, 939

**Physical dependence:** accommodation of the body to continued use of a drug, such that withdrawing the drug causes pronounced physical reactions (withdrawal symptoms)

Physical dependence *See* Drug abuse

Physical examination, 607–08, 828

for children, 127

*See also* Examinations

Physical fitness, 278, 1106–1223

for the elderly, 312, 317–19, 1214–23, *1215, 1217, 1218–20*

getting started, 1107–1110

middle age, 275–76, 278–81

space to exercise, 1109–10

teenagers, 210–12

*See also* Exercise; Individual sports by name, e.g., Golf

**Physical medicine:** branch of medicine utilizing physical procedures, such as heat, cold, massage, or mechanical devices, to diagnose disease or treat disabled patients, 827

**Physical therapist:** specialist in physical therapy

**Physical therapy/physiotherapy:** the treatment of disability, injury, or disease by external physical means, such as heat, massage, planned exercises, electricity, or mechanical devices, to restore function or aid rehabilitation

**Physicians:**

1. any authorized practitioner of medicine, 823

2. one trained in medicine, as distinguished from surgery

group practice, 997–98

partnerships, 997

office-based practices, 997

relationships with patient, 851–55

Physicians'-expense insurance

*See* Health insurance

**Pia mater:** the delicate, vascular, innermost membrane of the three membranes that envelop the brain and spinal cord

**Pica:** appetite for substances unfit to eat, 175

**Piebald skin:** vitiligo

**Pigeon breast/pectus carinatum:** congenital deformity in which the sternum protrudes

**Pigment:** substance that imparts coloring to tissue

Piles *See* Hemorrhoids

"The Pill" *See* Oral contraceptives

Pilocarpine, 1102

**Pimple/papule:** small, usu. inflamed swelling on the skin

Pinch test, 865

**Pineal gland/pineal body:** small, cone-shaped body of rudimentary glandular structure located at the base of the brain and having no known function, 79–80, *80*

**Pinkeye:** acute, contagious conjunctivitis, marked by redness of the eyeball, 768

*See also* Conjunctivitis

**Pinworm:** parasitic worm of the lower intestines and rectum, esp. of children, causing intense itching in the anal area

*See* Threadworms

**Pituitary gland/hypophysis cerebri/pituitary body:** small endocrine gland situated at the base of the brain, consisting of anterior and posterior lobes whose hormonal secretions stimulate the production of hormones in other glands and regulate vital body functions such as growth and metabolism, 72, *72, 73,* 498, *500,* 508

**Pityriasis rosea:** skin disease, esp. of children, marked by a rash, 180

PKU *See* Phenylketonuria

**Placebo:** any harmless substance given to humor a patient or as a test in controlled experiments on the effects of drugs

**Placenta:** the vascular structure in pregnant women that unites the fetus with the uterus, and through which the fetus is nourished via the umbilical cord, usu. expelled naturally immediately following birth (when it is called the *afterbirth*), 258–59

**Plague:**

1. any epidemic disease that is contagious and often deadly

2. contagious, often fatal disease caused by a bacterium transmitted by fleas from infected rats, and characterized by fever, chills, prostration, and often by buboes (hence the name *bubonic plague*)

Planned Parenthood Federation of America, 1007, 1013–14

**Plantar warts:** warts on the soles of the feet, caused by a virus, 714

**Plaque:** mucus containing bacteria that collects on teeth, 729

**Plasma:** the clear fluid portion of the blood, 35, 407

*See also* Lymph

**Plastic surgeon:** physician specializing in plastic or cosmetic surgery, 678

**Plastic surgery:** surgery that deals with the restoration or healing of lost, injured, or deformed parts of the body, mainly by the transfer of tissue, and with the improvement of appearance (cosmetic surgery), 322, 604–05, 677–84, 827

*See also* Cosmetic surgery

**Platelets/thrombocytes:** small, disk-shaped body found in blood that aids in clotting, 37, 409

Play, 111, 145, 146–47, 156

hobbies, 156

toys, 195

**Play therapy:** psychotherapy, esp. for patients who are children, in which toys or other playthings are made available for the patient to play with in the presence of the therapist, 923

**Pleura:** serous membrane that enfolds the lungs and lines the chest cavity, 478

**Pleural cavity:** the space between the two pleuras lining the lungs and chest cavity, 66–67

Pleural membranes, 66–67

**Pleurisy:** inflammation of the pleura, characterized by fever, chest pain, and difficulty in breathing, 67, 478

**Plexus:** interlacement of cordlike body structures, such as blood vessels or nerves, 30

Plexus block *See* Nerve block

PMS *See* Premenstrual Syndrome

**Pneumococcus:** bacterium that can cause pneumonia, 476

**Pneumoconiosis:** any of various lung disorders, such as silicosis or black lung disease, resulting from the inhalation of dust or other minute particles, 495–96

Pneumocystis carinii, 584, 586

Pneumoencephalography, 382

**Pneumoencephalogram:** X-ray picture of the brain taken after air or gas has been injected to partially replace the cerebrospinal fluid, 842

**Pneumoencephalography:** technique of producing pneumoencephalograms and interpreting them

**Pneumonia:** inflammation of the lungs, usu. bacterial in origin and acute in course, characterized by

**Pontic:** in dentistry, a part of a bridge serving as a substitute for a missing tooth

**Popliteal:** pertaining to the back part of the leg behind the knee

Pork,

  danger in undercooking, 466

Pornography, 186–87

**Portal vein:** vein that conveys blood from the intestines and stomach to the liver, 57

"Port wine stain" *See* Hemangioma

**Positive pressure breathing:** breathing of air or other gas mixture at pressure greater than the surrounding atmospheric pressure

Post-coronary exercise, 1183–88

Position emission tomography (PET), 445

**Posterior:** toward the rear

**Posterior lobe hypophysis:** the posterior part of the pituitary gland that produces hormones regulating kidney function and other vital processes, 72

Posterior pituitary gland, 508

**Posterior urethra:** prostatic urethra

**Postmenopausal:** being or occurring after menopause

**Postpartum:** after childbirth

Posture, 177, 833

  arthritis patients, 345, 355

  backache in pregnancy, 242

**Postural drainage:** the loosening and draining of lung secretions by assuming a prone position with the head lower than the feet

Potassium, 209, 1102

Potassium citrate, 542, 632

Potassium permanganate, 558

Potential acuity meter (PAM), 658

**Pott's disease:** tuberculosis or tissue destruction of the spinal vertebrae, causing angular, spinal curvature, 364

**PPD:** purified protein derivative

Precocity, 116

**Prediabetic condition:** diabetes, chemical

Prednisolone, 1102

Prednisone, 394, 1102

**Pre-eclampsia:** disorder of late pregnancy or following childbirth, 241. *See also* Toxemia of pregnancy.

**Preemie/premie:** premature infant

Preferred-provider organizations (PPOs), 981, 998

**Pregnancy:** condition or time of being pregnant, 238–54

  anemia, 413, 759

  amniocentesis, 246

  backaches, 242, 749

  chlamydia, 549

  delivery date, 250, 252

  dental care, 724–25

  diabetes, 511, 520

  diet, 239–41

  weight gain, 239–41

  drugs, 239

  ectopic, 248

  endometriosis, 805

  excessive noise, 966

  fetal position, 253–54

  hemorrhoids, 461, 651

  herpes simplex virus type 2, 713, 792–93

  hiatus hernia, 453

  home test, 855

  immunizations, 243–44

  influenza, 244

  leg cramps, 243

  lightening, 252–53

  nutrition requirements, 862, 1000

  pre-natal exams, 100

  rape, 821

**Prostatectomy:** surgical removal of all or part of the prostate gland, 626

**Prostatic urethra/posterior urethra:** the part of the male urethra that passes across the prostate gland

**Prostatitis:** inflammation of the prostate gland, characterized by painful and excessive urination, 770

acute: severe, relatively uncommon form of prostatitis, marked by painful and excessive urination, high fever, and a discharge of pus from the penis, 546

**Prosthesis** *(pl., prostheses)*/**prosthetic device:** artificial substitute for a missing or amputated part, as an arm or leg

impotence, 302–03

hip replacement, 376

**Proteins:** any of a class of highly complex organic compounds, composed principally of amino acids, that occur in all living things and form an essential part of animal food requirements

body composition, 857

deficiency, 369

nephrosis, 540

**Proteinuria:** excretion of protein through the urine, 241

**Prothrombin:** the inactive precursor of thrombin, an agent in the process of forming blood clots, 409

**Protozoa** *(sing., protozoon):* microscopic animal organisms that exist in countless numbers, including one-celled organisms and parasitic forms that cause malaria, sleeping sickness, and other diseases

**Proximal:** relatively near the center of the body or near a point considered as central. Compare *distal.*

**Proximal muscles:** those muscles closest to the trunk of the body, such as the shoulder-arm and hip-thigh muscles

**Pruritus:** localized or general itching

anal: intense itching in the area of the anus, 558, 708

Pseudoephedrine, 1103

**Pseudohypertrophic muscular dystrophy/Duchenne's muscular dystrophy:** disease characterized by the enlargement and apparent overdevelopment (hypertrophy) of certain muscles, esp. of the shoulder girdle, which subsequently atrophy

**Pseudotumor/pseudoneoplasm:** condition that has the appearance of a tumor but is not a tumor, such as an inflammation, 569

Psilocin, 951

**Psilocybin:** derivative of the mushroom *Psilocybe mexicana,* which produces hallucinations in the user, 951

**Psittacosis/parrot fever:** infectious disease of parrots and other birds that can be transmitted to humans and cause symptoms like those of influenza

**Psoralen:** chemical derived from a plant that is used in the treatment of psoriasis, 717

hair loss, 288

**Psoriasis:** a noncontagious chronic condition of the skin, marked by bright red patches covered by silvery scales, 357, 716–17

arthritis, 359

Psoriatic arthropathy, 359

**Psychiatrist:** physician specializing in psychiatry, 827, 911, 921

**Psychiatry:** the branch of medicine that treats disorders of the mind (or psyche), including psychoses and neuroses

Psychic determinism, 911

**Psychoanalysis:** system of psychotherapy originated by Sigmund Freud for treating emotional disorders by bringing to the attention of the conscious mind the re-

**Rabies/hydrophobia:** acute viral disease of the central nervous system transmitted to humans by the bite or saliva of an infected animal, as a dog, bat, or squirrel, invariably fatal unless treated before symptoms appear, 1060–61

*See also* Animal bites

Radiation,

*See also* Irradiation

**Radiation sickness:** illness caused by the body's absorption of excess radiation, marked by fatigue, nausea, vomiting, and sometimes internal hemorrhage and tissue breakdown

**Radiation therapy/radiotherapy:** treatment of disease by radiation, as by X rays or other radioactive substances

bladder cancer, 571

Hodgkin's disease, 580

leukemia, 416

radioactive phosphorus, 414

thyroid cancer, 579

Radiolabeled antibodies,

liver cancer, 576

**Radical:** of or involving procedures or treatment intended to go to the root of a disease and thereby eliminate it, as by excising an entire organ or part that is diseased

**Radiograph:** X-ray photograph

**Radiography:** X-ray photography

**Radiologist:** physician specializing in radiology, 827

**Radiology:** the branch of medical science that deals with radiant energy, such as X rays and energy produced by radium, cobalt, and other radioactive substances, esp. in the diagnosis and treatment of disease,

**Radiopaque:** impervious to X rays

**Radius *(pl., radii):*** the bone of the forearm on the same side as the thumb, thicker and shorter than the ulna bone, 7

fracture with metal plate, 375

Radon gas, 961, 1052–53

Rafampin, 1104

Radio therapy, 327, 565

Ragweed,

hay fever, 484

Rape Crisis Centers, 822

Rape, 820–22, 1085–86

**Rale:** abnormal sound heard in the chest with the aid of a stethoscope, indicating the presence of disease

Rashes, 179–81

juvenile rheumatoid arthritis, 355

treatment, 179

*See also* Chicken pox

**Raynaud's syndrome/Raynaud's disease:** condition characterized by spasms of small blood vessels when exposed to cold, esp. the fingers and toes, which become cyanotic (bluish) and then red,

**RBC:** red blood cell; *See* Erythrocyte

Reach-to-Recovery, 1010

Reading,

children, 181

later years, 333

Reading problems,

dyslexia, 143

*See also* Learning disabilities

Records, medical *See* Health records

**Recovery room:** hospital room or section for patients immediately following surgery, where their postoperative conditions can be closely monitored, 616–17

Rectal bleeding, 564

Rectal surgery,

diet, 621

**Rectocele:** hernia in which part of the rectum protrudes through the wall of the vagina, *797, 798*

tate gland by insertion into the urethra, 627

Reserpine, 1104

**Residency:** period of training in a hospital, usu. in a medical specialty, for physicians preparing for private practice

**Resident:** physician working and undergoing training (residency) in a hospital in preparation for private practice in a specialty

Residential care, 1005–06

alcoholism treatment, 935–36

Residue diet,

minimal, 907–08

minimal, menus, 907–08

**Resorb:** to reabsorb

**Respiration:** the process by which an animal or plant takes in oxygen from the air and gives off carbon dioxide and other products of oxidation

cellular, 63–64

checking at home, 985

diaphragm, 64–66

moisture, 63

oxygen exchange, 63–63

*See also* Breathing

Respiratory arrest, 1025–26

cocaine, 942

Respiratory disease, 472–86

air pollution, 957, 958, 960

diagnostic techniques, 849–50

infections, 744–45

steam inhalators, 992

voluntary agencies, 1019

*See also* Cystic fibrosis

Respiratory system, 60–69, 849

common disorders, 766–67

tuberculosis, 661–62

Rest,

middle age, 281–82

**Resuscitation:** mouth-to-mouth respiration

Retardation *See* Mental retardation

Retention cyst *See* Follicular cysts

**Reticulum:** network of cells or cellular tissue

Reticulum-cell sarcoma, 582–85

**Retina:** the inner membrane at the back of the eyeball, containing light-sensitive rods and cones which receive the optical image, 82, 83

*See also* Detached retina

**Retinoblastoma:** tumor of the eye, found esp. in children, 126

**Retinopathy:** diseased condition of the retina of the eye,

**Retinoscope:** special device for examining the retina, 850

Retirement, 331–42

leisure, 331–35

volunteer work, 334–35

selecting housing, 339–42

Retirement communities, 341

**Rhesus factor:** Rh factor

**Rheumatic fever:** acute infectious disease chiefly affecting children and young adults, characterized by painful inflammation around the joints, intermittent fever, and inflammation of the pericardium and valves of the heart, 182, 360, 425

causes, 440–41

symptoms, 441–42

treatment, 442–43

*See also* Rheumatic heart disease

**Rheumatic heart disease:** impairment of heart function as a result of rheumatic fever, 182, 425–26, 440–43

**Rheumatism:** painful inflammation and stiffness of muscles, joints, or connective tissue,

*See* Arthritis

**Rheumatoid arthritis:** chronic disease characterized by swelling and inflammation of one or more joints, often resulting in stiffness and eventual impairment of mobility, 326, 348–49, 352–53

**Rheumatoid arthritis, juvenile/ Still's disease:** form of rheumatoid arthritis affecting children, often characterized by fever, rash, pleurisy, and enlargement of the spleen as well as rheumatoid joint symptoms, 355–56

**Rheumatologist:** physician specializing in rheumatology, 825

**Rheumatology:** subspecialty of internal medicine concerned with the study, diagnosis, and treatment of rheumatism and other diseases of the joints and muscles, 825, 839

**Rh factor/rhesus factor:** protein present in the blood of most people (called Rh-positive) and absent from others (called Rh-negative). Under certain conditions the blood of a pregnant Rh-negative woman may be incompatible with the blood of her fetus, 36–37, 244–45, 414–15

**Rhinencephalon/"nose brain":** the part of the brain controlling the sense of smell, 91

**Rhinitis:** inflammation of the mucous membranes of the nose,

**Rhinoplasty:** plastic surgery of the nose, 286, 604, 678–80

**Rhythm method:** birth control method whereby sexual intercourse is avoided during the period of ovulation in the menstrual cycle, 268

**Rhytidoplasty/face lift/facial plasty:** plastic surgery to eliminate facial wrinkles, 286, 605, 681, *682*

**Rib cage/thoracic cage:** the part of the skeleton that encloses the chest, bound by the ribs and the spinal vertebrae,

birth defects, 346

fracture and injury, 378

**Riboflavin/vitamin B₂:** member of the vitamin B complex, found in milk, green leafy vegetables, eggs and meats

**Ribs:** one of the series of curved bones attached to the spine and enclosing the chest cavity,

Rice bran, 876

**Rickets:** early childhood disease characterized by softening of bones and consequent deformity, caused by deficiency of vitamin D, 368, 371

**Rickettsiae** *(sing., rickettsia):* parasitic microorganisms transmitted to humans by the bites of infected ticks, lice, and fleas, and causing Rocky Mountain spotted fever, Q fever, rickettsial pox, and typhus

**Rickettsial disease:** any of the diseases, as typhus or Rocky Mountain spotted fever, caused by rickettsiae,

**Rickettsial pox:** infectious disease, rickettsial disease, transmitted by mites which infest mice, and characterized by fever, chills, rash, headache, and backache

**Ringworm/tinea:** contagious fungus disease of the skin, hair, or nails marked by ring-shaped, scaly, reddish patches of skin, 711

**Rocky Mountain spotted fever:** infectious disease (rickettsial disease) transmitted by the bite of certain ticks and characterized by fever, chills, rash, headache, and muscular pain, 180–81, 589–90

*See also* Ticks

**Rod:** one of many rod-shaped bodies in the retina of the eye, sensitive to faint light and peripheral objects and movements. Compare *cone.* 82–83, *82*

**Roentgenogram:** X-ray photograph

**Roentgenologist:** physician specializing in the diagnosis and treatment of diseases with the application of X rays

**Roentgenology:** the branch of medical science dealing with the properties and effects of X rays

**Root canal:** the passageway of nerves and blood vessels in the root of a tooth leading into the pulp, 4

Root canal therapy, 732–33, *732*

**Roseola infantum:** childhood illness characterized by high fever followed by a body rash, 180

**Roughage:** food material containing a high percentage of indigestible constituents

**Roundworm/ascaris:** parasitic nematode worm, as the hookworm and pinworm, whose eggs hatch in the small intestines, 466–67

**Rubella/German measles:** contagious viral disease benign in children but linked to birth defects of children born of women infected in early pregnancy, 182–83

congenital heart disease, 444–45

deafness, 531

immunization, 159

mental retardation, 168

pregnancy, 244

Rubella arthritis, 358–59

**Rubeola:** measles

**Rubin's test:** tubal insufflation, 235

Runaway Hotline, 184

Runaways, 183–84

Running *See* Jogging

**Rupture:**

1. any breaking apart, as of a blood vessel

2. hernia

*See* Hernia

**Sabin vaccine:** live polio vaccine taken orally to immunize against polio, 176

**Sacral:** pertaining to the sacrum

**Sacroiliac:** pertaining to the sacrum or the ilium, or to the places on either side of the lower back where they are joined, 367

**Sacrum:** bone in the lower spine formed by the fusing of five vertebrae, constituting the rear part of the pelvis, 6

**Saddle block:** form of anesthesia used esp. for childbirth, in which the patient is injected in the lower spinal cord while in a sitting position, 256

Safety,

avoiding sexual abuse, 187

in the home, 1036–55

**Safety glass:** glass strengthened by any of various methods to reduce the likelihood of the glass shattering upon impact

Safety standards, 1008

**St. Vitus's dance** *See* Chorea,

**Saline amniocentesis/salting out:** technique of inducing abortion by injecting a saline solution into the amniotic fluid, 249

**Saliva:** fluid secreted by the salivary glands in the mouth that lubricates food and contains an enzyme (ptyalin) that begins to break down starch, 47–48, 450–51, 728–29

**Salivary glands:** glands located in the mouth which secrete saliva, 47, *47,* 48, 450–51

**Salk vaccine:** dead polio virus taken by injection to immunize against polio, 176

**Salmonella:** genus of aerobic bacteria that cause food poisoning and other diseases, including typhoid fever, 468, 1056

**Salmonella typhosa:** rod-shaped bacteria that cause typhoid fever, 457

**Salpingitis:**

1. inflammation of a Fallopian tube, a potential cause of sterility,

2. inflammation of a Eustachian tube

**Salt:** sodium chloride

iodine as an addititive, 78

restricted intake, 622

Salt-free diets, 875

chart, 898–901

**Saltiness:** taste of

**Salting out:** the injection of a saline solution into the amniotic fluid to induce labor and thus terminate a pregnancy

*See* Saline amniocentesis

Salt tablets,

heat cramps, 751

Sanatoriums, 480

Sandflies,

Leishmaniasis, 593–95

**Saphenous vein:** either of two large, superficial veins of the leg, a common site of varicosity

**Sarcoidosis/Boeck's sarcoid/sarcoid:** disease of unknown cause with symptoms resembling those of tuberculosis, marked by the formation of nodules, esp. on the skin, lungs, and lymph nodes, 482

**Sarcoma:** malignant tumor that arises in the connective tissue (bones, cartilage, tendons), 561

**Saturated:** (of fats) tending to increase the cholesterol content of the blood, 858

**Saucerization:** procedure of forming a shallow depression by scraping away tissue to assist healing, 632–33

Saunas,

after exercise, 1119

**Scabies/the itch:** contagious inflammation of the skin caused by a mite and characterized by a rash and intense itching, 711

**Scan:** to measure for diagnostic purposes the concentration in a particular area of a radioactive material that has been introduced into the body.

*See* Computerized tomography

**Scapula:** shoulder blade, 5, 403

**Scarlet fever:** contagious disease caused by streptococci and characterized by a scarlet rash and high fever, 184–85

Scarlet fever, 184–85

Scars,

surgery to reduce, 683

**Schistosomiasis/bilharziasis:** tropical disease caused by a fluke worm (trematode) whose larvae penetrate the skin and invade the circulatory system, 571, 598–601

**Schizoid:**

1. describing a personality disorder in which the individual is withdrawn from and indifferent to other people, 917

2. pertaining to or resembling schizophrenia

**Schizophrenia:** 167, 918–19

catatonic: schizophrenia marked by motor disturbances, such as maintenance of fixed, often awkward, position with muscles rigid,

hebephrenic: schizophrenia marked by delusions, hallucinations, and regressed or childish behavior,

paranoid: schizophrenia marked by variable delusions of persecution or grandeur, often with hallucinations and behavioral deterioration

**Schizophrenic:** of or pertaining to schizophrenia

**Schizophrenic reaction/schizophrenia:** psychosis characterized by withdrawal from external reality and a retreat into a fantasy life, with deterioration of behavior,

School *See* Education

School and college health program, 999

**Sciatic nerve:** nerve of the lower spine that traverses the hips and runs down the back of the thigh of each leg

**Sclera:** the firm outer coat of the eye continuous with the cornea, visible as the white of the eye, 85

**Sclerose:** to harden and thicken, as tissue

**Sclerosis:** abnormal thickening and hardening tissue, as of the lining of arteries

**Scoliosis:** spine, lateral curvature, 363, *364,* 670, *670*

amyotrophic lateral/Lou Gehrig's disease: disease characterized by increasing muscle weakness (atrophy) or paralysis, caused by the progressive degeneration of motor nerve cells in the brain and spinal cord, 30

Scorpion stings, 1086

**Scratch test:** skin test for allergic response to different substances by applying suspected allergens in diluted form to scratches,

**Scrofula:** tuberculosis of the lymph nodes, esp. of the neck

Scopolamine,

labor, 255

Scratch test, 779

**Scrotum:** pouch that contains the testicles, 99, 203, 504,

tumors, 628

**Scrub nurse:** operating room nurse authorized to handle sterilized equipment in assisting the surgeon, 611

**Scurvy:** disease characterized by livid spots under the skin, swollen and bleeding gums, and prostration, caused by lack of vitamin C, 863

Seat belts,

chest injuries, 378

**Sebaceous cyst:** hard, round, movable mass contained in a sac, resulting from accumulated oil from a blocked sebaceous gland duct, 714–15

**Sebaceous gland:** gland within the dermis that secretes oil (sebum) for lubricating the skin and hair, 20, 22, 690

**Seborrhea:** abnormal increase of secretion from the sebaceous skin glands

**Sebum:** fatty lubricating substance secreted by the sebaceous glands, 22

Secobartital, 1104

**Secondary:** produced as an effect or complication of another condition, as distinguished from *primary*

Secondary care, 996

**Secondary disease:** disorder of a target gland caused by an excess or deficiency of a stimulating hormone supplied by the anterior pituitary gland

**Sedation:** reduction of sensitivity to pain, stress, etc., by administering a sedative

pre-operative, 610

**Sedative:** medicine for allaying irritation or nervousness,

Seizures, 144–45

*See also* Epilepsy

Self-testing,

diagnostic tests, 855

**Semen:** thick, whitish fluid containing spermatozoa that is ejaculated by the male at orgasm, 228

infertility exam, 234–35

**Seminal vesicle:** one of two small pouches on either side of the prostate gland that serve to store spermatozoa temporarily, 204, 228

Senile dementia *See* Dementia

**Senile macula degeneration:** visual defect affecting the elderly, 327

**Senile psychosis/senile dementia:** mental disorder of the aged characterized by progressive deterio-

**Sigmoidoscope:** surgical instrument for examining the interior of the sigmoid, 565, 645

**Sign (of disease):** observable or objective manifestation, as distinguished from symptoms reported by the patient,

**Silica:** extremely hard mineral, the chief constituent of quartz and sand

pneumoconioses, 495

Silicone and breast enlargement, 681

**Silicosis:** lung disorder, a form of pneumoconiosis, caused by inhaling silica dust, as of stone or sand,

Silver nitrate,

new borns eyes, 1013

**Simple fracture:** closed fracture, 1078

Single photon emission, computed tomography, 422

**Sinoatrial node:** sinus node

**Sinus:** opening or cavity, as in bone, or a channel or passageway, as for blood

**Sinusitis:** inflammation of a sinus, 69, 475

**Sinus node/sinoatrial node:** small mass of nerve tissue in the right atrium of the heart that triggers heart contractions and regulates heartbeat, thus serving as cardiac pacemaker, 43

**Sitz bath:** hot bath taken in a sitting position,

**Skeletal muscle/voluntary muscle:** striated muscle attached to bones and joints, used chiefly in voluntary action, 11. Compare *smooth muscle.*

abdomen, *11*

back, *12*

thorax, *11*

back, *12*

Skeletal system, 2–7

diseases of, 345–79

Skeleton, 1–10, *2, 347, 840*

appendicular: the bones of the arms, hands, legs, and feet, 3, 6–8

axial: the bones of the head and the trunk, 3–6

Skiing, 279

Skilled nursing facilities, 1006

**Skin/integument:** the outer, membranous covering of the body, consisting of an outer layer (epidermis) and inner layer (dermis), 18–23, *19,* 81–82, 92–93, 689–93, 705–06

acne, 715–16

aging, 320–22, 692

allergies, 777

anatomy, *690*

boils, 712

chapping, 752–53

color, 21, 691

cosmetics, 694–96

functions, 19

heat flush, 22–23

grafting, 685

granulomas (nodules), 482

itching, 321

problems in later years, 320–22

sunlight and aging, 692

sun-tan lotions, 696

test-tube skin for burns, 1068

types, 693, 702

*See also* Sunburn; Suntan

Skin cancer, 565–66

basal cell, 321

squamos cell, 321

Skin care,

adolescents, 206–07

aging, 285–86

creams for dryness, 322

hearing aids, 323

runaways, 184

sexual abuse, 189

single parents, 310

**Social workers:** person trained to work in a clinical, social, or recreational service for improving community welfare or aiding the rehabilitation or emotional adjustment of individuals, 922

**Sociopathic/psychopathic:** describing a personality disorder in which the individual characteristically lacks a sense of personal responsibility or morality and may be disposed to aggressive and violent behavior, to self-destructive behavior, or to sexual deviation, 917

Sodium,

restricted diets, 875

restricted diets (chart), 898–901

restricted diet, menus, 901

teenage diet, 209

*See also* Salt

**Sodium amytal:** chemical used as sedative for soldiers in World War I, 924

Sodium bicarbonate, 1093

Sodium pentothal, 256, 943

Soft contact lenses *See* Contact lenses

Soft diets

chart, 895–98

**Soft spots:** fontanels

**Soldiers' disease:** morphinism

Solvents, 953–54

Somatrophin, 72–73

**Soot-wart:** name for cancer of the scrotum that afflicted 18th-century chimney sweeps,

*See* Cancer, scrotum

Sore throats, 190

**Spasm:** involuntary convulsive contraction of muscles, called *clonic*

when alternately contracted and relaxed, and *tonic* when persistently contracted

**Spastic:** of or characteristic of spasms

**Spasticity:** the condition of having spasms, 383

Special perils insurance *See* Health insurance

Specialities,

medical and surgical, 823–27

**Specimen:** sample, as of blood, sputum, etc., for laboratory analysis

**Speculum:** instrument that dilates a passage of the body, as for examination, 783, 807

Speech,

eating, 50

strokes, 422

toddlers, 110

Speech *See also* Language development

Speech defects, 190

*See also* Talking

Speech disorders,

dyslexia, 143

Speech pathology, 190

**Speech reading:** lip reading, 324

Speech therapy, 190

Speedwalking, 1179

**Sperm** *See* Spermatozoa

**Spermatozoa** *(sing., spermatozoon)/* **sperm/sperm cells:** male reproductive cells or gametes, one of which must fertilize an ovum to produce an embryo, 203, 228, 424–25

**Sperm cell:** the male reproductive cell, one of the spermatozoa

**Sperm ducts:** vas deferens

**Spermicide:** contraceptive substance that destroys sperm, 266, 267, 268

**Sphincter(s):** ringlike muscle surrounding an opening or tube that serves to narrow or close it, 16, 97

anal, 51, 59

cardiac, 51

pyloric, 51

**Sphygmomanometer:** device for measuring arterial blood pressure, 44, 438, 833

Spider bites,

black widow, 1063

recluse spider, 1066

Spinal,

fractures, 671

fusion, 356, 669–70, *669*

infections, 364

tumors, 364–65

**Spinal anesthesia/spinal:** form of anesthesia in which the patient is injected in the region of the spinal cord, 615–16

**Spinal arthritis:** arthritis of the spine, found esp. in the elderly, 350, 356

**Spinal column/backbone/spine:** the series of segmented bones (vertebrae) which enclose the spinal cord and provide support for the ribs, 3–7

disorders, 362–67, 667–70

fusion, 364, 366

infections, 364

injuries, 378–79

psoriatic arthropathy, 359

tumors, 364–65

**Spinal cord:** the part of the central nervous system enclosed within the spinal column,

**Spinal fluid exam:** spinal tap, 842

Spinal meningitis,

bacteria and arthritis, 359

Spinal nerves, 27

syphilis, 554

**Spinal puncture** *See* Spinal tap

**Spinal reflex:** reaction to an outside stimulus that originates in the

spinal cord and bypasses the brain, 31

**Spinal tap/lumbar puncture/spinal fluid exam/spinal puncture:** needle puncture and withdrawal of cerebrospinal fluid from the lower spinal column for diagnostic examination,

*See* Lumbar puncture; Spinal fluid exam

Spinal tuberculosis, 364

**Spirochete:** any of various spiral-shaped bacteria, some of which cause syphilis and yaws

Spirochete, 553

**Spleen:** vascular, ductless organ located near the stomach that produces red blood cells in infancy and modifies blood composition, 411

producer of white blood cells, 38

white blood cells, 415

Splinters, 758, 1088

**Splints:** appliance for supporting or immobilizing a part of the body, as a fracture bone, 1078

**Spondylitis:** inflammation of the vertebrae of the spine

rheumatoid/ankylosing spondylitis: chronic disease characterized by inflammation of the spine and resulting in the fusing (ankylosing) of the spinal joints, 356

**Spondylolisthesis:** forward displacement of one of the lower vertebrae over the vertebra below it or over the sacrum, causing severe pain in the lower back, 366–67, 670

**Spontaneous abortion** *See* Miscarriage

**Sporadic:** characterized by scattered cases, as of a disease, rather than by concentration in one area

**Spore:** single-celled reproductive body of a flowerless plant, capable of developing into an independent organism

**Sprains:** the stretching or rupturing of ligaments, usu. accompanied by damage to blood vessels, 1088

Spurs *See* Osteophytes

**Sputum:** expectorated matter, as saliva, sometimes mixed with mucus, 475, 493

**Sputum exam:** bacteriological, chemical, and microscopic testing of sputum for presence of disease, 849–50

Squamous cell,

carcinoma, 566

Stabismus *See* Crossed eyes

Stab wounds, 603

Stamp test, 303

**Stapedius:** small muscle in the tympanum of the middle ear whose function is to dampen loud sounds,

**Stapes** *See* stirrup,

**Staphylococcus** *(pl., staphylococci)/* **staph:** parasitic bacterium that can cause boils and other infections

aureus: bacterium that causes food poisoning

**Startle response/startle reflex:** complex involuntary reaction to sudden noise occurring esp. in infancy, where it is marked by a sudden jerk of the arms and legs, 100–02

Stasis dermatitis, 322

**Static exercises:** isometrics,

*See* Exercises

**Status epilepticus:** series of epileptic seizures, occuring virtually without interruption, 389

STD *See* Sexually transmitted diseases

Steam Baths,

after exercise, 1119

Steam inhalators, 992

**Stenosis:** the narrowing of a duct or canal in the body

valvular, 442, 443

Stepchildren, 308–09

**Sterile:**

1. being incapable of producing offsring

2. being free of germs

**Sterility:**

1. condition of being incapable of producing offspring

2. condition of being free of germs

**Sterilization:** the process of destroying reproductive capacity by surgical means, as by tying the Fallopian tubes of a woman (tubal ligation) or by tying the seminal duct of a man (vasectomy), 269–70

voluntary agencies, 1021

*See also* Tubal ligation; Vasectomy

Sternum,

fracture, 378

**Steroid(s):** any of a group of organic compounds occuring naturally and produced synthetically, including the sex hormones, the bile acids, oral contraceptives, and many drugs, 354

hair loss, 287

nephrosis, 540

purpura, 410–11

sarcoidosis, 482

**Stethoscope:** diagnostic device that conducts sounds produced within the body, as the heartbeat, to the ear of the examiner,

Stiffness,

arthritis, 352,

**Stiff toe:** pain and stiffness in the joint of the big toe,

Stilbestrol *See* Diethylstibestrol

Still's disease *See* Rheumatoid arthritis, juvenile

**Stimulant:** drug or other substance that increases or agitates the physiological processes of body or mind, 939–42. Compare *Depressant.*

teenagers, 213–19

**Stimulus** *(pl., stimuli):* that which initiates an impulse or affects the activity of an organism

Sting ray, 1088–89

**Stirrup/stapes:** the innermost of the three ossicles of the middle ear, the bone between the anvil and the cochlea, 87, 90

**Stokes-Adams syndrome:** sudden unconsciousness and sometimes convulsions caused by heart block, 447

**Stoma:** small opening in a surface, as in a membrane or wall of a blood vessel

Stomach, 51–53

aches, 190–91

Stomach,

chemicals, 53

food processing, 52–53

Stomach cancer, 567–69, 642–44

Stones,

salivary glands, 451

**Stool exam:** laboratory analysis of feces, as for presence of blood or parasitic organisms, 847

**STP:** DOM,

**Strabismus/squint:** disorder of the eye muscles in which one eye drifts so that its position is not parallel with the other, 657

**Strains:** excessive stretching of a muscle, tendon, or ligament, 1089

Strangulated hernia, 462

Strangulation,

emergency treatment, 1032–34

**Stratum corneum:** the outermost layer of the epidermis, consisting of horny, lifeless cells, 21

"Strawberry mark" *See* Hemangioma

**Strep throat:** streptococcal infection of the throat, 195

nephritis, 538–39

**Streptococcal:** of or relating to the streptococcus bacterium, 538

erysipelas, 713

impetigo, 712

Streptococcal infections, 185, 190, 426

rheumatic fever, 440–41

**Streptococcus:** kind of bacteria including some forms that cause diseases, as pneumonia and scarlet fever, 182, 360

Stress, 913

children, 120

delayed puberty, 201

heart disease, 325, 435

herpes attacks, 551

infertility, 232

middle age, 276, 277

nervous habits, 171

noise, 966

onset of menstruation, 199

physiological effect, 1121

posture, 177

toxemia of pregnancy, 241

vomiting, 170–71

ways to handle it, 1120–21, 1158–59

**Stress fracture:** tiny crack in a bone caused by repeated stress,

Stretch marks, 252

Stretcher, 1056

**Striated:** striped, as certain muscle

**Stripping:** surgical removal of lengths of varicose veins, exp. one of the saphenous veins of the leg, 288–89, 665–66

*See also* Varicose veins

**Stroke/apoplexy:** attack of paralysis caused by the rupture of an artery and hemorrhage into the brain, or by an obstruction of an artery, as from a blood clot, 326, 421–22, 1089–90

alcohol use, 932

atherosclerosis, *420*

STP, 952

**Stupor:** condition in which the senses and faculties are suspended or greatly dulled, as from shock, drugs, etc.

Stuttering *See* Speech defects

**Sty:** small, inflamed swelling of a sebaceous gland on the edge of the eyelid, 768, 1090

**Subacute:** intermediate between *acute* and *chronic:* said of a disease

Subacute bacterial endocarditis *See* Endocarditis

**Subarachnoid:** situated or occuring between the middle layer (arachnoid) and the innermost layer (pia mater) of the brain

**Subcutaneous:** situated or applied beneath the skin, 20

**Subcutaneous injection:** an injection given in the subcutaneous tissue beneath the skin, 513

**Subcutaneous tissue:** layer of fatty tissue below the skin (dermis) which acts as an insulator against heat and cold and as a shock absorber against injury, 691

**Subdural:** situated or occuring between the outermost layer (dura mater) and the middle layer (arachnoid) of the brain

Subdural hematoma, 377

**Subjective:** (of symptoms) of a kind that only the patient is aware of. Compare *objective.*

**Sublingual gland:** either of a pair of salivary glands located beneath the tongue, 47

**Submandibular gland:** submaxillary gland

**Submaxillary gland/submandibular gland:** either of a pair of salivary glands located under each side of the lower jaw, 47

Substance abuse, 926–55

*See also* Alcohol abuse; Drug abuse

**Subtotal:** less than total, as a surgical procedure involving the excision of an organ or part

Sucking, 109

pacifiers, 174

Suction lipectomy, 681–82

**Sudden infant death syndrome/crib death/SIDS:** death of an infant, usu. between one and six months of age and without any preceding sign of distress and of undetermined cause, 191

Sugar *See* Glucose

Suicide, 219–20, 913

**Sulfa drug:** any of a group of organic compounds used in the treatment of a variety of bacterial infections,

Sulfamethoxazole, 1104

Sulfisoxazole, 1104

Sulfiting agents, 968

**Sulfonamide(s):** any of a group of chemical compounds including the sulfa drugs, used in the treatment of bacterial infections

allergic reactions, 776

**Sulfonylurea:** drug used to treat diabetes, 516

Sulfur,

teenage diet, 209

Sulfur dioxide, 958

Sunburns, 21, 751, 1090

Sun exposure, 690

lip cancer, 652

skin aging, 286, 692

skin cancer, 565, 566

sun screens, 322, 696

tanning, 21, 696

**Sunstroke/heatstroke:** condition marked by an acutely high fever and the cessation of perspiration, caused by prolonged exposure to heat and sometimes leading to convulsions and coma, 752

*See also* Heatstroke

tuberculosis, 661–62

types, 602–06

ulcers, 460

ureter stones, 631

urgent, 603–04

urinary tract, 544

varicose veins, 288–89

vascular system, 664–66

vasectomy, 629–30

vesical stones, 632

water loss, 622

*See also* Laser surgery; Operating room

**Surgical:** of or relating to surgery

**Surgical diathermy:** electrosurgery

Surgical insurance *See* Blue Cross/ Blue Shield; Health Insurance

Surgical team, 610–11

Surrogate motherhood, 238

**Suture:**

1. to sew together cut or separated edges, as of a wound, to promote healing

2. the thread, wire, gut, etc., used in this process

**Suture line:** line formed by the edges of the separate bones of a baby's skull, 4

Swallowing, 49–50

difficulties, 454

foreign bodies, 191–92, 458

transition to breathing, *49*

*See also* Eating

Swearing, 192

Sweat *See* Perspiration

**Sweat gland/sudoriferous gland:** any of numerous glands that secrete sweat, found almost everywhere in the skin except for the lips and a few other areas, 20, 22–23

**Swimmer's itch:** mild form of schistosomiasis in which parasitic fluke worm larvae invade the skin of swimmers, causing dermatitis, 600

Swimming, 192, 279, 318

Swollen glands, 40

**Sycosis/barber's itch:** bacterial infection of the hair follicles, marked by inflammation, itching, and the formation of pus-filled pimples, 713

**Sympathetic nervous system:** the part of the autonomic nervous system that controls such involuntary actions as the dilation of pupils, constriction of blood vessels and salivary glands, and increase of heartbeat, 28. Compare *Para-sympathetic nervous system.*

**Symptom:** change in one's normal feeling or condition of well-being, indicating the presence of disease, 829

**Symptomatic:** having observable symptoms of a disease or condition. Compare *Asymptomatic.*

**Symptomatology:** the combined symptoms of a disease

Synanon, 948

**Synapse:** the junction point between two neurons, across which a nerve impulse passes from the axon of one neuron to the dendrite of another, 30–31

**Syncope:** temporary loss of consciousness; fainting

**Syndrome:** set of symptoms occurring at the same period and indicating the presence or nature of a disease

**Synovia/synovial fluid:** viscid, transparent fluid secreted as a lubricating agent in the interior of joints and elsewhere,

**Synovial aspiration/synovial fluid exam:** laboratory analysis of synovia, withdrawn from joints by needle, in order to diagnose gout or certain forms of arthritis, 839

**Synovial fluid:** synovia

**Thalamus:** round mass of gray matter at the base of the brain that transmits sensory impulses to the cerebral cortex

**Thalassemia/Cooley's anemia:** form of anemia caused by inherited abnormality of red blood cells, often fatal in utero, 824

Thalidomide, 239, 246

**THC:** tetrahydrocannabinol, 952

Theophylline, 485, 1104

**Therapy:** treatment of a disease by a prescribed method or medicine, 923

speech, 190

*See also* Marriage counseling

Thermometers, 985–86

**Thermogram:** measurement of the surface temperature of a region of the body such as the breast, with an infrared sensing device,

**Thermography:** technique of measuring the surface temperature of a region of the body, such as the breast, with an infrared sensing device, 813–14

**Thiamine/vitamin B₁:** vitamin found in cereal grains, green peas, liver, egg yolk, and other sources, and also made synthetically, that protects against beriberi

Thiopental, 614, 943

**Thoracic:** of or relating to the thorax, or chest cavity

Thoracic cavity, 66

disease, 474

lung collapse, 497

**Thoracic surgeon:** surgeon specializing in thoracic surgery, having to do with the chest cavity, 827, 842

**Thoracic surgery:** branch of surgery having to do with the chest cavity and its organs, the heart and lungs, and large blood vessels

**Thorax:** Chest, 472

abnormal, 363

muscles, *11*

Threadworms, 466

**Thrombin:** enzyme present in the blood that reacts with fibrinogen to form fibrin in the process of clotting, 409

**Thrombocytes** *See* Platelets

**Thromboembolism:** obstruction of a blood vessel by a blood clot (thrombus) that has broken away from the place where it was formed, 265

**Thrombophlebitis:** formation of a blood clot (thrombus) in the wall of an inflamed vein (phlebitis), 418, 496

**Thromboplastin:** substance found in blood platelets that helps to convert prothombin into thrombin in the clotting process, 409

**Thrombosis:** formation of a blood clot (thrombus) in a blood vessel, resulting in the partial or complete blocking of circulation, 421, 430

atherosclerosis, *420*

**Thrombus:** stationary blood clot within a blood vessel, 421, 422

Thorazine, 296

**Thrush:** fungus infection in the mouth, esp. of infants, characterized by white patches that become sores, 452, 586, 791

Thumb-sucking, 171

**Thymectomy:** surgical removal of the thymus, 406

Thymosin Alpha 1, 549

**Thymus:** glandlike, lymphoid organ located near the base of the neck, believed to play a role in the body's immunological responses, 79–80, *80*

Thyroid cancer, 579

iodine concentration, 971

Thyroid disease,

hair loss, 287

**Thyroid gland:** endocrine gland located at the neck just below the larynx, extending around the front and to either side of the trachea (windpipe), and secreting the hormone thyroxin, which is vital to growth and metabolism, 73–74, 77–78, 77, 498, *655*

disorders, 501–02

Thyroid gland,

enlargement, 502

infertility, 235

miscarriage, 247

myasthenia gravis, 405–06

pregnancy, 247

surgery, 654

Thyroid preparations, 1105

**Thyroid-stimulating hormone/TSH:** hormone secreted by the anterior lobe of the pituitary gland which stimulates the production of hormones in the thyroid gland, 72

Thyrotrophin *See* TSH

**Thyroxin:** hormone secreted by the thyroid gland, vital to growth and metabolism, 73, 77, 501, 1105

**Tibia:** the shin bone, the inner and larger of the two bones of the lower leg,

**Tic:** involuntary, recurrent muscle twitch or spasm

Tick bites, 162, 1090–91

*See also* Lyme disease; Rocky Mountain Spotted Fever

**Tinea:** ringworm

**Tinnitus:** ringing, buzzing, hissing, or clicking sound in the ears, not caused by external stimuli, 531, 769

Tissues,

alcohol consumption, 931

compatibility, 684–85

grafts, 685

Toddlers

development, 110–11

independence, 160–61

punishment, 111

*See also* Children

Toenails,

ingrown, 284

*See also* Nails

Toes,

hammer toe, 284

stiff toe, 284

Toilet training, 193–94

Tolbutamide, 1105

**Tolerance:** the ability of the body to adjust to increasingly larger doses of a drug through habitual use,

*See also* Drug abuse

**Tomography:** radiography of a section of the body

**Tone/tonicity:** the normal tension of muscle tissue

Tongue, 81

coated, 762

digestive process, 48–49

role in taste, 92

**Tonic:** of or characteristic of tonus

**Tonic phase:** the period during a grand mal epileptic convulsion when the body is rigid, 388

**Tonometer:** device for measuring pressure, as of the eyeball, 850

**Tonsillectomy:** surgical removal of the tonsils, 653–54

**Tonsillitis:** inflammation of the tonsils, 190, 194–95, 653

**Tonsils:** either of two small round, lymphoid organs at each side of the back of the throat, 653

**Tonus:** muscular spasm characterized by persistent contraction. Compare *clonus.*

Toothaches, 1091

Tooth decay, 723, 724, 728–33

fillings, 724

halitosis, 451

**Trematode:** any of a class of parasitic flatworms, as the flukes, causing various diseases such as schistosomiasis, 598

**Tremor:** any involuntary quivering or trembling, as of a muscle,

syphilis, 554

*See also* Parkinson's disease

**Trench foot:** foot condition resembling frostbite, due to exposure to continued dampness and cold,

**Trench mouth/Vincent's angina/ Vincent's disease:** painful infection of the gums (called necrotizing ulcerative gingivitis) and sometimes of the pharynx and palate, characterized by the formation of ulcers and necrosis,

Trench mouth *See* Gingivitis

Treponema, 553

**Trichina:** Trichinella spiralis

**Trichinella spiralis/trichina:** the parasitic worm that causes trichinosis, 466

**Trichinosis:** disease caused by a parasitic worm (Trichinella spiralis) that enters the body via undercooked or raw meat, esp. pork, invading the intestines and muscles and provoking gastrointestinal symptoms initially and muscle stiffness and pain later, 466

**Trichomonas:** genus of protozoa that cause vaginal infections in women, 791–92

**Trichomoniasis:** vaginal infection by the trichomonas organism, 552, 791–92

Tridihexethyl, 1105

**Triglyceride:** glycerol compound containing one to three acids

**Trimester:** period of three months, used to identify the progress of a pregnancy which consists of three such periods

Trimethadione, 391

Trimethoprim, 1105

Triplets, 196

Triprolidine, 1105

Trips (hallucenogenic), 949, 950

**Trivalent:** pertaining to a form of the Sabin polio vaccine in which each dose gives protection against three strains of polio, 176. Compare *monovalent.*

**Trophoblast:** layer of cells developing around a fertilized ovum and contributing to the formation of the placenta, 248

**Trophoblastic disease:** disease of the trophoblast in a pregnant woman, marked by the degeneration of the placenta into a mass of grapelike cysts *(hydatidiform mole)*, 248–49

Tropical diseases, 590–601

True skin *See* Dermis

**Trypanosomiasis:** sleeping sickness, 595–97

**Trypsin:** enzyme in the pancreatic juice that breaks up proteins for digestion

Truancy *See* Runaways

Tsetse flies, 595

**TSH:** thyroid-stimulating hormone, 72

**Tubal insufflation/Rubin's test:** the injection of carbon dioxide gas, or sometimes ordinary air into the uterus to check for obstruction in the Fallopian tubes, 235–36

**Tubal ligation:** the typing or binding of a tube, especially of the Fallopian tubes as a method of sterilization, 270, *270*

Tubal pregnancies *See* Ectopic pregnancies

**Tubercle:** small nodule or tumor formed within an organ, as that produced by the bacillus causing tuberculosis

**Tubercle bacillus:** rod-shaped bacterium that causes tuberculosis,

**Tuberculin:** liquid containing substances extracted from weakened (attenuated) tubercle bacilli, used a test for tuberculosis

**Tuberculin test:** skin test for determining whether tuberculosis bacteria are present, used esp. for children, 481

**Tuberculoid:** of or resembling a tubercle or tuberculosis

Tuberculoid leprosy, 601

**Tuberculosis:** infectious, communicable disease caused by the tubercle bacillus and characterized by the formation of tubercles within some organ or tissue, often the lungs (pulmonary tuberculosis), 67, 478–82,

arthritis, 358

adrenal gland hormones, 502

skeletal system, 358, 364

surgical treatment, 661–62

treatment, 480

voluntary agencies, 1019

**Tubule(s):** very narrow, minute tube or duct of kidney, 538

**Tularemia:** acute bacterial infection that can be transmitted to humans from infected rabbits, squirrels, or other animals, by the bite of certain flies, or by direct contact, 588–89

**Tumor:** mass of tissue growing independently of surrounding tissue and having no physiological function, sometimes confined to the area of origin (benign) and sometimes invading other cells and tissue and causing their degeneration (malignant), 125–26

fibroid: benign tumor composed of fibrous tissue, usu. attached to the wall of the uterus

*See also* Fibroids

Tumors,

benign, 803–04

bladder cancer, 570

bone, 371–72

brain, 577

intestinal obstruction, 456

jaundice, 469

ovaries, 507

salivary glands, 451

skin cancer, 566

spine, 364–65

testicular hyperfunction, 505

urinary tract, 544

*See also* Sarcomas

**Turbinate:** one of the thin, curved bones on the walls of the nasal passages, 69

Twins, 195–96

Tympanic membrane, 87, 528, 964

**Tympanum:**

1. the cavity in the middle ear lined with the tympanic membrane (eardrum) and containing the ossicles

2. eardrum

**Typhoid fever/enteric fever:** acute infectious disease caused by a Salmonella bacterium and characterized by diarrhea, fever, eruption of bright red spots on the chest and abdomen, and physical prostration, 457–58

**Typhus:** acute disease caused by a rickettsial microorganism that is transmitted to humans by the bite of certain lice and fleas, and is characterized by high fever, severe headaches, and a red rash,

Uric acid,

gout, 356–58

**Ulcer(s):** open sore with an inflamed base on an external or internal body surface, 459–60

gastric, 53

perforated, 603

special diets, 874

symptoms, 459

**Ulcerative colitis:** colitis accompanied by ulcerated lesions on the colon, characterized by bloody diarrhea and abdominal pain, 464

with the spermicide nonoxynol-9, 266–67

Vaginal ulcers, 791

**Vaginitis:** inflammation of the vagina

**Vagotomy:** surgical procedure of cutting the vagus nerves, 64

**Vagus:** the tenth cranial nerve, which originates in the brain and extends branches to the lungs, heart, stomach and intestines, 27

Valley fever *See* Coccidioidomycosis

Value systems,

children, 147

**Valve:** membranous structure inside a vessel or other organ, as the heart, allowing fluid to flow in one direction only

Valves of hearts

*See* Heart valves

Vaporizers, 196, 493–94

Varices, 452–53

**Varicose:** abnormally dilated, as veins

**Varicose ulcer:** ulcer resulting from varicose veins, usu. on the inner side of the leg above the ankle

**Varicose vein/varix:** swollen and contorted vein, often in the leg, 243, 288–89, 418–19, *419,* 759–60

blood clots, 497

surgery, 665

vaginal area, 798–99, *799*

*See also* Stasis dermatitis

Varicose ulcers, 289

**Varicosity:**

1. condition of being varicose

*See* Varicose vein

**Varix** *(pl., varices):* varicose vein

**Vascular:** of, involving or supplied with vessels, as blood vessels

**Vascularization:** process of becoming vascular

**Vascular surgeon:** surgeon specializing in vascular surgery, having to do with the blood vessels, 842

**Vascular surgery:** branch of surgery having to do with the operative treatment of diseases of the blood vessels,

Vascular trauma, 380–81

**Vas deferens:** duct in males that conveys semen from the testicles to the seminal vesicles, 99

**Vasectomy:** surgical removal of part of the vas deferens or sperm duct of the male, thus rendering him sterile by preventing semen from reaching the seminal vesicles, 99, 269, *269,* 629–30

**Vasoconstrictor:** medicine that causes the blood vessels to contract, thus restricting blood flow

**Vasodilator:** medicine that causes the blood vessels to dilate, thus producing greater blood flow

**Vasomotor:** producing contraction or dilation of the blood vessels

**Vasopressin:** hormone secreted by the posterior lobe of the pituitary gland that raises blood pressure and increases peristalsis, known also as antidiuretic hormone because of its action on the kidneys to stimulate the reabsorption of water, 72, 508

**Vectorcardiogram:** graph indicating the magnitude and direction of the electrical currents of the heart, 844

Vegetarians, 878–79

**Vein(s):** any of a large number of muscular, tubular vessels conveying blood from all parts of the body to the heart, 33–34, *34,* 42

pulmonary: vein that delivers oxygen-rich blood from the lungs to the heart

**Velum:** soft palate

**Vena cava:** either of two large veins that bring blood to the heart from the upper part of the body (superior vena cava) and lower part of the body (inferior vena cava),

**Venereal disease:** any of those diseases transmitted by sexual intercourse, such as syphilis and gonorrhea, 230

arthritis, 358, 360

infertility, 234

*See also* Gonorrhea; Sexually transmitted diseases; Syphilis

**Venereal wart/condyloma acuminatum:** wart caused by a virus and occurring in the anal and genital areas, transmitted by sexual contact and by other means, 552–53

**Venom:** poison secreted by certain reptiles, insects, etc., transferred to a victim by a bite or sting

**Venous:** having to do with or carried by the veins

**Ventral:** toward, near, or in the abdomen.

Ventral hernia, 462

**Ventricles:** any of various body cavities, as of the brain, or chambers, esp. either of the two lower chambers of the heart, which receive blood from the atria and pump it into the arteries, 41

Ventricular fibrillation, 433–34

**Ventriculography:** technique of X raying the brain after the removal of cerebrospinal fluid and the injection of air into the ventricles, 382

**Venule:** small vein continuous with a capillary, 34

**Vermiform appendix/appendix vermiformis:** the worm-shaped appendage attached to the cecum of the large intestine; *See* Appendix vermiformis

**Vermifuges:** Any drug or remedy that destroys intestinal worms, 465

**Vernix caseosa:** cheesy substance sometimes covering a newborn baby's skin, 100

**Vertebrae:** one of the segmented bones that make up the spinal column,

cervical, 4

herniating disc, 365–66

lumbar region, 4–5

processes, 4–5

slipped disc, 365–66

thoracic/thoracic spine: the vertebrae to which the ribs are attached, 4

Vertebral column, *363*

**Vertebrate:** any animal having a backbone

**Vertigo:** disorder in which a person feels as if he or his surroundings are whirling around, 531

**Vesical:** of or pertaining to the bladder

**Vesicle:** small bladderlike cavity, or a small sac containing fluid

Vesical stones, 632

**Vestibular nerve:** the part of the auditory nerve leading from the vestibule of the inner ear to the brain, controlling equilibrium, 90

**Vestibule:** space or cavity, as within the labyrinth of the inner ear, 90

**Vestigial:** of the nature of a remnant of an organ that is no longer functional

Veterans Administration hospitals, 1001

**Viable:** capable of living and developing normally, as a newborn infant

**Vibrissae** *(sing., vibrissa):* hairs that grow in the nasal cavity, 69

**Villi** *(sing., villus):* minute, hairlike structures on the mucous membrane of the small intestine that absorb nutrients, 55–56, 60

Vinca alkaloid, 582

Vincristine sulfate, 582

Viral pneumonia *See* Walking pneumonia

**Virulent:**

1. severe and rapid in its progress, as a disease

2. highly infectious, as a disease-causing microorganism

**Viruses:** any of a large group of particles too small to be seen by an ordinary microscope, that are typically inert except when in contact with certain living cells, and that can cause a variety of infectious diseases

arthritis, 360

common cold, 475

Hodgkin's disease, 580

rheumatoid arthritis, 352–53

tropical diseases, 590–601

**Viscera:**

1. the internal organs of the body, as the stomach, lungs, heart, etc.

2. the intestines

**Visceral:** pertaining to the viscera

**Visceral leishmaniasis** *See* Kala-azar

**Viscid:** sticky or adhesive

**Viscous:** semifluid or gluelike in texture

Vision

children, 146

correction with contact lenses, 527

correction with glasses, 524

diseases affecting, 528

optic nerve, 83–84

peripheral, 83

seeing color, 83

Visiting Nurses Association, 1011

home health care, 1002

**Visual purple:** reddish purple protein found in the rods of the retina, esp. important to night vision, 83

**Visual radiations:** smaller nerve bundles that split off from the optic nerve and enter the occipital lobes of the brain, 84

**Vitalometer:** device for measuring sensitivity of a tooth, 732

**Vital signs:** measurement of body temperature, pulse rate, and respiration,

after surgery, 617, 618

home nursing care, 984–86

**Vitamins:** any of a group of complex organic substances found in minute quantities in most natural foods and closely associated with the maintenance of normal physiological functions,

deficiencies, 452, 456

food additives, 968

in middle years, 296

role in diet, 858

**Vitamin A:** vitamin found in green and yellow vegetables, dairy products, liver and fish liver oils, that prevents atrophy of epithelial tissue and protects against night blindness,

hair loss, 287

vision, 83

**Vitamin B$_1$:** thiamine

thrush, 452

**Vitamin B$_2$:** riboflavin

Vitamin B$_6$, 788

**Vitamin B$_{12}$:** vitamin extracted from liver and believed to protect against pernicious anemia, 412

**Vitamin B complex:** group of water-soluble vitamins including thiamine and riboflavin,

**Vitamin C/ascorbic acid:** white, odorless, crystalline compound found in citrus and other fresh fruits and green leafy vegetables, and also made synthetically, that prevents scurvy, 1105

colds, 745, 876

**Vitamin D:** vitamin that protects against rickets, found in fish liver oils, butter, egg yolks, and specially treated cow's milk, and also produced in the body on exposure to sunlight, 19

muscle spasms, 78

rickets, 371

**Vitamin E:** vitamin found in whole grain cereals, legume seeds, corn oil, egg yolks, meat, and milk, sometimes called the anti-sterility vitamin because its absence in rats causes sterility,

**Vitamin K:** vitamin that promotes the clotting of blood and is found in green leafy vegetables, 409

**Vitiligo/piebald skin:** skin disorder characterized by a loss of pigment in sharply defined areas, 321, 718

**Vitreous humor:** the transparent, jellylike tissue that fills the posterior chamber or ball of the eye and is enclosed by the hyaloid membrane, 86

**Vocal cords/vocal folds:** two bands of ligaments extending across the larynx which, when tense, are made to vibrate by the passage of air, thereby producing voice,

**Voice box** See Larynx

**Void:** excrete waste, esp. urine

Voiding cystometrics, 851

Voluntary Health Agencies, 1002

health screening, 1000

See also Health agencies

Voluntary muscles See Muscles

Volunteers,

health agencies, 1008

**Volvulus:** obstruction of the intestines caused by twisting, 456, *456*

Vomiting, 170–71, 190

stomach cancer, 568

See also Morning sickness

**Vomitus:** vomited substance

**Vulva:** the external genitals of the female, located beneath the front part of the pelvis

Walking,

as exercise, 318, 1179–82

speedwalking, 1179

**Walking pneumonia:** mild viral pneumonia that does not confine the patient to bed, 478

**Walleye:** strabismus characterized by a tendency of the eyes to turn outward away from the nose. Compare *crossed eyes.*

**Warts:** small, usu. hard, benign growth formed on and rooted in the skin, caused by a virus, 714

**Wasserman test:** blood test for the presence of the organism causing syphilis

Waste material *See* Feces; Urine

Water,

body composition, 859

**Water blister:** blister beneath the epidermis that contains lymph

**"Water-pills"** *See* Diuretics

Water pollution, 961–62

chemicals, 961

fish, 964

oil spills, 964

Weather discomforts, 708–10, 751–54

Weight,

averages for men and women (chart), 893

boys and girls (chart), 154–55

desirable weights for men and women (chart), 892

Weight control, 750–51, 864, 868–69

children, 164

diabetes, 512

exercise, 278

heart disease, 325, 435, 436–37

hernia prevention, 18

later years, 314–15, 320

middle years, 297

pregnancy, 239–40, 241

sexual maturity, 205